Annals of Tropical Medicine and Parasitology

Editorial Board, Chairman: W. Peters
Senior Editor: W.N. Beesley
Publication Six issues per year
Subscription Volume 72, 1978, £24.00/$31.00 (overseas)
prices include postage

The *Annals of Tropical Medicine and Parasitology,* the journal of the Liverpool School of Tropical Medicine started publication in 1902. It is now published by Academic Press and for the first time is a bimonthly publication rather than a quarterly. From its first issue it has been a key international journal in the fields of tropical medicine, medical parasitology, veterinary parasitology, entomology, the systematics of parasites and experimental parasitology with considerable cover of the fields of chemotherapy and immunology.

(Available from Academic Press (Inc.) London Ltd.)

Tropical Doctor

A Journal of Modern Medical Practice Published by the Royal Society of Medicine and distributed by Academic Press

Editors: A.W. Woodruff and L.J. Bruce-Chwatt
Publication Quarterly
Subscription Volume 8, 1978, £6.00(UK), £8.80 (overseas)
prices include postage

Tropical Doctor aims primarily to provide practical down-to-earth instruction for doctors working in developing countries, especially those in relatively isolated locations where the more elaborate hospital facilities are not always available. The journal covers all aspects of medicine, since in such hospitals and health centres the doctor may have to turn his hand not only to routine medical treatment, but also to emergency surgery, obstetrics, preventive medicine and basic laboratory techniques.

(Available from Academic Press (Inc.) London Ltd.)

Journal of the Royal Society of Medicine

Editor: Victor Bloom
Publication Monthly
Subscription Volume 7l, 1978, £22.00/$27.00 (overseas) $54.50 (USA)
prices include postage

The *Journal of the Royal Society of Medicine* appeared for the first time in January 1978. It replaces the *Proceedings* which has been the principal publication of the Royal Society of Medicine since 1907. A selective approach to the publication of papers read at Society meetings has now been adopted so that only papers of outstanding interest are published.

Academic Press

London   New York   San Francisco
A Subsidiary of Harcourt Brace Jovanovich, Publishers
24-28 Oval Road, London NW1, England
111 Fifth Avenue, New York, NY 10003, USA

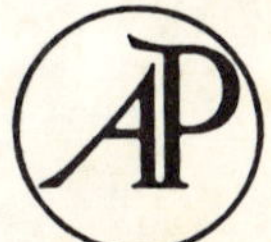

LEWIS'S PUBLICATIONS

CLINICAL RADIOLOGY OF THE EAR, NOSE AND THROAT
2nd Edition by ERIC SAMUEL and GLYN A. S. LLOYD   £15·00 net.

BAILEY AND LOVE'S SHORT PRACTICE OF SURGERY.
17th Edition revised by A. J. HARDING RAINS and H. DAVID RITCHIE.
£17·50 net

1001 MULTIPLE CHOICE QUESTIONS AND ANSWERS IN SURGERY
(*Based on BAILEY AND LOVE'S SHORT PRACTICE OF SURGERY*)
By A. J. HARDING RAINS   (Nearly Ready)

A SHORT TEXTBOOK OF GENERAL PRACTICE.
By DENIS CRADDOCK, M.D., F.R.C.G.P., D.Obst. R.C.O.G. Third Edition.
756 pages.   £12·50 net.

SURGICAL DIAGNOSIS.
By GEORGE QVIST, F.R.C.S. 867 illustrations.   £15·00 net.

A HANDBOOK OF RADIOGRAPHY.
By JOHN A. ROSS and R. W. GALLOWAY. 4th Edition.   £8·50 net.

A SYNOPSIS OF PHYSICAL SIGNS IN MEDICINE.
By H. FULD, M.D., F.R.C.P.Ed. 2nd Edition.   £6·00 net.

WOLFF'S ANATOMY OF THE EYE AND ORBIT.
7th Edition revised by R. WARWICK.   £14·00 net.

ROXBURGH'S COMMON SKIN DISEASES.
14th Edition by PETER BORRIE. 528 pages, 239 illustrations.   £7·00 net.

MEDICAL OFFICERS OF SCHOOLS ASSOCIATION—HANDBOOK OF SCHOOL HEALTH.
15th Edition.   £3·00 net.

OPERATIVE SURGERY REVISION.
By JOHN J. SHIPMAN, M.S., F.R.C.S. Third Edition.   £5·00 net.

WE ALSO STOCK A COMPREHENSIVE SELECTION OF THE MULTIPLE CHOICE QUESTION REVIEW BOOKS

Particulars on request

H. K. LEWIS & Co. Ltd.,
136 Gower Street, London, WC1E 6BS
Telephone: 01-387 4282

Current Topics in Immunology Series

Edited by John Turk

1. The Practice of Clinical Immunology *Second Edition*

R. A. Thompson

'It is so good that it will undoubtedly create interest and anticipation of
the volumes to follow' – *On Call*

Probable publication September   Paper £9.95 approx

2. Cancer and the Immune Response

G. A. Currie

'. . . an interesting and stimulating review of the field.' – *Medical
Laboratory Technology*

Paper £4.25   120 pages   12 illustrations

3. Blood Group Topics

Barbara E. Dodd and P. J. Lincoln

'. . . this topic makes a particularly relevant contribution to the present
series.' – *British Medical Journal*

Paper £5.45   156 pages   13 illustrations

4. Organ Grafts

R. Y. Calne

'The book is well produced and illustrated with clear line drawings . . .'
– *The Lancet*

Paper £2.75   80 pages   40 illustrations

5. Allergic Drug Reactions

H. E. Amos

'This book is recommended for dermatologists, embryo immunologists,
and clinicians alike.' – *British Journal of Hospital Medicine*

Paper £4.95   144 pages   41 illustrations

6. Immunodeficiency

A. Hayward

'One can confidently recommend this book for all medical and technical
staff.' – *Archives of Disease in Childhood*

Paper £5.50   140 pages   26 illustrations

7. Immunology of the Rheumatic Diseases:
Aspects of Autoimmunity

R. N. Maini, D. N. Glass and J. T. Scott

'. . . this book is timely' – *The Lancet*

Paper £5.95   160 pages   9 illustrations

8. Immunology of Gastrointestinal and Liver Disease

Ralph Wright

'. . . well worth having ' – *British Medical Journal*

Paper £4.75   140 pages   23 illustrations

'. . . each one of this series is both academic and clinical, authoritative
without being verbose, practical as well as basic, and a joy to read . . .'
– *British Journal of Hospital Medicine*

Edward Arnold
41 Bedford Square, London WC1B 3DP

1978 **Oxford University Press**

Growth Kinetics of Tumours
Cell Population Kinetics in relation to the Growth and Treatment of Cancer
G. Gordon Steel

Starting with a review of the rate of growth of tumours in animals and man, this book provides a comprehensive summary of information on the underlying cell proliferation processes. The properties of tumour stem-cells are reviewed, and the book concludes with a discussion of the relevance of cell population kinetics to tumour therapy. £15

Dermatology in Clinical Medicine
Sam Shuster

This is an up-to-date account of dermatology as it occurs in general medicine and is based on the author's wide experience as a teacher, clinician, and researcher. It covers all the common dermatological conditions a physician is likely to encounter.
Paper covers £4.25 *Oxford Medical Publications*

Brain's Clinical Neurology
Revised by Sir Roger Bannister

For the new edition of this successful textbook, the reviser has added new sections on computerized axial tomography, disconnection syndromes, prolactin-secreting tumours, drug-induced dyskinesias, autonomic neuropathies, and carcinomatous syndromes.
Fifth edition £10 paper covers £5.50 *Oxford Medical Publications*

Diagnostic ENT
G. D. L. Smyth

Medical students studying ENT lack a concise text which firmly concentrates on problem solving, the real basis of otorhinolaryngology. This new textbook fills this need. It is illustrated throughout and will be useful to nurses, junior hospital doctors in paediatrics, neurology, neurosurgery, and ENT, and ENT consultants.
Illustrated   paper covers £3 *Oxford Medical Publications*

THE MEDICAL ANNUAL

THE YEAR-BOOK OF TREATMENT

Editors: **Sir Ronald Bodley Scott** GCVO, MA, DM, FRCP

Sir James Fraser BT, BA, CHM EDIN, FRCS

Ninety-sixth year

BRISTOL · JOHN WRIGHT

ISBN 0 7236 0509 2

PRINTED IN GREAT BRITAIN BY HENRY LING LIMITED,
AT THE DORSET PRESS, 23 HIGH EAST STREET, DORCHESTER DT1 1HD

The Editors' Preface

Every year we have to report some changes amongst our contributors: on this occasion Dr P. Carson and Dr K. M. Citron have found that other commitments force them to retire from the *Medical Annual*. Both have provided us with excellent articles and it is with regret that we lose them. We are greatly in their debt for the support they have given over the past years. Dr B. L. Pentecost of the United Birmingham Hospitals follows Dr Carson in contributing the section on Cardiovascular Diseases; he will be known to many of our readers as one of the leading cardiologists in the Midlands. Dr Citron is succeeded by Dr John Collins of St Bartholomew's and the Brompton Hospitals, an association which guarantees the continued high standard of the chapter on chest disease. We welcome them both with pleasure and in the certain anticipation of reviews of the quality our readers have come to expect.

We also welcome Mr J. Gilmore of St Bartholomew's Hospital who this year has provided the section on General Surgery. Mr Gilmore is well known for his continuing contributions to the complex field of surgical infection and to the problems of wound healing. His contributions will undoubtedly be of great interest to all surgeons.

Following the initial enthusiasm for resuscitation after cardiac arrest many physicians have begun to question the long term results. They have started to wonder how many are salvaged and of these how many are physically or intellectually impaired. Answers to some of their questions are to be found in the valuable special article by Dr M. W. McNicol and Dr R. C. Peatfield on the long term results of resuscitation. The second special article has been contributed by Dr A. Milford Ward of the Department of Immunology at the Hallamshire Hospital Medical School, Sheffield. It is a useful review of that form of immunopathy now known as 'immune complex disease'. Mr Ian Burn provides the third special article. In this he discusses the highly topical and still controversial subject of cancer screening. Using as his model cancer of the cervix and breast cancer he underlines some of the economic and logistic factors that might seem to be insuperable obstacles to an effective national screening programme. However, he does confirm that, especially in regard to breast cancer, screening is the most likely means by which the at present unhappy situation in this curable disease can be improved.

It is always difficult to select points for special mention from the different sections. There are, however, two cautionary tales worthy of note. Dr G. Kazantzis draws our attention to the risks to health faced by those working in medical laboratories. The incidence of pulmonary tuberculosis in laboratory technicians is five times that of the general population. Marburg disease was first described in a laboratory worker, and the last epidemic of smallpox in this country started in a research laboratory. If we are to advise on public health it is more than ever vital to put our own pathological house in order.

Professor J. H. Middlemiss devotes the whole of this section to discussing the question, 'Is your X-ray examination really necessary?' In the present economic blizzard, the answer to this question is doubly important and the 'code of efficacy' he quotes could with advantage be applied throughout the National Health Service.

The cost effectiveness of hospital treatment is also discussed by Mr J. L. Monro with particular reference to cardiac surgical operations. Although in the United Kingdom each individual procedure may cost from £1 500 to £2 500 and by some may be regarded as an unjustifiable luxury for a National Health Service, Mr Monro points out that in terms of benefit to the patient and ultimate cost to the State the returns on this investment are considerable.

The adult respiratory distress syndrome or 'shock lung' has only been recognized within the last ten years and only now is its frequency and importance becoming appreciated. Dr John Collins has long been interested in the condition and his review of the subject will be of great value to readers.

Clinical measurement as applied to urology is similarly a relatively new development but both its application and its importance have increased dramatically in the past few years. This development is especially true in urodynamics and the section by Roger Feneley and P. H. Abrams, while providing an up to date review, confirms that a technique previously regarded as a research tool has now become part of a routine service investigation.

It is not easy to arouse enthusiasm for vital statistics in the generality of our profession. Nevertheless, they do reveal trends which can easily be overlooked and Dr Michael Clarke makes some interesting points. The crude birth rate at 11·9 per thousand persons living for 1976 was the lowest ever recorded and contrasts sharply with that of 18·6 only 12 years previously. When taken with the fact that 17% of the population are over the retiring age and indeed 5% over the age of 75 years this figure shows how the nation is becoming progressively more elderly. This trend is likely to become even more evident when the oral contraceptive for males, alpha-chlorohydrin, of which Professor H. Schnieden writes, is perfected and freely available.

1st July, 1978

Contents

xviii Contents

Contributors and Contributions

P. H. Abrams FRCS

Urogenital tract, surgical (jointly), 313.

S. J. Arnott FRCSE, FRCR

Senior Lecturer, Department of Radiotherapy, University of Edinburgh.

Radiotherapy (jointly), 245.

J. Bonnar MA, MD, FRCOG

Professor and Head of Obstetrics and Gynaecology, University of Dublin, Trinity College Medical School, Rotunda Hospital.

Gynaecology and obstetrics, 154.

J. I. Burn FRCS (ENG)

Consultant Surgeon, Charing Cross Hospital, Fulham Palace Road, London.

Screening in cancer, 17.

M. Clarke MB, DPH, MFCM

Senior Lecturer in Community Health, Department of Community Health, University of Leicester.

Vital and morbidity statistics, 328.

R. S. J. Clarke BSC, MD, PHD, FFARCS

Reader in Anaesthetics, Queen's University of Belfast; Consultant Anaesthetist, Northern Ireland Hospitals.

Anaesthesia and analgesia, 57.

J. Collins MD, MRCP

Brompton Hospital, Fulham Road, London.

Respiratory tract, medical, 251.

J. Cunningham BM, MRCP

Lecturer in Medicine, The London Hospital Medical College, Whitechapel, London.

Urogenital tract, medical (jointly), 303.

A. A. Dawson MD, FRCP (EDIN), MRCPATH

Consultant Haematologist, Aberdeen Royal Infirmary; Senior Lecturer in Haematology, University of Aberdeen.

Recent advances in haematology (jointly), 64.

A. S. Douglas DSC, MD, FRCP (LOND, EDIN, GLASG), FRCPATH

Regius Professor of Medicine, University of Aberdeen; Honorary Consultant Physician, Aberdeen Royal Infirmary and Woodend Hospital, Aberdeen.

Recent advances in haematology (jointly), 64.

W. Duncan FRCPE, FRCSE, FRCR

Professor of Radiotherapy, University of Edinburgh.

Radiotherapy (jointly), 245.

C. J. Earl MD, FRCP

Physician, Neurological Department, The Middlesex Hospital, National Hospital, Queen Square, and Moorfield's Eye Hospital, London; Neurologist, King Edward VII Hospital for Officers, London.

Neurology: medical, 187.

H. H. G. Eastcott MS, FRCS

Consultant Surgeon, St Mary's Hospital, London.

Peripheral vascular disease: surgical, 89.

A. N. Exton-Smith MA, MD, FRCP

Barlow Professor of Geriatric Medicine, University College Hospital Medical School, London; Consultant Physician, Geriatric Department, University College Hospital; Honorary Physician, Hospital of St John and St Elizabeth and Whittington Hospital, London.

Geriatrics, 147.

R. C. L. Feneley MChir, FRCS

Consultant Urological Surgeon to the United Bristol Hospitals and Southmead General Hospital.

Urogenital tract, surgical (jointly), 313.

Sir James Fraser BT, BA, CHM (EDIN), FRCS

Professor of Clinical Science in Surgery, University of Southampton; Honorary Consultant Surgeon, Southampton Hospital Group.

Oesophagus, stomach and small intestine: surgical, 32.

O. J. A. Gilmore MS, FRCS, FRCS Ed.

Consultant Surgeon, Royal Hospital of St Bartholomew, London, and Hackney Hospital, London.

General surgery, 286.

J. C. Goligher CHM, FRCS

Professor of Surgery, University of Leeds; Surgeon, General Infirmary, Leeds.

Colon, rectum and anus: surgical, 38.

Huw B. Griffith MA, BM, BCH, MRCP (LOND), FRCS (ENG)

Consultant Neurosurgeon, United Bristol Hospitals and South West Regional Hospital Board.

Neurology: surgical, 194.

John Groves FRCS

Consultant Ear, Nose and Throat Surgeon, The Royal Free Hospital, London.

Ear, nose and throat diseases (jointly), 117.

C. W. H. Havard MA, DM, FRCP

Consulting Physician, Royal Northern Hospital and Royal Free Hospital, London.

General medicine, 172.

J. D. Jessop MD, FRCPI, MRCP

Consultant Physician, Department of Rheumatology, University Hospital of Wales, Cardiff.

Chronic rheumatic diseases (jointly), 267.

Ivan D. A. Johnston MCH, FRCS

Professor of Surgery, University of Newcastle upon Tyne; Consultant Surgeon, Royal Victoria Infirmary, Newcastle upon Tyne.

Endocrine glands: surgical, 121.

Sir Francis Avery Jones CBE, MD, FRCP

Consulting Physician, Gastro-enterological Department, Central Middlesex Hospital; Consulting Gastro-enterologist, St Mark's Hospital, London, and to the Royal Navy.

Oesophagus, stomach and small intestine: medical, 22.

G. Kazantzis MB, BS, PHD, FRCS, MRCP, MFCM

Senior Lecturer and Consultant Physician, Department of Community Medicine, The Middlesex Hospital Medical School, London.

Occupational health, 210.

J. D. E. Knox MD, FRCP, FRCGP

Professor of General Practice, University of Dundee.

General practice, 135.

Richard E. Lea FRCS

Consultant Thoracic Surgeon, Hampshire Area Health Authority (Teaching), Wessex Cardiac and Thoracic Centre, Southampton Western Hospital, Southampton.

Respiratory tract: surgical, 262.

Nicholas Lyell MA

Barrister.

Legal decisions and legislation, 169.

J. I. McGill MA, D PHIL, FRCS

Consultant Ophthalmologist, Hampshire Area Health Authority, Southampton Eye Hospital and Southampton Group of Hospitals.

Eye diseases, 127.

M. W. McNicol MB, FRCP (GLASG), FRCP (EDIN) FRFPS (GLASG)

Cardiothoracic Department, Central Middlesex Hospital, Acton Lane, London.

The long term results of resuscitation (jointly), 1.

D. O. Maisels FRCS (EDIN)

Consultant Plastic Surgeon, Liverpool Regional Hospital and United Liverpool Hospitals; Clinical Lecturer in Plastic Surgery at Liverpool University.

Plastic surgery, 230.

J. H. Middlemiss CMG, MD, FRCP, FRCR

Director, Department of Diagnostic Radiology of the Bristol United Hospitals; Professor of Radiodiagnosis, University of Bristol.

Radiodiagnosis, 242.

Ralph E. Midwinter BSC, MD, MFCM, DPH, DCH

Consultant Senior Lecturer in Community Medicine, University of Bristol, and Specialist in Community Medicine, South Western Regional Health Authority.

Community medicine and epidemiology, 111.

J. P. Mitchell TD, MS, FRCS, FRCSE

Professor of Surgery (Urology), University of Bristol; Urological Surgeon, United Bristol Hospitals and Southmead General Hospital.

Urogenital tract, surgical (jointly), 311, 319.

C. J. E. Monk MCH ORTH, FRCS (EDIN), FRCS (ENG)

Consultant Orthopaedic Surgeon, Liverpool Area Health Authority (Teaching), Central and Southern District.

Orthopaedics and traumatology, 217.

J. L. Monro FRCS

Consultant Cardiac Surgeon and Senior Lecturer, Southampton University Hospitals; Member of the Cardiac Society.

Heart and major vessels: surgical, 82.

A. G. Morgan BSC, MD, MRCP

Lecturer in Medicine, The London Hospital Medical College.

Urogenital tract: medical (jointly), 301

G. Nuki MRCP

Senior Lecturer, Department of Medicine, Welsh National School of Medicine, and Hon. Consultant Physician, University Hospital of Wales, Cardiff.

Chronic rheumatic disorders (jointly), 267.

Major-General W. O'Brien OBE, MD, FRCP

Consultant Physician to the Army.

Tropical diseases, 290.

R. C. Peatfield MB, MRCP

Medical Registrar, Cardiothoracic Department, Central Middlesex Hospital, Acton Lane, London.

The long term results of resuscitation (jointly), 1.

B. L. Pentecost MD, FRCP

Central Birmingham Health District, The General Hospital, Birmingham.

Cardiovascular disease, 76.

J. S. Price DM, MRCP, MRCPSYCH, DPM

Consultant Psychiatrist to the Northwick Park Hospital and the Clinical Research Centre, Harrow, Middlesex.

Mental disease, 180.

J. R. S. Rendall MB, BS, MRCP

Senior Registrar, Department of Dermatology, University College Hospital, London.

Skin diseases (jointly), 276.

Trevor Robinson MA, MB, FRCP

Part-time Senior Lecturer at the Medical School, Consultant Dermatologist and Lecturer in Dermatology, University College Hospital, London; Part-time Consultant Dermatologist, Edgware General Hospital.

Skin diseases (jointly), 276.

H. Schnieden MD, MSC

Leech Professor of Pharmacology, Materia Medica and Therapeutics of the University of Manchester.

Pharmacology and toxicology, 223.

Ivan M. Sharman PHD, FRIC

Member of the Scientific Staff, Dunn Nutritional Laboratory, University of Cambridge, and the Medical Research Council.

Nutrition and vitamins, 199.

V. L. Sharman MA, MB, BChir, MRCP

Senior Registrar in Nephrology, Medical Unit, The London Hospital Medical College, Whitechapel, London.

Urogenital tract, medical, 308.

Sheila Sherlock MD, FRCP, FRCP (EDIN), FRCCP (HON), FACP (HON)

Professor of Medicine, University of London (Royal Free Hospital Medical School).

Liver and pancreas: medical, 46.

Hillas Smith MA, MD, FRCP

Consultant Physician, Royal Free Hospital, London; Department of Infectious Diseases, Coppets Wood Hospital, Muswell Hill, London; Consultant in Infectious Diseases, Neasden Hospital, London.

Infectious diseases, 160

M. O. Symes MD

Consultant Immunologist to the United Bristol Hospitals and Senior Lecturer in Immunology, University of Bristol.

Urogenital tract, surgical, 325.

R. N. T. Thin MD, FRCP (EDIN)

Consultant Venereologist, Royal Hospital of St Bartholomew, London.

Sexually transmitted diseases, 271.

J. E. Trapnell MA, MD, FRCS

Consultant Surgeon, Royal Victoria Hospital, Bournemouth.

Gallbladder and pancreas: surgical, 50.

M. J. VandenBurg BSc, MB, BS, MRCP

Lecturer in Medicine, The London Hospital Medical College, Whitechapel, London.

Urogenital tract, medical, 306.

A. Milford Ward MA, MB (CAMB), BChir

Hon. Consultant in Clinical Immunology Sheffield AHA, Senior Lecturer in Immunology, University of Sheffield.

Immune complex diseases, 7.

Brian Webb MD, FRCP, DCH

Consultant Paediatrician, Taunton and Somerset Hospitals; Postgraduate Medical Tutor, University of Bristol; Previously WHO Professor of Paediatrics and Child Health, University of Khartoum.

Children's diseases: medical, 96.

A. W. Wilkinson CHM (EDIN), PRCSE, FRCS, FAAP (HON), FRACS (HON)

Nuffield Professor of Paediatric Surgery, Institute of Child Health, University of London; Surgeon, Hospital for Sick Children, Great Ormond Street, London.

Children's diseases: surgical, 103.

Our Books Last for Generations.

Medical students and practitioners have relied on these Appleton texts since the First Edition . . .

Maingot: Abdominal Operations/*Sixth Edition*

From its first publication in 1940, Rodney Maingot's two-volume text quickly established itself as the authoritative work on the techniques of abdominal surgery. Today, with 111 chapters from younger as well as senior surgeons in each subspecialty, this revision can claim to reflect approved practice throughout the U.S.A. and Great Britain. As the *British Medical Journal* observed, 'The latest edition taxes even the most hard-bitten reviewer for sufficient superlatives to praise adequately the superb quality of text, illustrations, and production.'   1974 2,240pp 2 vols. illus. £66·15

Harvey: The Principles and Practice of Medicine/*Nineteenth Edition*

This Appleton classic, inspired by Sir William Osler's famous lectures at Johns Hopkins, puts its main emphasis on the patient rather than the disease. A primary text, reference and research tool, it has been described as 'A readable, up-to-date and fully comprehensive book containing a vast amount of information' for the clinical years and beyond, by the *Medical Textbook Review*.   1976 1,892pp illus. £24·85 c **International Student Edition** £15·00 p

Cole & Puestow: Emergency Care/*Seventh Edition*

This broadly-based book, in print since 1942, has been frequently updated to provide physicians and paramedical personnel with the medical and surgical information they need for both emergent and definitive care of traumatic injuries, including military casualties and civilian accidents. 1972 438pp illus. £10·15

Gallagher *et al:* **Medical Care of the Adolescent**/*Third Edition*

'The authors take on the formidable task of dealing with all aspects of medical care which involves the adolescent and succeed in a most readable way . . . It is, of course, a large volume, but then it performs the function of several textbooks rolled into one...every group that deals with adolescents, such as a student health service, should have a copy.'– *The Practitioner*. 1975 672pp illus. £25·55

Prices may be subject to change without notice.

Appleton-Century-Crofts/Medical publishers since 1825
66 Wood Lane End Hemel Hempstead Herts HP2 4RG 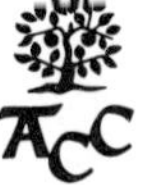

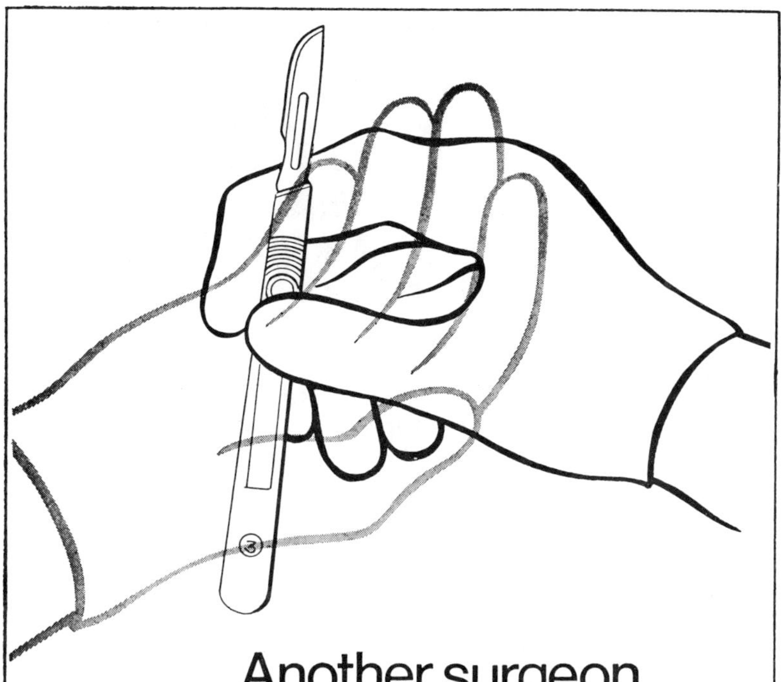

Another surgeon is about to use one of the world's finest surgical blades.... ....this happens thousands of times every day!

It happens because the blades are by Swann-Morton,
the people who meet the highest requirements in surgical knives.
We need say very little about our superiority.
The world's surgeons have proved it for us!

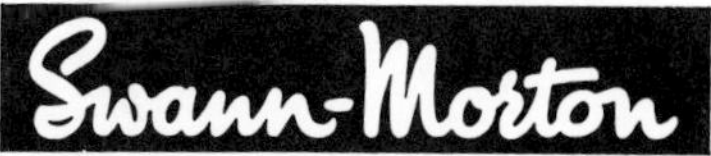

SWANN-MORTON (SALES) LIMITED
PENN WORKS, OWLERTON GREEN,
SHEFFIELD S6 2BJ, ENGLAND.

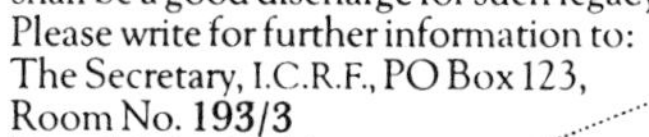
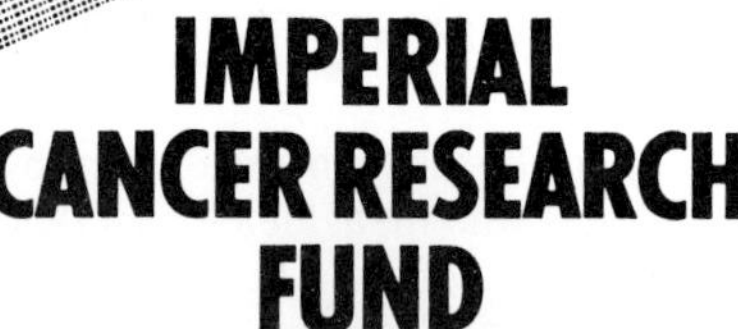
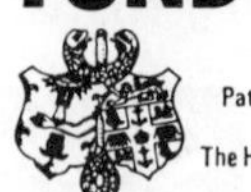

THE LONG TERM RESULTS OF RESUSCITATION

M. W. McNICOL MB, FRCP
R. C. PEATFIELD MB, MRCP

Attitudes to resuscitation have changed considerably in the last 30 years. Its development followed the introduction of defibrillation and external cardiac massage in the 1950s (Beck et al., 1956; Kouwenhoven et al., 1960), and during the 1960s the techniques became widely established as part of the routine service in every acute hospital in the developed world. In the present decade this initial enthusiasm has been replaced by some scepticism. More critical evaluation is now possible and results of attempted resuscitation in large series of patients are now reported.

The proportion of hospital deaths which are the subject of a cardiac arrest procedure is seldom disclosed. Resuscitation was attempted in 9·3 per cent of hospital deaths in the series of Peatfield et al. (1977), but they excluded special care areas such as coronary and intensive care units, unlike Coskey (1971) and Lemire and Johnson (1972), who had attempted resuscitation rates of 13 and 20 per cent respectively. Although the long term success rate in these series was higher than that of Peatfield et al. (1977), it is probable that this difference was largely accounted for by the inclusion of the special care areas, and that it is not likely that increasing the number of attempts at resuscitation except in these areas will lead to any improvement in the results.

Although the immediate results of resuscitation may be good, up to 90 per cent of the subjects successfully resuscitated initially will die within a few days (Johnson et al., 1967; Peschin and Coakley, 1970; Peatfield et al., 1977). Long term success rates are thus relatively low, ranging from 3·7 per cent (Peschin and Coakley, 1970) to 23 per cent (Dupont et al., 1969). There are a few exceptions to these poor overall results—long term survival in catheter laboratories may approach 100 per cent (Johnson et al., 1967; Coskey, 1971), and in coronary and intensive care units, where arrhythmias are common, results are also good (Hill et al., 1977). The inclusion of arrests from these locations is usually associated with the more optimistic reports of overall results (Coskey, 1971). There is no doubt that particularly energetic resuscitation should be mandatory in these high care areas, whatever reservations may apply elsewhere.

FACTORS INFLUENCING THE SURVIVAL RATE

Our conclusions are based on the series of Johnson et al. (1967), Coskey (1971), Jeresaty et al. (1973) and Peatfield et al. (1977). The most important factor is the patient's original diagnosis. The best results (15 − 23 per cent survival) are seen in myocardial infarction. Studies dealing exclusively with cases of myocardial infarction in coronary care units have shown that patients with primary ventricular fibrillation have a 13 per cent mortality, whereas those with ventricular fibrillation complicating cardiac failure or hypotension have a 70 per cent mortality (Goble et al., 1966; Lawrie et al., 1967). The prognosis is particularly poor in cardiac arrests complicating cardiogenic shock — Goble et al. (1966) had no survivors in 7 cases. Resuscitation seems to be more likely to be successful inside a coronary care unit (Hill et al., 1977). In ischaemic heart disease without evidence of infarction the prognosis does not seem any worse (Coskey, 1971). Drug overdose and anaesthetic arrests also carry a prognosis of at least 20 per cent survival, reflecting the good response usually seen to prompt restoration of ventilatory function.

In contrast, cardiac arrest complicating traumatic and neurological disease carries a recovery rate of less than 2 per cent (Johnson et al., 1967; Peatfield et al., 1977). The precise cause of the arrest in successful cases is often in doubt, and may actually be a reversible cardiac or pulmonary catastrophe. The distinction between cardiac arrest as a potentially reversible complication of the patient's illness and as cessation of the heart secondary to irreversible failure of another vital system, such as the brain, is a compelling explanation for these differences.

The nature of the rhythm disturbance is also influential. Ventricular fibrillation, par excellence a complication of myocardial infarction, is a much more favourable rhythm than asystole, which probably follows it in untreated cases and occurs de novo in patients with overwhelming disease (Restieaux et al., 1967; Lawrie et al., 1967; Dupont et al., 1969; Hollingsworth, 1969; Peschin and Coakley, 1970).

The location of the arrest within the hospital also influences the outcome, and this is independent of the distribution of patients by diagnosis (Peatfield et al., 1977). Up to one-third of cardiac arrests occur in the casualty department, and the results there tend to be better than on wards (Coskey, 1971; Peatfield et al., 1977), no doubt reflecting different degrees of vigilance and the presence of more easily reversible complications at the onset of illnesses such as myocardial infarction and drug overdose.

Perhaps more surprising is the finding in many surveys that results in older subjects are no worse, and indeed patients less than 40 years old tend to have a higher mortality, reflecting the greater proportion with traumatic, neurological and other less favourable diagnoses (Hollingsworth, 1969; Peatfield et al., 1977). Results in any single large category, such as myocardial infarction, are totally independent of the age of the subject (Peatfield et al., 1977). The natural tendency to persist more energetically in younger subjects is probably unjustified.

The promptness with which restoration of some circulation by external cardiac massage and artificial ventilation is started after the arrest is also very important (Pederson et al., 1965), although there have been many cases responding well after cardiac arrest long before arrival in hospital (Pantridge and Geddes, 1967; Adgey et al., 1969; Liberthson et al., 1974). A prolonged period of external cardiac massage, however, has been shown to be prognostically unfavourable (Pederson et al., 1965), and coma soon after resuscitation carries a poor prognosis for life (Willoughby and Leach, 1974; Bell and Hodgson, 1974).

QUALITY OF THE SURVIVORS

Concern has been expressed since the beginnings of resuscitation that the survivors may be physically or neurologically damaged by their experience. It is easy to accumulate a small series of obviously damaged subjects, but seldom is the number of undamaged patients surviving at the same time made clear. It is notoriously difficult to provide satisfactory objective criteria comparing each survivor with this state before the event, but those most often used are the semi-quantitative grading of exercise tolerance of the New York Heart Association (1964), and the number of subjects returning to work — a crude criterion only applicable to about half the survivors. The New York Heart Association Gradings of a sample of 36 of their 230 survivors by Lemire and Johnson (1972) showed that 27 of the 36 did not change grades, 2 dropped one class, and only 3 patients dropped by more than one. Four patients showed an improvement which was associated with cardiac surgery or the insertion of a pacemaker. Of 74 patients graded by Peatfield et al. (1977), only 4 patients declined to Grade III or lower as a result of their arrest; 2 of these were dead within 3½ months of the arrest, and all were dead within 3 years of it. McNamee et al. (1970) found that of 65 eligible survivors of ventricular fibrillation complicating myocardial infarction, 86 per cent were fit for work and 68 per cent were actually at work after a period of convalescence. Kushnir et al. (1975) compared the recovery of 28 survivors of ventricular fibrillation due to myocardial infarction with 90 uncomplicated cases: 70 per cent of the former and 86 per cent of the latter were back at work after ten months. This difference is not statistically significant, though the figures when assessed at four months were significantly different. Lawrie (1969) found that 92 per cent of 25 males with myocardial infarction eligible for work had returned to work one year after cardiac arrest: 70·5 per cent of the 17 previously employed patients of Minuck and Perkins (1969) and 68 per cent of the 41 surviving patients of Jeresaty et al. (1973) returned to work.

More sophisticated approaches seem of little value. Binnie et al. (1970) described a complex computer-based electroencephalographic method of predicting crude survival which makes little mention of patients permanently damaged or any correlation with coma in the early stages. It must be concluded that those patients who survive to discharge from hospital do extremely well thereafter.

In large series reported in their entirety significantly brain-damaged subjects discharged from hospital are uncommon. There were 4 in the 230 survivors of Lemire and Johnson (1972), and 2 in the 93 survivors of Peatfield et al. (1977). Many authors emphasize the poor prognosis for life in such patients, so that survivors living for many years are seldom significantly affected (Johnson et al., 1967; Hollingsworth, 1969; Coskey, 1971; Norris and Chandrasekar, 1971; Ruosteenoja et al., 1972; and Bell and Hodgson, 1974). Willoughby and Leach (1974), in a prospective study, showed that formal neurological assessment, particularly of conscious level one hour after cardiac arrest, was a reliable way of predicting the outcome. Eight of their 34 survivors, who were all deeply unconscious when assessed at one hour, had neurological damage, and 3 of these died within three months of the arrest. Bell and Hodgson (1974) described the progress of 284 patients admitted to an intensive care unit immediately after cardiac arrest with reference to the conscious level once initial resuscitation was complete: 48 per cent of the subjects were comatose and 81 per cent of these died in the unit. Only 10 patients (3·5 per cent) were discharged with brain damage and all those were comatose on admission. Two recovered fully later, 3 had focal neurological deficits (2 of which preceded arrest) and only 5 had intellectual impairment. They concluded that full recovery from coma of more than three days' duration was exceptional.

Other authors have concentrated exclusively on patients with residual brain damage. The problem seems to be commoner in neonates (Steiner and Neligan, 1975), and in those suffering their cardiac arrest outside hospital (Coskey, 1971; Bell and Hodgson, 1974; and Yarnell 1976). It has been stated that the brain can survive indefinitely on external cardiac massage and oxygen (Gilston and Resnekov, 1971), suggesting that the problem is delayed or inadequate first aid rather than choice of subject. Norris and Chandrasekar (1971) reviewed the literature and described 7 brain-damaged patients surviving for more than 6 weeks, all of whom were comatose and decerebrate on transfer to a chronic care hospital. One of these remained unconscious and the others were demented and/or had a focal neurological disturbance. Five died within a year of the arrest, 1 recovered completely and returned to work, and only 1, with ataxia and myoclonic jerking, remains in hospital. Yarnell (1976) described a series of 9 brain-damaged patients drawn from 137 cardiac arrests, but his total survival rate is not stated. All these patients had collapsed outside hospital and 4 of the 9 died within 6 months of the arrest; 3 were ultimately assessed as being 'independent but unemployable'.

Other authors have concentrated on the emotional and psychological aspects of the experience of being resuscitated. Druss and Kornfeld (1967) reported that 9 of 10 patients showed reactions varying from anxiety to manifest psychosis, though many of them were only assessed 6 weeks after the cardiac arrest. The symptoms tended to subside with time, and were little different from those in subjects treated for uncomplicated myocardial infarction. Dobson et al. (1971), in a similar study of 20 patients with assessment after at least 6 months, found that initial anxiety was common, but this tended to subside over the first 3 months and only 5 of the 20 showed unsatisfactory social and psychological rehabilitation. Jeresaty et al. (1973) reported 5 cases of depression and one of personality disorder among 59 survivors.

PROGNOSIS FOR THE SURVIVORS

Many reports have outlined prognosis for life once the survivors have left hospital, using actuarial methods (Lemire and Johnson, 1972; Jeresaty et al., 1973; Peatfield et al., 1977). In some studies this is done separately for subjects with myocardial infarction and for those with other diagnoses (Lemire and Johnson, 1972; Jeresaty et al., 1973), and the survival curves are little different. Neither of them differ significantly from studies of men with uncomplicated myocardial infarction (Pell and D'Alonzo, 1964; Beard et al., 1967; Lawrie, 1969; McNamee et al., 1970). Interestingly, in three studies with follow-up of up to ten years (Lemire and Johnson, 1972; Jeresaty et al., 1973; Peatfield et al., 1977), the mortality curve seems to level out after the first 4 – 6 years, but the numbers of subjects are low and this may well turn out to be coincidental. Peatfield et al. (1977) showed that this was not due to any one diagnostic category (such as young patients arresting during surgery) surviving disproportionately well.

CONCLUSIONS

It is possible to define certain categories of patients or locations where the results of cardiac resuscitation are particularly good. These are:

1. Cardiac arrest as a complication of cardiac catheterization, cardiac pacing or cardiac or thoracic surgery.
2. Primary ventricular fibrillation in coronary or intensive care units.
3. Ventricular fibrillation in the casualty department.
4. All anaesthetic and postoperative cases.
5. Cardiac arrest secondary to drug overdose.
6. Cardiac arrest complicating ischaemic heart disease without evidence of myocardial infarction.

Concentration of effort on these groups of patients is likely to produce the greatest improvement in results and the greatest reduction in 'preventible' deaths. More attempts at resuscitation elsewhere are unlikely to increase the return. A more selective approach will not only improve the results, but will also tend to reduce the suffering of patients and their relatives when inevitable death is merely being postponed.

Detailed examination of one aspect of particular concern, the long term survival of the severely damaged patient, indicates that this is not a major problem. Although there are many individual reports of such cases, their number in total is small, as is the proportion of them with prolonged survival. Clearly concern about the survival of potential cripples need not inhibit attempts at resuscitation. The quality of life and the expectation of life of those who survive is generally good.

REFERENCES

Adgey A. A. J., Scott M. E., Allen J. D., Nelson P. G., Geddes J. S., Zaidi S. A. and Pantridge J. F. (1969) Management of ventricular fibrillation outside hospital. *Lancet* **1**, 1169 – 1171.

Beard O. W., Hipp H. R., Robins M. and Verzolini V. R. (1967) Initial myocardial infarction among veterans: Ten-year survival. *Am. Heart J.* **73**, 317 – 321.

Beck C. S., Weckesser E. C. and Barry F. M. (1956) Fatal heart attack and successful defibrillation. *J.A.M.A.* **161**, 434 – 435.

Bell J. A. and Hodgson H. J. F. (1974) Coma after cardiac arrest. *Brain* **97**, 361 – 372.

Binnie C. D., Prior P. F., Lloyd D. S. L., Scott D. F. and Margerison J. H. (1970) Electroencephalographic prediction of fatal anoxic brain damage after resuscitation from cardiac arrest. *Br. Med. J.* **4**, 265 – 268.

Coskey R. L. (1971) A resuscitation program in a community hospital: five-year experience. *Geriatrics* **26**, 66 – 72.

Dobson M., Tattersfield A. E., Adler M. W. and McNicol M. W. (1971) Attitudes and long-term adjustment of patients surviving cardiac arrest. *Br. Med. J.* **3**, 207 – 212.

Druss R. G. and Kornfeld D. S. (1967) The survivors of cardiac arrest. *J.A.M.A.* **201**, 291 – 296.

Dupont B., Flensted-Jensen E. and Sandøe E. (1969) The long-term prognosis for patients resuscitated after cardiac arrest. *Am. Heart J.* **78**, 444 – 449.

Gilston A. and Resnekov L. (1971) Cardio-respiratory resuscitation. London, Heinemann.

Goble A. J., Sloman G. and Robinson J. S. (1966) Mortality reduction in a coronary care unit. *Br. Med. J.* **1**, 1005 – 1009.

Hill J. D., Holdstock G. and Hampton J. R. (1977) Comparison of mortality of patients with heart attacks admitted to a coronary care unit and an ordinary medical ward. *Br. Med. J.* **2**, 81 – 83.

Hollingsworth J. H. (1969) The results of cardiopulmonary resuscitation: a 3-year University Hospital experience. *Ann. Intern. Med.* **71**, 459 – 465.

Jeresaty R. M., Liss J. P. and Basu S. K. (1973) Long-term follow-up of 122 patients who survived cardiac arrest. *Resuscitation* **2**, 191 – 198.

Johnson A. L., Tanser P. H., Ulan R. A. and Wood T. E. (1967) Results of cardiac resuscitation in 552 patients. *Am. J. Cardiol.* **20**, 831 – 835.

Kouwenhoven W. B., Jude J. R. and Knickerbocker G. G. (1960) Closed-chest cardiac massage. *J.A.M.A.* **173**, 1064 – 1067.

Kushnir B., Fox K. M., Tomlinson I. W., Portal R. W. and Aber C. P. (1975) Primary ventricular fibrillation and resumption of work, sexual activity, and driving after first acute myocardial infarction. *Br. Med. J.* **4**, 609 – 611.

Lawrie D. M. (1969) Long-term survival after ventricular fibrillation complicating acute myocardial infarction. *Lancet* **2**, 1085 – 1087.

Lawrie D. M., Goddard M., Greenwood T. W., Harvey A. C., Donald K. W., Julian D. G. and Oliver M. F. (1967) A coronary-care unit in the routine management of acute myocardial infarction. *Lancet* **2**, 109 – 114.

Lemire J. G., and Johnson A. L. (1972) Is cardiac resuscitation worthwhile? *N. Engl. J. Med.* **286**, 970 – 972.

Liberthson R. R., Nagel E. L., Hirschman J. C. and Nussenfeld S. R. (1974) Prehospital ventricular defibrillation. *N. Engl. J. Med.* **291**, 317 – 321.

McNamee B. T., Robinson T. J., Adgey A. A. J., Scott M. E., Geddes J. S. and Pantridge J. F. (1970) Long-term prognosis following ventricular fibrillation in acute ischaemic heart disease. *Br. Med. J.* **4**, 204 – 206.

Minuck M. and Perkins R. (1969) Long-term study of patients successfully resuscitated following cardiac arrest. *Can. Med. Assoc. J.* **100**, 1126 – 1128.

New York Heart Association (1964) *Diseases of the Heart and Blood Vessels.* London, Churchill, pp. 110 – 113.

Norris J. R. and Chandrasekar S. (1971) Anoxic brain damage after cardiac resuscitation. *J. Chronic Dis.* **24**, 585 – 590.

Pantridge J. F. and Geddes J. S. (1967) A mobile intensive-care unit in the management of myocardial infarction. *Lancet* **2**, 271 – 273.

Peatfield R. C., Sillett R. W., Taylor D. and McNicol M. W. (1977) Survival after cardiac arrest in hospital. *Lancet* **1**, 1223 – 1225.

Pedersen J. E. P., Brams L., Buchmann G., Friis Fl. U. and Guldmann N. (1965) Closed chest cardiac compression administered to 177 patients. *Dan. Med. Bull.* **12**, 93 – 98.

Pell S., and D'Alonzo C. A. (1964) Immediate mortality and five-year survival of employed men with a first myocardial infarction. *N. Engl. J. Med.* **270**, 915 – 922.

Peschin A. and Coakley C. S. (1970) A five-year review of 734 cardiopulmonary arrests. *South. Med. J.* **63**, 506 – 510.

Restieaux N., Bray C., Bullard H., Murray M., Robinson J., Brigden W. and McDonald L. (1967) 150 patients with cardiac infarction treated in a coronary unit. *Lancet* **1**, 1285 – 1289.

Ruosteenoja R., Inkovaara J. and Koskinen P. J. (1972) Long-term prognosis after ventricular fibrillation in acute myocardial infarction. *Acta Med. Scand.* **191**, 229 – 232.

Steiner H. and Neligan G. (1975) Perinatal cardiac arrest. *Arch. Dis. Child.* **50**, 696 – 702.

Willoughby J. O. and Leach B. G. (1974) Relation of neurological findings after cardiac arrest to outcome. *Br. Med. J.* **3**, 437 – 439.

Yarnell P. R. (1976) Neurological outcome of prolonged coma survivors of out-of-hospital cardiac arrest. *Stroke* **7**, 279 – 282.

IMMUNE COMPLEX DISEASES

A. MILFORD WARD MA, MB, BChir, MRCPath

Humoral antibodies have a protective role and are produced to effect the neutralization or removal of antigenically foreign material. This reaction, although usually advantageous to the host, may on occasions have deleterious effects. This may be because the antibody—usually IgE—is tissue-bound and on complexing with antigen causes release of vasoactive amines or other pharmacologically active compounds. Other immunoglobulin classes are only rarely bound to cell membrane and the resultant antigen – antibody complexes have no such tissue affinity. Rare exceptions to this rule are recognized, such as the Stibophen – IgM antibody complex which binds to erythrocyte membranes and causes an anaemia and the quinine – IgC antibody complex which binds to platelets causing thrombocytopenia (Shulman and Rall, 1963).

Immune complexes are macromolecular aggregates of antigen and antibody, the size of the aggregates depending on the number and proportion of antigen and antibody molecules complexed together. The complexes may be soluble or insoluble, soluble complexes being formed in antigen excess and insoluble complexes being formed at the point of equivalence of the antigen – antibody reaction. Insoluble complexes, by precipitating at the site of their formation, give rise to local lesions, whereas soluble complexes enter the circulation and may be distributed throughout the intravascular and extra-vascular fluid compartments giving rise to more systemic disease.

Immune complexes occur frequently, in infectious diseases and in many autoimmune diseases. Immune complex disease or a tissue damaging reaction induced by the presence of circulating immune complexes is a less common situation.

BIOLOGICAL PROPERTIES OF IMMUNE COMPLEXES

The biological properties of immune complexes are determined by their interaction with humoral or cellular receptors. The binding of complexes to the classic humoral receptor, the first component of complement (C1q), will activate the complement cascade and its effector systems (Müller-Eberhard, 1975). Immune complexes may also become bound to lymphocyte membranes by means of specific antigen receptors (Warner, 1974) or non-specific Fc receptors (Nussenzweig, 1974). Cellular recognition of immune complexes and complement activation stimulates their phagocytosis by polymorphonuclear leucocytes (Nydegger, Anner et al., 1974).

Most immune complexes in the circulation are cleared rapidly by the mononuclear phagocytic system and particularly by the Kupffer cells (Weigle, 1961), and as such the clearance of immune complexes may represent a physiological mechanism for the elimination of antigen. Only relatively small complexes in antigen excess can persist in the circulation for any length of time and in these circumstances they may become deposited on vascular endothelium in small vessels or on filtration membranes giving rise to local inflammatory reactions.

Immune complexes formed in the extravascular spaces are not cleared so rapidly and are more likely to initiate local inflammatory reactions.

RECOGNITION OF IMMUNE COMPLEX DISEASE

Although the 'immune complex diseases' are of considerable current interest, the basic concept was first voiced more than seventy years ago. Friedemann (1909) demonstrated the anaphylactic properties of experimentally induced antigen and antibody complexes, and in so doing he created the situation for von Pirquet (1911) to propose that immune complexes could cause disease in man. In his studies on serum sickness he proposed that the coexistence of foreign antigen and its homologous antibody in the circulation resulted in the production of toxic compounds which were the cause of the characteristic vascular, renal, cardiac, cutaneous and joint lesions developing in the absence of an immunological relationship between the tissue and the initiating antigen. Here the concept rested for almost fifty years before Dixon et al. (1958) explained the pathogenesis of serum sickness and demonstrated immune complexes in the circulation.

LOCAL IMMUNE COMPLEX DISEASE

The Arthus reaction is an example of tissue injury resulting from insoluble immune complexes (Cochrane, 1967). The localized Arthus reaction with vasculitis is produced when antigen is introduced to a previously sensitized host. The pre-existing antibody combines with antigen to form complexes which precipitate and localize along the vascular basement membrane. Complement activation, polymorph chemotaxis and lysosome release are the immediate mediators of the local vasculitis and tissue injury.

SYSTEMIC OR CIRCULATING IMMUNE COMPLEX DISEASE

The systemic or circulating immune complex diseases induced by soluble complexes occur in a state of antigen excess. The classic situation is that of serum sickness. When an excess of foreign protein is injected there is an initial induction period or lag phase before antibody production occurs. The antibody produced combines with antigen in an initial gross antigen excess giving rise to small soluble complexes which persist in the circulation and give rise to inflammatory lesions in multiple sites with a characteristic lowering of the serum complement.

The conditions necessary for a circulating immune complex disease may arise acutely, as with serum sickness, or subacutely, but in all cases the antigen is present in the circulation before an antibody response begins. Many of the diseases are chronic and the failure to effect proper antigen elimination may be genetically determined, either by the production of low affinity antibody (Steward et al., 1973) or as a result of defects in the complement system (Lachmann, 1976). Microbial antigens persisting in chronic infectious states may also provide a nucleus for persistent antigenaemia. The demonstrations of immune complexes in infective diseases (Oldstone and Dixon, 1970; Zuckerman, 1975) and the demonstration of immune complexes involving HB-

Ag in the vascular lesions of polyarteritis nodosa (Gocke et al., 1971) has prompted many workers to search for such complexes in other diseases where the aetiology is obscure.

CLINICAL INVESTIGATION OF IMMUNE COMPLEX DISEASE

Two main approaches have been made towards the identification of immune complexes in human disease. The examination of biopsy material by immunohistochemical techniques allows the demonstration of immuno-globulin deposits often with associated complement components and some identified antigens in a pattern that suggests complex formation (Wilson and Dixon, 1974). Similar appearances have also been demonstrated by electron microscopy where the typical morphological features of immune complex glomerulonephritis equate with the appearances described in the experimentally produced lesion (Dixon, 1963). Whilst the identification of immunoglobulin and complement components deposits can be made fairly readily in biopsy material and has become a routine practice in the examination of renal and certain other biopsies, the identification of antigen presents rather more of a problem. The limited number of antigens positively identified in immune complex disease by immunofluorescent microscopy is illustrated in *Table* 1.

Table 1. ANTIGENS DETECTED BY IMMUNOFLUORESCENT MICROSCOPY

Site	Antigen	Disease	Reference
Glomeruli	DNA	Systemic lupus	Koffler et al., 1967
	HB Ag	Post transfusion glomerulonephritis	Combes et al., 1971
	IgG	Mixed cryoglobulinaemia	Feizi and Gitlin, 1969
	Heterophile reactive	Infectious mononucleosis	Peters, 1967
	Streptococcal	Poststreptococcal glomerulonephritis	Zabriskie, 1971
	Staphylococcal	Shunt nephritis	Kaufman and McIntosh, 1971
	Plasmodium malariae	Quartan malarial nephropathy	Hendrickse et al., 1972
Skin	Candida	Vasculitis	Parish, 1971
	Streptococcal	Vasculitis	Parish, 1971
	Staphylococcal	Vasculitis	Parish, 1971
	Mycobacterium tuberculosis	Vasculitis	Parish, 1971
	IgG	Mixed cryoglobulinaemia	Cream, 1971
Muscle	HBAg	Polyarteritis nodosa	Gocke et al., 1971

The second approach is the direct examination of plasma or other body fluid for the presence of complexes or for the presence of serological changes that are often associated with the formation of immune complexes. Many methods have been developed over the years and none is entirely satisfactory. Not all the methods detect the same complexes and a method which may be satisfactory in one clinical situation may not be so in another. Almost all of the methods suffer from the major disadvantage that aggregated or altered IgG will give positive results even when this aggregation is an artefactual or *in vitro* phenomenon.

METHODS OF DETECTION OF SOLUBLE IMMUNE COMPLEXES

The methods of detection of circulating immune complexes may be divided into—

1. Antigen independent methods:
    a. Physicochemical properties
    b. Biological properties
        i. Free molecule receptors
        ii. Cellular receptors
2. Antigen specific methods
3. Indirect serological methods

The antigen independent methods are all liable to major problems of specificity and sensitivity and require rigorous control to exclude non-specific reactions obscuring the true interpretation. The methods do not usually allow the identification of antigen or antibody class in the complex.

The antigen specific methods may be useful in specific clinical instances where the antigen is defined. With the multiplicity of possible antigens in most disease states, the widespread adoption of these techniques would seem an unlikely proposition.

Immune complexes formed *in vivo* usually activate the complement system by the classic pathway. Indirect evidence as to the presence of immune complexes may be obtained from the plasma complement analysis with particular reference to the presence or absence of *in vivo* activation products C3c and C3d.

Antigen independent methods

a. PHYSICOCHEMICAL

The production of immune complexes results in the formation of particles that differ from free antibody in their molecular size, solubility and electric charge.

Analytical ultracentrifugation has been used to demonstrate the presence of complexes in sera and other body fluids, but the technique is not specific and sensitivity is low. 22s IgG – IgM complexes and 9 – 17s IgG – IgG complexes have been demonstrated in rheumatoid arthritis (Franklin et al, 1957; Kunkel et al., 1961). Similar results can be achieved by *sucrose density gradient centrifugation* or by *molecular sieving in gels*. These two techniques offer the advantage that the complexes can be collected and analysed by immuno-chemical techniques demonstrating not only antibody class but also the presence of complement components.

Macromolecular components containing C3 have been demonstrated in various immune complex disorders following gel chromatography (Soothill and Hendrickse, 1967).

Some separation techniques for normal serum proteins can also be used to precipitate immune complexes and large molecules whilst leaving free immunoglobulin molecules in solution. *Precipitation with polyethylene glycol* (PEG MW 6000) has been used in the clinical identification of immune complexes (Creighton et al., 1973). Precipitation of serum proteins by PEG is proportional to PEG concentration and molecular size (Zubler et al., 1977), at low PEG concentration high molecular weight proteins and immune complexes are preferentially precipitated. Decreased solubility of immune complexes under defined conditions of temperature has also been extensively demonstrated. The *cryoprecipitation* of proteins from a serum sample is perhaps the simplest technique that may be used to demonstrate the presence of immune complexes, but monoclonal immunoglobulins and many other proteins may also exhibit cryoprecipitability. Extensive immunochemical investigation of the cryoprecipitate including identification of antibody and complement components is required before a cryoglobulin can be considered as an immune complex (Bronet et al., 1974).

b. BIOLOGICAL

The presence of aggregated immunoglobulin or immune complexes allows the recognition of the structurally altered immunoglobulin by specific receptors either on free molecules or on cell surface receptors. The free molecule receptors used are almost exclusively complement (C1q), antiglobulin or immunoconglutinin, whilst the cell surface receptors are Fc receptors or C3 receptors on isolated or cultured blood and tissue cells.

i. *Free molecule receptor methods*

One of the oldest techniques for the demonstration of immune complexes involving complement interaction is the measurement of *anticomplementary activity* (Shulman and Barker, 1969). The method is a standard complement fixation reaction and all substances that can interfere with the complement reaction can give false positive results. Recent refinements have been added to the test restricting action to the C1q step of the reaction to give the *C1q deviation test* (Sobel et al., 1975). This modification is extremely sensitive and is not subject to interference by substances activating the alternate pathway of complement activation. The direct demonstration of C1q binding by the immune complexes may be demonstrated by precipitation in gel—*C1q agarose precipitation test* (Agnello et al., 1970)—or by binding in the fluid phase using radio-labelled C1q as a trace substance to identify the complex—*C1q binding test* (Nydegger, Lambert et al., 1974). This latter technique is sensitive and allows quantitation of the immune complexes but does require heat inactivation of the patient's own C1q, a step which can decrease specificity by aggregating immunoglobulin. Heat inactivation can be avoided by the addition of EDTA, a step which also prevents the possible interference of C-reactive protein. More recent developments of the technique include the *solid phase C1q binding tests* in which the C1q is bound to the wall of polystyrene test tubes (Hay et al., 1976).

The interaction between rheumatoid factor and immune complexes has been demonstrated by various techniques. Monoclonal rheumatoid factor is used as a precipitant of immune complexes in *direct precipitation in agarose gel* (Winchester et al., 1971) and the *agglutination inhibition reaction* (Luthra et al., 1975). Neither of these methods is applicable to sera containing rheumatoid factor and the heat inactivation step may produce aggregation of immunoglobulin. Immunoglobulin concentration also influences the test result because normal monomeric immunoglobulin may react with rheumatoid factor.

Immunoconglutinins are immunoglobulins which react with complement components bound to immune complexes. These, and bovine conglutinins, represent an additional potential reagent for the demonstration and detection of immune complexes.

ii. Cell surface receptor methods

The use of living cells as the substrate for laboratory tests makes standardization difficult and renders the test liable to interference by substances which modify cell metabolism. The techniques described do, however, reveal important information as to the biological effect of immune complexes.

The *platelet aggregation test* (Pentinnen et al., 1975) and the *inhibition of antibody dependent cell mediated cytotoxicity* (Jewell and MacLennan, 1973) are dependent on Fc receptors, whilst the *Raji cell immunoassay* (Theofilopoulos et al., 1974) and the *inhibition of complement dependent lymphocyte rosettes* (Ezer and Hayward, 1974) are dependent on C3 receptors.

Antigen specific methods

Except in certain well defined situations methods dependent on knowing the antigen concerned in an immune complex disorder have little practical application. The one good example is the morphologic identification of hepatitis B antigen by electron microscopy (Almeida and Watson, 1969).

A variation of the antigen specific methodology is the measurement of specific antibody before and after removal of antigen. This has been successfully applied to the detection of DNA-antibody complexes (Harbeck et al., 1973) and insulin-antibody complexes (Jayarao et al., 1973).

Indirect serological methods

Most immune complexes will activate the complement system by the classic activation pathway. When large amounts of such complexes are formed there is marked depletion of plasma C4 and C3 levels with resultant hypocomplementaemia. This situation holds for the more gross immune complex diseases such as systemic lupus erythematosus and glomerulonephritis, but in many other situations the changes in the complement profile may be masked by the acute phase response. This increased synthesis of complement components in inflammation renders the complement profile inconclusive (Ruddy et al., 1972). Demonstration of complement hypercatabolism (Charlesworth et al., 1974) suggests consumption by immune complexes, but metabolic studies of this nature are not of immediate practical value in clinical diagnosis.

An alternative to this metabolic approach is to examine plasma for the presence of complement breakdown products. During activation by $C\overline{42}$ (C3 convertase) the native C3 molecule is converted into the active molecule C3b. Inactivation of this component produces two breakdown products, C3c and C3d. C3c, by virtue of its faster electrophoretic mobility, can be distinguished from the native molecule by *antigen-antibody crossed electrophoresis* (Laurell, 1965). The proportion of C3 present in plasma as the inactive C3c is a measure of C3 activation *in vivo* and presumptive evidence of immune complex formation. The technique requires strict attention to factors which might promote C3 conversion *in vitro* and the use of EDTA as an anticoagulant to prevent coagulation-induced C3 cleavage. An alternative approach is to precipitate native C3 and inactive C3c with PEG and to estimate the concentration of C3d in the plasma sample with a specific antiserum (Perrin et al., 1975). This latter technique has been shown to correlate well with the amount of immune complexes present as detected by other methods.

CIRCULATING IMMUNE COMPLEXES IN CLINICAL MEDICINE

Two distinct clinical patterns of disease associated with circulating immune complexes are recognized: widespread multifocal vasculitis and isolated glomerulonephritis. In reality, however, these represent the opposite ends of a spectrum of diseases which have a common pathogenic mechanism although diverse initiating factors.

Iatrogenic disease: Serum sickness is the classic example of an iatrogenic immune complex disorder, but one which is rarely encountered in modern clinical practice. Drug sickness commonly associated with penicillin therapy, although also encountered with insulin therapy, is the nearest modern equivalent.

Infections: The clinical finding of myalgia, arthralgia, haematuria, albuminuria and fleeting skin rashes in many infections can be ascribed to the presence of circulating immune complexes as well as to the toxic effect of the infective agent.

Viral infections: Circulating immune complexes have been described in *hepatitis B infection* (Alpert et al., 1971) during the phase of polyarthralgia and urticaria which is often associated with hypocomplementaemia. Gocke et al. (1971) have described hepatitis B antigen and immune complexes in *polyarteritis nodosa*. The acute haemorrhage shock of *Dengue haemorrhagic fever* is probably due to the presence of massive amounts of immune complexes (Sobel et al., 1975) and immune complexes have been demonstrated in *mycoplasma pneumonia* (Biberfeld and Norberg, 1974) and *measles* (Myllyla et al., 1971).

Bacterial infections: The glomerulonephritis occurring in patients with *infected ventriculo-atrial shunts (shunt nephritis)* and in *bacterial endocarditis* are of immune complex aetiology. The skin lesions of *erythema nodosum* have been ascribed to an Arthus phenomenon but the associated arthralgia and glomerulonephritis are of circulating immune complex aetiology (Moran et al., 1972). Moderate levels of circulating immune complexes have been shown in *leprosy* (Bjorvatn et al., 1976).

Parasitic infections: Circulating immune complexes have been demonstrated in *schistosomiasis* (Butterworth et al., 1976) and may be involved in the mechanism by which the parasite evades the consequences of the immune response. In *malaria* immune complexes are responsible for the rare nephrotic complication but may also be relevant in the cerebral complications (Lambert and Houba, 1974).

Collagen vascular disorders

Circulating immune complexes are intimately associated with the evolution, manifestation and pathogenesis of *systemic lupus erythematosus* (Agnello et al., 1970). The quantitation or indirect evaluation of the level of circulating complexes has a practical value in the clinical management of patients with SLE. The level of complexes is closely correlated with disease activity. Similar observations have been made in *rheumatoid arthritis* (Winchester et al., 1970) although the level of immune complexes is usually somewhat lower and may in part be restricted to the synovial fluid. Complexes have also been demonstrated in association with the vasculitis of *Wegener's granulomatosis* (Howell and Epstein, 1976).

Other conditions in which immune complexes have been described include *inflammatory bowel disease* (Jewell and MacLennan, 1973), *Crohn's disease* and *coeliac disease* (Doe et al., 1973), *chronic liver disease* (Pentinnen, 1972), *sarcoidosis* (Hedfers and Norberg, 1974), *Hashimoto's disease* (Barkas et al., *1976), dermatitis herpetiformis* (Mowbray et al., 1973) and *amyotrophic lateral sclerosis* (Oldstone et al., 1976).

Neoplasia

Circulating immune complexes have been demonstrated between tumour antigens and antibody in experimental animals, but the relevance of this to disease in man is not yet explained. It is possible that the presence of immune complexes may limit the host's response to the tumour and limit his ability to control the cancer by cell mediated cytotoxicity. Increased levels of immune complexes have been demonstrated in various forms of *cancer, Hodgkin's disease* and *leukaemia,* but as yet correlation with the clinical course is incomplete.

REFERENCES

Agnello V., Winchester R. J. I. and Kunkel H. G. (1970) Precipitin reactions of the C1q component of complement with aggregated gammaglobulin and immune complexes in gel diffusion. *Immunology* **19**, 909 – 919.

Almeida J. D. and Watson A. P. (1969) Immune complexes in hepatitis. *Lancet* **2**, 983 – 986.

Alpert E., Isselbacher K. J. and Schur P. H. (1971) The pathogenesis of arthritis associated with viral hepatitis. *N. Engl. J. Med.* **285**, 185 – 189.

Barkas T., Al-Khatab S. F., Irvine W. J. et al. (1976) Inhibition of cell mediated cytotoxicity as a means of detection of immune complexes in the sera of patients with thyroid disorders and bronchogenic carcinoma. *Clin. Exp. Immunol.* **25**, 270 – 279.

Biberfeld G. and Norberg G. (1974) Circulating immune complexes in mycoplasma pneumonial infections. *J. Immunol.* **112**, 413 – 415.

Bjorvatn B., Barnetson R. S., Kronvall G. et al. (1976) Immune complexes and complement hypercatabolism in patients with leprosy. *Clin. Exp. Immunol.* **26**, 388 – 396.

Bronet J. C., Clauvel J. P., Danon F. et al. (1974) Biologic and clinical significance of cryoglobulins. *Am. J. Med.* **57**, 775 – 788.

Butterworth A. E., Sturrock R. F., Houba V. et al. (1976) *Schistosoma mansoni* in baboons: antibody-dependent cell mediated damage to ^{51}Cr-labelled schistosomata. *Clin. Exp. Immunol.* **25**, 95 – 102.

Charlesworth J. A., Williams D. G., Sherington E. et al. (1974) Metabolic studies of the third component of complement and glycine rich betaglycoprotein in patients with hypocomplementaemia. *J. Clin. Invest.* **53**, 1578 – 1587.

Cochrane C. G. (1967) Mediators of the arthus and related reactions *Prog. Allergy* **11**, 1 – 35.

Combes B., Stastney P., Shorey J. et al. (1971) Glomerulonephritis with deposition of Australia antigen and antibody complexes in the glomerular basement membrane. *Lancet* **2**, 234 – 237.

Cream J. J. (1971) Immunofluorescent studies of the skin in cryoglobulinaemic vasculitis. *Br. J. Dermatol.* **84**, 48 – 53.

Creighton W. D., Lambert P. H. and Meischer P. A. (1973) Detection of antibodies and soluble antigen antibody complexes by precipitation with polyethylene glycol. *J. Immunol.* **111**, 1219 – 1227.

Dixon F. J. (1963) The role of antigen-antibody complexes in disease. *Harvey Lect.* **58**, 21 – 52.

Dixon F. J., Vasquez J. J. and Weigle W. O. (1958) Pathogenesis of serum sickness. *Arch. Pathol.* **65**, 18 – 28.

Ďoe W. F., Booth C. C. and Brown D. L. (1973) Evidence of complement binding immune complexes in adult coeliac disease, Crohn's disease, and ulcerative colitis. *Lancet* **1**, 402 – 403.

Ezer G. and Hayward A. R. (1974) Inhibition of complement dependent lymphocyte rosette formation: a possible test for activated complement products. *Europ. J. Immunol.* **4**, 148 – 150.

Feizi T. and Gitlin N. (1969) Immune complex disease of the kidney associated with chronic hepatitis and cryoglobulinaemia. *Lancet* **2**, 873 – 876.

Franklin E. C., Holman H. R., Müller Eberhard H. J. et al. (1957) An unusual protein component of high molecular weight in the serum of certain patients with rheumatoid arthritis. *J. Exp. Med.* **105**, 425 – 438.

Friedemann U. (1909) Weitere untersuchungen uber dan mechanisms de anaphylaxie. *Z. Immun. Allergie forset.* **2**, 591.

Gocke D. J., Hsu K., Morgan C. et al. (1971) Vasculitis in association with Australian antigen. *J. Exp. Med.* **134**, Suppl. 330.

Harbeck R. J., Bardana E. J., Kouler P. F. et al. (1973) DNA – anti-DNA complexes: their detection in systemic lupus erythematosus sera. *J. Clin. Invest.* **52**, 789 – 795.

Hay F. C., Mineham L. J. and Roitt I. M. (1976) Routine assay for the detection of immune complexes of known immunoglobulin class using solid phase C1q. *Clin. Exp. Immunol.* **24**, 396 – 400.

Hedfers E. and Norberg R. (1974) Evidence for circulating immune complexes in sarcoidosis. *Clin. Exp. Immunol.* **16**, 493 – 496.

Hendrickse R. G., Glasgow E. F., Adeniyi A. et al. (1972) Quartan malarial nephrotic syndrome. *Lancet* **1**, 1143 – 1148.

Howell S. B. and Epstein W. V. (1976) Circulating immune complexes in Wegener's granulomatosis. *Am. J. Med.* **60**, 259 – 268.

Jayarao K. S., Faulk W. P., Karam J. H. et al. (1973) Measurement of immune complexes in insulin treated diabetics. *J. Immunol. Methods* **3**, 337 – 346.

Jewell D. P. and MacLennan I. C. M. (1973) Circulating immune complexes in inflammatory bowel disease. *Clin. Exp. Immunol.* **14**, 219 – 226.

Kaufman D. B. and McIntosh R. (1971) The pathogenesis of the renal lesion in a patient with streptococcal disease, infected ventriculo-atrial shunt, cryoglobulinaemia and nephritis. *Am. J. Med.* **50**, 262 – 268.

Koffler D., Schor P. H. and Kunkel H. G. (1967) Immunological studies concerning the nephritis of systemic lupus erythematosus. *J. Exp. Med.* **126**, 607 – 623.

Kunkel H. G., Müller Eberhard H. J., Fudenberg H. H. et al. (1961) Gammablobulin complexes in rheumatoid arthritis and certain other conditions. *J. Clin. Invest.* **40**, 117 – 129.

Lachmann P. (1976) Clinical effects of complement deficiencies. In: Peters D. K. (ed.), *Advanced Medicine,* vol. 12, London, Pitman Medical.

Lambert P. H. and Houba V. (1974) Immune complexes in parasitic diseases. In: Brent L. and Holborow J. (ed.), *Progress in Immunology* II, vol. 5. Amsterdam, North-Holland, pp. 57 – 67.

Laurell C. B. (1965) Antigen-antibody crossed electrophoresis. *Anal. Biochem.* **10**, 358 – 361.

Luthra H. S., McDuffie F. C., Hunder G. G. et al. (1975) Immune complexes in sera and synovial fluids of patients with rheumatoid arthritis — Radio immunoassay with monoclonal rheumatoid factor. *J. Clin. Invest.* **56**, 458 – 466.

Moran C. J., Ruder G., Turk J. L. et al. (1972) Evidence for circulating immune complexes in lepromatous leprosy. *Lancet* **2**, 572 – 573.

Mowbray J. F., Hoffbrand A. V., Holborrow E. J. et al. (1973) Circulating immune complexes in dermatitis herpetiformis. *Lancet* **1**, 400 – 402.

Müiler-Eberhard H. J. (1975) Complement. *Ann. Rev. Biochem.* **44**, 697 – 724.

Myllyla G., Vaheri A. and Pentinnen K. (1971) Detection and characterisation of immune complexes by the platelet aggregation test: 2, Circulating complexes. *Clin. Exp. Immunol.* **8**, 399 – 408.

Nussenzweig V. (1974) Receptors for immune complexes on lymphocytes. *Adv. Immunol.* **19**, 217 – 258.

Nydegger U. E., Anner R. M., Gerebtzoff A. et al. (1974) Polymorphonuclear leucocyte stimulation by immune complexes: assessment of the nitro blue tetrazolium dye reduction. *Europ. J. Immunol.* **3**, 465 – 470.

Nydegger U. E., Lambert P. H., Gerber H. et al. (1974) Circulating immune complexes in the serum in systemic lupus erythematosus and in carriers of hepatitis B antigen: quantitation by binding to radiolabelled C1q. *J. Clin. Invest.* **54**, 297 – 309.

Oldstone M. B. A. and Dixon F. J. (1969) Pathogenesis of chronic disease associated with persistent lymphocytic choriomeningitis viral infection. *J. Exp. Med.* Part I, **129**, 483 – 505. Part II, 1970, **131**, 1 – 19.

Oldstone M. B. A., Wilson C. B., Perrin L. H. et al. (1976) Evidence for immune-complex formation in patients with amyotrophic lateral sclerosis. *Lancet,* **2**, 169 – 172.

Parish W. E. (1971) Studies on vasculitis. *Clin. Allergy* **1**, 97 – 109.

Pentinnen K. (1972) Platelet aggregation test in the study of hepatitis. *Am. J. Dis. Child.* **123**, 418 – 420.

Pentinnen K., Wagner O., Rasanen J. A. et al. (1975) Platelet aggregation and Cryo IgM in the study of hepatitis and immune complex status. *Clin. Exp. Immunol.* **15**, 409 – 416.

Perrin L. H., Lambert P. H. and Miescher P. A. (1975) Complement breakdown products in plasma from patients with systemic lupus erythematosus and patients with membranoproliferative or other glomerulonephritis. *J. Clin. Invest.* **56**, 740 – 750.

Peters J. H. (1967) Heterophile reactive antigen in infectious mononucleosis. *Science* **157**, 1200 – 1202.

Ruddy S., Gigli I. and Austen K. F. (1972) The complement system of man. *N. Engl. J. Med.* **287**, 642 – 646.

Shulman N. R. and Barker L. F. (1969) Virus-like antigen, antibody and antigen-antibody complexes in hepatitis measured by complement fixation. *Science* **165**, 304 – 306.

Shulman N. R. and Rall J. E. (1963) *Trans. Assoc. Am. Physicians* **76**, 72.

Sobel A. T., Bokisch V. A. and Müller-Eberhard H. J. (1975) C1q deviation test for the detection of immune complexes, aggregates of IgG, and bacterial products in sera. *J. Exp. Med.* **142**, 139 – 150.

Soothill J. F. and Hendrickse R. G. (1967) Some immunological studies of the nephrotic syndrome of Nigerian children. *Lancet* **2**, 629 – 632.

Steward M. W., Petty R. E. and Soothill K. F. (1973) Low affinity antibody: its possible immunopathological significance. *Int. Arch. Allergy Appl. Immunol.* **45**, 176 – 179.

Theofilopoulos A. N., Wilson C. B., Bokisch V. A. et al. (1974) Binding of soluble immune complexes to human lymphoblastoid cells. 2, Use of Raji cells to detect circulating immune complexes in animal and human sera. *J. Exp. Med.* **140**, 1230 – 1244.

von Pirquet C. E. (1911) Allergy. *Arch. Intern. Med.* **7**, 259 – 288.

Warner N. L. (1974) Membrane immunoglobulins and antigen receptors on B and T lymphocytes. *Adv. Immunol.* **19**, 67 – 216.

Weigle W. O. (1961) Fate and biological activity of antigen-antibody complexes. *Adv. Immunol.* **1**, 283 – 317.

Wilson G. B. and Dixon F. J. (1974) Diagnosis of immunopathological renal disease. *Kidney Internat.* **5**, 389 – 401.

Winchester R. J., Agnello V. and Kunkel H. G. (1970) Gammaglobulin complexes in synovial fluids of patients with rheumatoid arthritis. Partial characterisation and relationship to lowered complement level. *Clin. Exp. Immunol.* **6**, 689 – 706.

Winchester R. J., Kunkel H. G. and Agnello V. (1971) Occurrence of gammaglobulin complexes in serum and joint fluid of rheumatoid arthritis patients: use of monoclonal rheumatoid factors as reagent for their demonstration. *J. Exp. Med.* **134**, 286s – 295s.

Zabriskie J. B. (1971) The role of streptococci in human glomerulonephritis. *J. Exp. Med.* **134**, Suppl. 180.

Zubler R. H., Perrin L. H., Creighton W. D. et al. (1977) The use of polyethylene glycol (PEG) to concentrate immune complexes from serum and plasma samples. *Ann. Rheum. Dis.* **36**, Suppl. 1, 23 – 25.

Zuckerman A. J. (1975) Viral hepatitis: current studies and future prospects. *Monogr. Allergy* **9**, 196 – 216.

Special Article

SCREENING IN CANCER

IAN BURN FRCS

In our attempts to cure cancer during the first half of this century, the task was an almost impossible one because of the very high proportion of patients presenting with advanced disease when first seen by a doctor. In this context the term 'advanced' implies that the cancer had progressed beyond the scope of excisional surgery, either because of the involvement of the vital local structures or because of metastatic spread. Unfortunately, cancer in its early stages usually results in relatively trivial symptoms and only the most obvious surface lesions provoke a response from the patient.

During the past 25 years the proportion of treated early cancers has gradually increased. This has been due to a certain amount of effective publicity and, in the United Kingdom, to the availability of early consultation with a specialist in the N.H.S. This has resulted in some improvement in cure rates, but certainly not enough to justify any sense of satisfaction.

For cure of the common cancers, such as stomach, large intestines, breast, lung, cervix, bladder and skin, it is imperative that the disease is diagnosed while still confined to its site of origin, and small enough to enable the surgeon to excise widely and safely—safely, that is to say, in respect both of inadvertent dissemination of the disease during operation and of reconstruction of the residual defect. The presence of progressive metastic disease makes cure impossible. Endocrine therapy, cytotoxic therapy and most certainly immunotherapy cannot eradicate metastic disease totally, although appropriate use of the two first-named methods has certainly lengthened the survival of many thousands of patients with incurable malignant disease.

This somewhat lengthy preamble is deliberate in order to emphasize the continuing need for the early diagnosis of cancer. At the present time, there is no other realistic way in which we may hope to improve *cure* rates. Continued publicity and sensible investigation of trivial, but persistent symptoms will unquestionably improve the situation. The fact has to be faced, however, that malignant disease in general will never produce symptoms early enough for any major improvement to occur if we continue to adopt the conventional approach of 'waiting for trouble'.

How far should we depart from this conventional approach and begin to search meticulously for occult lesions, which perhaps are years away from causing symptoms if allowed to develop unchecked? It would be helpful if we had a 'spot' test, haematological, urine or dermal, which could identify unequivocally any individual harbouring an unsuspected malignancy. There is nothing, however, to suggest that such a test will be forthcoming in this century. Many ideas, mainly based on immunotesting, have been explored, but no convincing accurate test has emerged.

This means, therefore, that search for occult cancer has to be carried out on specific organs. The thought is daunting, especially in terms of economics, logistics and human emotions. What makes the problem *more* difficult is the fact that modern technology has now provided the methods for diagnosis of very small cancers in most areas of the body. Breast, intestine, brain, lung, bone, urinary tract, pelvic organs and skin are all now amenable to the most minute scrutiny through the media of isotope scanning, ultrasonics, thermography, high calibre radiology, cytology and fibre-optic endoscopic examination. Much of this is highly expensive, of course, and realistically screening must be considered only in the context of those cancers which are most prevalent and most likely to cause premature death. These are cancer of the lung, stomach and large intestines in both men and women, and cancer of the breast and cervix in women.

In Japan, where cancer of the stomach is perhaps that nation's most dominant health problem, a determined effort has been made to identify the disease at an early stage by screening the population. Mostly this screening consists of clinical examination and meticulous radiology of the upper gastro-intestinal tract. Latterly, widespread use of fibre-optic gastroscopy has increased the accuracy of detection of very early gastric cancer. The impact of this national programme, forced upon the Japanese by the massively high incidence of the disease, has already been reflected in the survival rate after treatment. Japan now has a 5-year postoperative survival rate, which is infinitely superior to any other nation in the world.

The Japanese experience with gastric cancer is unique. No other country has felt the need to screen for any malignant disease on the same scale. Routine chest X-rays in many countries have revealed occasional early lung cancers, but there has been no defined attempt at screening for this prevalent disease. Many health screening centres in the U.S.A. include barium enema and sigmoidoscopy in their routine general screening programme, influenced by the high incidence of colo-rectal cancer in that country. However, to date there has been no national or even regional attempt to screen the adult population definitively for cancer of the large intestine in the U.S.A.

The malignant disease which has received most screening attention internationally is cervical cancer, and attempts at population screening have been made in many countries.

CERVICAL SCREENING

It is now 30 years since the Papanicolaou smear became available for detecting early cancer of the cervix. It has been claimed that carcinoma of the uterine cervix and endometrium are eradicable diseases—'by means of the cytologic techniques known to us today'. Although this is perhaps a rather extravagant claim, it expresses the optimism which is justified by continued use of this investigation.

One of the first countries to appreciate the potential of cervical cytology was Canada. Screening services started in British Columbia in 1949 and subsequently have extended across Canada. In less than a decade the incidence of invasive cancer of the cervix in Vancouver was reduced by 30 per cent, due entirely to the recognition of the pre-invasive stages of the disease in asymptomatic women and the institution of appropriate treatment. Canada is now in the process of establishing an official task force which will make recommendations on cervical screening, presumably on a national basis.

In the U.S.A. it has been estimated that over 30 million tests are carried out each year, and the advisability of regular screening has been accepted in that country to a large extent. In Britain, where cervical cancer kills 2000 women each year, a nation-wide screening programme was inaugurated in 1964, and it is estimated that over 2·5 million smears are now examined annually, through the services of family doctors, hospital clinics and a variety of local health clinics, including mobile units.

Basically screening for cervical cancer employs meticulous examination of cytological specimens which may be obtained by various methods. Preferably the specimens should be obtained by skilled medical personnel, trained to expose the cervix and fornices accurately when taking the material for examination. Recently 'do-it-yourself' kits were utilized in mass screening in Denmark, the women making their own smears at mid-cycle by use of irrigation cyto-pipettes. It is doubtful, however, if such self-conducted methods can ever be as reliable as smears made by trained personnel.

Examination of cervical cytology specimens will reveal the presence of normal, atypical or frankly malignant cells. The recognition of either of the last 2 categories is always an indication for further action as determined by the gynaecologist. The pathologist's contribution to cervical screening has been a major one, with the defining and better understanding of dysplastic states, carcinoma-in-situ and micro-invasive cancer. Women with carcinoma-in-situ are younger on the average by a decade than those with frankly invasive cancer, and this is one area of cancer screening which must start in the young.

In general screening should start in women in their 20s and be repeated at intervals of 5 years if the test is technically reliable and the result normal. In older women, after the age of 35 years, it is advisable that screening should then continue on a 3-yearly basis.

The success of cervical screening is dependent on the co-operation of women. Unfortunately, there still remains a reluctance on the part of those who historically are at greater risk, namely multiparous women over the age of 35 whose husbands are employed in semi-skilled or unskilled occupations. Much still has to be done to encourage greater participation by women of these social groups. Nevertheless, cervical screening undoubtedly is a success story and a major advance in health care.

MAMMARY SCREENING

The striking difference in the curability of small, confined carcinomas of the breast (stage $T_1N_0M_0$) compared with all other clinical stages emphasizes the advantage of early diagnosis. According to *Hansard* on 30th November, 1976, there were 19 952 new cases of breast cancer registered in the British Isles in the year 1970 and 11 775 deaths. It is now a disease of formidable proportions and all the evidence points to a gradual but definite increase in incidence of the disease throughout the world.

Evidence that screening of asymptomatic women for evidence of mammary cancer can result in a reduction in mortality from the disease has already been provided by the controlled trial carried out in New York. Initiated in the early 1960s under the auspices of the Health Insurance Plan of Greater New York, the study involved 62 000 women aged between 40 and 65 years who were randomly allocated to 2 groups. One group were offered annual screening consisting of clinical examination and mammography, the other group were not. After 9 years of the investigation, there was no difference in the results of treatment of those who developed cancer of the breast in the 2 groups under the age of 50 years, but there was a 40 per cent reduction in mortality in women over the age of 50 years whose cancers were detected on screening. This study has come under considerable scrutiny recently and in particular by a working group set up by the National Cancer Institute in Bethesda, on behalf of the U.S. Department of Health, Education and Welfare. Nevertheless, the study was perhaps one of the most important ever carried out and has pioneered the way to population screening for breast cancer.

Inspired by the New York study and a growing awareness of the development of individual mammary screening clinics in Britain, a Working Group on Breast Cancer Screening was set up by the Department of Health in 1971. As a result, 3 official pilot studies were designed to investigate many of the problems involved in mammary screening. One of these was sited in West London and involved deliberate screening of a volunteer section of the female population in the London Borough of Ealing. The study started in 1973, women over the age of 40 being invited to attend for clinical examination and mammography annually, with interval clinical examination at 6 months. By the end of April 1977, 2,484 women had enrolled and 29 cancers had been detected by screening. Preliminary results from this study confirmed the New York experience, namely that cancers detected by screening were frequently very early in clinical terms, and those detected solely by mammography were unlikely to be associated with involved regional lymph nodes, this latter fact carrying the implication of an excellent prognosis with adequate treatment.

Effective mammary screening requires meticulous clinical examination combined with low-dose mammography. Techniques such as mammary thermography, ultrasonics and nipple suction cytology have yet to prove their value. Mammography is vital, however, and concern about its safety is more theoretical than real if the technique is restricted to women over the age of 40, and all the available precautions, such as the use of intensifying screens, are taken to keep the radiation dose to the breast tissue below 1 rad per examination.

There are still innumerable problems associated with mammary screening. Interpretations of mammographic findings are far from accurate as yet and much work needs to be done to correlate these with subsequent histology. In particular mammography can be difficult to interpret in pre-menopausal women, and this fact probably accounted for its limited use in the under 50s in the New York study. Nevertheless, unless mammography is included in the screening programme, probably about one-third of existing early asymptomatic cancers will be missed.

If we can ever envisage mammary screening on a national scale, there would be massive problems over training staff to carry out the work proficiently as well as deciding such vital questions as the optimum intervals for screening and the most suitable publicity for encouraging women to attend. In this latter context, however, mammary screening has one great advantage over cervical screening. Cancer of the breast occurs most commonly in the upper socio-economic classes of women, who already have been shown to be most amenable to attend regularly for screening procedures.

There are also the problems of deciding whether screening should be reserved for the apparently high-risk groups and of defining those groups precisely. This has aptly been described as a 'Catch-22' situation, for those women who are at massive risk are few and highly atypical. Finally, as with any health screening programme, there must be a rapid facility for specialist opinion for those women in whom an abnormality is detected: not an easy prospect in an already overloaded hospital system, but not insuperable given the necessary facilities and goodwill.

Despite all the many problems, of all the many worth while areas of screening for early cancer, that for cancer of the breast probably has most to offer. Early cancer of the breast is a curable disease. Its present tragedy is the high proportion of women who only first notice the disease when it is already advanced and beyond cure.

ALIMENTARY DISEASE

SIR FRANCIS AVERY JONES
CBE, MD, FRCP
SIR JAMES FRASER Bt, BA,
ChM (Edin), FRCS
J. G. GOLIGHER ChM, FRCS
SHEILA SHERLOCK MD, FRCP,
FRCP (Edin), FRCCP (Hon),
FACP (Hon)
J. E. TRAPNELL MA, MD, FRCS

Oesophagus, stomach and small intestine: medical

SIR FRANCIS AVERY JONES CBE, MD, FRCP

ACUTE HAEMORRHAGIC GASTRITIS

Simonian and Curtis (1976) report beneficial treatment of acute haemorrhagic gastritis by massive antacid treatment. The study consisted of 49 patients with documented acute gastric mucosal haemorrhage. The diagnosis was based on endoscopic findings in all patients and it was confirmed at surgery in five. There were 35 men and 14 women. The total blood transfusion requirements per patient were 1 500 – 7 500 ml, with a mean of 4 200 ml. Excluded were patients with less than 1 500 ml blood transfusion requirement. The bleeding was associated with surgery, trauma, sepsis and excess intake of alcohol. Patients whose bleeding was secondary to peptic gastric or duodenal ulcers or to oesophageal varices or to associated coagulopathy were excluded. Treatment consisted of removal of blood clots from the stomach, iced saline lavage, followed by instillation of antacid-buffer (magaldrate, Riopan) into a nasogastic tube until the pH of the nasogastric aspirate was returned to 7. In each patient the amount of buffer required per hour to raise and maintain the intragastric pH at 7 was titrated as follows: a nasogastric tube was passed into the stomach; the gastric contents were aspirated as completely as possible and emptied into a basin by the bedside; using phenaphthazine pH paper (Nitrazine), the pH of the intragastric contents was measured and recorded. In most patients the pH was 5 or below 5. Sixty ml of antacid was instilled into the stomach by gravity drainage and was allowed to mix for 15 minutes with the nasogastric tube clamped. At the end of 15 minutes the stomach was re-aspirated. If the pH was below 7, an additional increment of 30 ml of antacid (total volume of antacid 90 ml) was instilled. Again, 15 minutes was allowed for mixing before the next pH measurement was taken. This procedure was continued until the amount of antacid required per 15 minutes to raise and maintain the intragastric pH at 7 was determined, usually in less than an hour. Thereafter, clamping of the nasogastric tube was prolonged to hourly intervals and the predetermined volume of antacid was instilled and reaspirated from the stomach to return the pH to 7. Titration was carried out by a nurse in the intensive care unit, and the measured volumes of antacid and pH value taken at the end of each hour were recorded on the bedside chart. In the majority of patients, the volume of antacid required to completely inactivate the gastric hydrochloric acid at a pH of 7 was 60 – 180 ml per hour.

Control of bleeding was usually achieved 4 – 24 hours after neutralizing gastric hydrochloric acid. If at the end of 24 hours there was clinical evidence that the bleeding had stopped (as indicated by blood-free nasogastric aspirate, cessation in blood transfusion requirements, and stabilization of haematocrit and vital signs), the frequency of antacid instillation and nasogastric tube clamping was reduced to 2-hourly intervals and continued for another 24 hours. If after 24 hours there was no further evidence of bleeding, the frequency of instillation and clamping was further decreased to every 4 hours for another 12 – 24 hours. The nasogastric tube was removed on the fourth day. Of the 44 patients treated and controlled by inactivation of gastric acid with antacid, three had rebleeding within 7 days after neutralization was discontinued. They required a second series of instillations of antacid and neutralization for control of the haemorrhage. Apparently a pH of 7 is necessary to control the haemorrhage, because two patients in whom the bleeding stopped at that pH had rebleeding when the pH was allowed to drift to 5. When the intragastric pH in these patients was raised back to 7 with additional antacid, haemorrhage ceased. The mechanism of action of controlled intragastric pH of 7 in the treatment of acute mucosal haemorrhage appears to involve: complete neutralization of gastric HCl; inhibition of back diffusion of hydrogen ions; and inhibition of pepsin action.

REFERENCE
Simonian S. J. and Curtis L. E. (1976) Treatment of haemorrhagic gastritis by antacid. *Ann. Surg.* **184**, 429.

CAMPYLOBACTER ENTERITIS

In an important paper Skirrow (1977) describes a new recognized cause of acute abdominal pain and diarrhoea: *Campylobacter enteritis.* The term 'campylobacter' (Greek, a curved rod) was proposed by Sebald and Véron in 1963 as a generic name for the microaerophilic vibrios on the grounds that these organisms differed from the classic cholera and halophilic groups in certain fundamental respects. Selective techniques for culturing campylobacters were used for examining routine faecal samples received in this laboratory over 18 months. These were performed in addition to the methods used for detecting known pathogens — salmonellae, shigellae, enteropathogenic *Escherichia coli* (in children less than 2 years old), and, when relevant, protozoa and food poisoning organisms. Viruses were not looked for routinely. The groups studied are shown in *Table* 1.

Table 2 shows the age distribution of all patients with *C.enteritis*. Although half of the patients were aged 15 – 44 years, the incidence was highest in the very young.

In about two-thirds of the patients the onset of diarrhoea was preceded by a period of fever and malaise lasting up to 24 hours, or, exceptionally, for a few days (longest four days). Sometimes the illness began with a rigor, and three patients experienced a short period of delirium. Other symptoms present at this stage were headache, backache, aching of the limbs, and colicky abdominal pains. Many complained of nausea but few were troubled by vomiting. The diarrhoea began gradually in some and explosively in others; but in both cases faeces became fluid, offensive, often bile-stained, and, finally, watery. Several patients observed blood in their stools and inflammatory cellular exudate was observed microscopically in 18 samples (this is almost certainly an underestimate for not all samples were submitted during the acute stages of the disease). Patients did not complain of tenesmus

Table 1. RESULTS OF FAECAL CULTURES

	No. tested	No. positive for Campylo-bacter	No. with Campylo-bacter as sole pathogen	No. positive for other pathogens
Patients with diarrhoea (unselected)	803	57 (7·1%)	54 (6·7%)	50 (6·2%)
Controls*	194	0	0	
Contacts of patients with campylobacter enteritis	113 (29 house-holds)	19 (12 house-holds)		

*Normal people and patients without gastrointestinal symptoms

Table 2. AGE DISTRIBUTION OF PATIENTS WITH CAMPYLOBACTER ENTERITIS

Age (years):	<1	1 – 4	5 – 14	15 – 44	45 – 64	⩾65	Total (all ages)
No. of patients	5	11	9	37	8	1	71
Incidence per 10 000 of the population*	13·0	9·5	2·5	4·3	1·6	0·32	3·2

*Worcester district

but rather of incontinence, particularly if they changed position in bed. One patient gave a vivid description of an attack of tetany (probably caused by a combination of electrolyte loss and over-breathing) at the end of a night of misery shut in a lavatory that she dared not leave for fear of soiling the house. This stage of profuse diarrhoea lasted from one to three days, after which the bowel actions became less frequent and the faeces semi-formed. Despite the easing of the diarrhoea, however, many patients continued to feel ill and were troubled for several more days by the persistence of intermittent central or upper abdominal pain. Indeed, throughout the illness many patients were more distressed by the pain than the diarrhoea. In some patients the illness followed a biphasic course with one or two days of relative calm in the middle. Recovery was often protracted, especially in adults; children tended to get better more quickly. Many found that a premature return to solid foods precipitated a recurrence of symptoms, and several patients stated that they lost over 6·5 kg. The illness lasted from a few days to three weeks and on average patients were away from work for 10–14 days. The incubation period, as judged by circumstantial evidence, ranged from 2–11 days. The most severely affected patient, a 33-year-old housewife with profuse watery diarrhoea, underwent an emergency laparotomy for suspected bowel perforation on account of the intensity of her abdominal pain. No perforation was found, but most of her ileum was inflamed and oedematous, there was some free fluid in the peritoneal cavity, and many large fleshy mesenteric lymph nodes were seen. A blood culture was negative but a profuse growth of campylobacters was subsequently obtained from the diarrhoeal fluid.

The close association between the presence of campylobacters in faeces and the occurrence of a distinctive clinical enteritis alone suggests that these organisms are pathogens. The site of the infection seems to be the ileum and jejunum. In conclusion, it seems that campylobacters (*C. jejuni* and *C. coli*) are an important addition to the growing list of known enteric pathogens.

REFERENCES

Sebald M. and Véron M. (1963) Teneur en bases de l'ADN et classification de vibrions. *Ann. Ins. Pasteur (Paris)* **105**, 897.
Skirrow M. B. (1977) Campylobacter enteritis: a 'new' disease. *Br. Med. J.* **2**, 9–11.

STEATORRHOEA IN OLDER PATIENTS

Price et al. (1977) reviewed all patients aged over 50 with steatorrhoea who had presented in the past ten years and who had had faecal fat concentrations estimated. Steatorrhoea was defined as more than 5 g of faecal fat a day on a 100-g fat diet. The Lundh test was performed and tryptic activity was assayed by a modification of Wiggins's method. A value of less than 4 units/ml/minute was considered to indicate pancreatic insufficiency. Jejunal

Table 3. CAUSES OF STEATORRHOEA IN 47 PATIENTS

	Age		
	Under 65	**Over 65**	Total
Coeliac disease	12	4	16
Pancreatic insufficiency:			
Carcinoma	4	0	4
Other	3	7	10
Postgastrectomy	6	2	8
Jejunal diverticula	1	1	2
Tropical sprue	0	2	2
'Collagen' disease	1	0	1
Diabetes mellitus	1	0	1
Scleroderma	1	0	1
Whipple's disease	1	0	1
Undetermined	1	0	1

biopsies were obtained just distal to the duodenojejunal junction by using the Crosby capsule. Of the 47 patients who were over 50 when steatorrhoea was diagnosed for the first time, 16 had coeliac disease and 14 had pancreatic insufficiency (*see Table* 3). A possible cause for pancreatic insufficiency was found in 8 of the 14 patients. Three gave a history of chronic alcoholsim, 1 had definite surgical trauma to the pancreas, but only 4 had carcinoma of the pancreas. Eight patients had steatorrhoea after a partial gastrectomy. The 3 postgastrectomy patients who had a faecal fat excretion greater than 12 g a day, however, had an additional reason for malabsorption—either a gastrocolic fistula, bacterial overgrowth in the afferent loop, or extrahepatic biliary obstruction. Only 2 patients with jejunal diverticula had documented steatorrhoea, but at least 6 other such patients admitted for the investigation of a classic history of pale, floating, bulky, offensive motions, which were difficult to flush, failed to have steatorrhoea confirmed biochemically, possibly because their diarrhoea had settled before investigated. The intermittent nature of fat malabsorption in bacterial overgrowth with jejunal diverticula was noted. (*See Fig.* 1.)

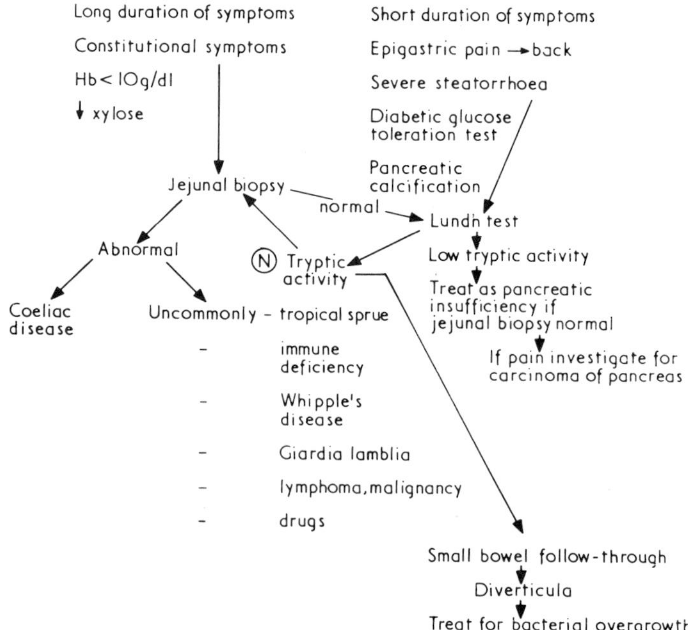

Fig. 1 Flow chart for investigating steatorrhoea. (By kind permission of the *British Medical Journal.*)

The commonest cause of steatorrhoea varied with age, being coeliac disease in those under 65 but pancreatic insufficiency in the geriatric age group (*Table* 3). Pancreatic insufficiency was the most frequent cause of steatorrhoea in the men (9 out of 30), whereas 10 of the 17 women had coeliac disease. Eleven of 17 patients with coeliac disease had had symptoms for more than two years before diagnosis, and 4 had had a history of anaemia as children. All patients with pancreatic insufficiency except 1 had complaints of less than two years' standing. While almost all patients with coeliac disease (14 of 16) gave a history of diarrhoea, only 7 had classic steatorrhoea stools. Every patient with pancreatic insufficiency complained of diarrhoea, which suggested steatorrhoea in all but 3. Characteristically, the diarrhoea began suddenly and was rapidly disabling in the group with idiopathic pancreatic insufficiency. Pain in the epigastrium sometimes radiating to the back was relieved by change of posture in all the 4 patients with pancreatic carcinoma but in only 4 of the 10 with non-neoplastic pancreatic insufficiency. Similar pain was rare in other patients, being found in 2 of those with coeliac disease and in 1 patient with partial gastrectomy. Anorexia and general malaise were found in most (12 of 16) patients with coeliac disease but in only 4 of 10 patients with non-neoplastic pancreatic insufficiency.

Despite the multiplicity of potential diagnoses, in practice only coeliac disease and pancreatic insufficiency were common causes of steatorrhoea in the series, though bacterial over-growth in jejunal diverticula is probably also an important but intermittent cause of steatorrhoea in the elderly. The periodic and variable malabsorption in bacterial overgrowth emphasizes the importance of timing the investigation of such patients. Thus the typical triad of vitamin B_{12} malabsorption, steatorrhoea associated with bile-salt deconjugation, and disordered amino-acid metabolism may occur together or independently, perhaps depending on the type and strain of organisms predominating at the time. It is often only possible to know if diarrhoea is caused by bacterial overgrowth by investigating patients during a symptomatic relapse. Otherwise erroneous conclusions that may lead to inadequate management can result. Others have noted the finding that if severe steatorrhoea is found after gastric surgery another cause must be looked for. Minor steatorrhoea is common after a partial gastrectomy. Coeliac disease was the commonest cause of steatorrhoea, emphasizing again that this life-long disease may first present in an older group. However, the frequency of coeliac disease as a cause of steatorrhoea was less than in other series of adults, partially because faecal fat concentrations have recently not been routinely estimated in such patients while in others steatorrhoea was not present. Another reason, however, is that pancreatic insufficiency was a common cause of steatorrhoea in elderly patients in contrast to a previous study in which steatorrhoea was not attributed to pancreatic insufficiency. Surprisingly, carcinoma of the pancreas was not the most common cause of pancreatic insufficiency in this series and in many the cause is unexplained. Some studies have suggested that pancreatic function deteriorates slightly with age. As a considerable reduction in pancreatic exocrine function is needed before steatorrhoea occurs, however, atrophy of the pancreas due to normal ageing is unlikely to explain the severe failure of pancreatic function. Coeliac disease and pancreatic insufficiency could often be distinguished clinically and by simple laboratory tests. The patients with coeliac disease often had symptoms for many years before diagnosis and felt generally unwell at the time of presentation. On the other hand, patients with pancreatic disease generally had short histories and usually were free of constitutional symptoms. Patients with pancreatic insufficiency, however, often had a characteristic pancreatic pain, which was rare in other diseases associated with steatorrhoea. Patients with pancreatic disease often experienced a sudden onset of disabling diarrhoea. As expected anaemia was common in coeliac disease and often quite severe compared to pancreatic disease. Haemoglobin values of less than 10 g/dl occurred in none of the patients with pancreatic insufficiency nor in any of those in a previous series. Malabsorption of folic acid is almost invariable in coeliac disease and, as in this series, nearly all untreated patients have a low red cell or serum folate concentration. Impaired xylose absorption was present in most coeliac patients, but is said to be rare in pancreatic disease. In the elderly the serum xylose concentration is preferable. A glucose tolerance test was valuable in that the result was diabetic almost exclusively in patients with pancreatic disease. Pancreatic calcification seen on plain X-ray film of the abdomen appeared only in patients with benign pancreatic insufficiency. A jejunal biopsy and Lundh test, together with a barium follow-through to exclude diverticula of the small bowel, will correctly diagnose the cause of steatorrhoea in most elderly patients. Such procedures may be instrumental in restoring severely disabled patients to a normal active life.

REFERENCE
Price H. L., Gazzard B. G. and Dawson A. M. (1977) Steatorrhoea in the elderly. *Br. Med. J.* **1**, 1582.

POSTVAGOTOMY DIARRHOEA

Allan and Russell (1977) have studied cholestyramine in the treatment of postvagotomy diarrhoea, in a double-blind controlled trial. Vagotomy and drainage is at present the most common operation for duodenal ulcer. Continuous diarrhoea, which produces considerable upset in working and social life, is a major side effect in about 1 per cent of patients. Such patients with severe, continuous postvagotomy diarrhoea excrete excessive amounts of bile acids in the faeces, the principal bile acid present being chenodesoxycholic acid. The cathartic action of these bile acids on the colon may be a major factor in causing the diarrhoea.

REFERENCE
Allan J. G. and Russell R. I. (1977 Cholestyramine in treatment of postvagotomy diarrhoea—double-blind controlled trial. *Br. Med. J.* **1**, 674 – 676.

BILE-ACID BINDING OF ALUMINIUM HYDROXIDE

Sali et al. (1977) draw attention to the bile-acid-binding properties of aluminium hydroxide, which have now been investigated in vivo and applied to the treatment of patients with choleraic diarrhoea. The enterohepatic circulation of bile-acids is maintained by active absorption from the terminal ileum, and normally less than 5 per cent of the circulating bile-acids enter the colon each cycle. If an excess of bile acid enters the colon diarrhoea may result. This symptom, sometimes referred to as 'choleraic diarrhoea', has been described in Crohn's disease of the terminal ileum and after ileal resection and truncal vagotomy and drainage. Patients with choleraic diarrhoea are often significantly incapacitated, both socially and at work, by urgent 'explosive' diarrhoea. The most successful treatment for this symptom is the bile-acid-binding resin cholestyramine. However, cholestyramine is expensive, has an unpleasant taste, and can cause nausea and vomiting. In vitro studies have shown that aluminium hydroxide has bile-acid-binding properties comparable with those of cholestyramine. Eight patients with severe choleraic diarrhoea were treated with aluminium hydroxide suspension: bowel motion became less frequent and daily faecal weight fell. The reduction in motions was dramatic, averaging from seven to two per day. In 5 patients the diarrhoea was best controlled by twice daily ingestion of aluminium hydroxide. This was given in a dosage of 30 – 40 ml first thing in the morning and before going to bed at night. The other 3 patients required medication three times a day before their diarrhoea could be controlled. No significant abnormalities were noted in the haematological and biochemical indices studied before and during the treatment with aluminium hydroxide. Hypophosphataemia, a possible complication of high-dose, long-term aluminium hydroxide therapy, has not been observed so far.

The most likely explanation is bile-acid binding to the aluminium ion (which is not absorbed). In vitro aluminium hydroxide binds bile acids as efficiently as does cholestyramine. It has long been known that aluminium hydroxide may produce constipation. The choleraic diarrhoea seemed to be best controlled when aluminium hydroxide was given first thing in the morning and on retiring at night. They recommend a starting dose of 30 ml twice a day. Bile salts accumulate in the gallbladder overnight, and it is not surprising that the bile-salt-binding capacity of aluminium hydroxide was most efficient when aludrox was present in large quantities in the bowel first thing in the morning.

[Any help in treatment for this difficult condition is most welcome. Aluminium hydroxide gel is another possibility as this also adsorbs bile salts. — F. A. J.]

REFERENCE
Sali A., Murray W. R. and MacKay C. (1977) Aluminium hydroxide in bile-salt
    diarrhoea. *Lancet* **2**, 1051.

GIARDIASIS INFESTATION

Forty adult Caucasians with giadiasis, 26 males and 14 females, were studied by Wright and his colleagues (1977). Half were young adults who had acquired the infection during overland travels in Africa, in India or in other parts of Asia. Three subjects were infected on brief trips to Leningrad. The remainder were businessmen, academics, or technical assistance personnel who had worked in Africa or Asia. These 40 subjects represent a consecutive series of patients with giardiasis initially investigated because they had profuse diarrhoea of undetermined cause or severe diarrhoea and giardiasis or symptoms that suggest malabsorption. Patients were investigated in a metabolic ward so that particular attention was paid to obtaining complete collections for absorption tests. After initial assessment they were treated with metronidazole 2·0 g as a single dose on three successive days, or mepacrine 100 mg thrice daily for 10 days, or tetracycline 250 mg four times daily for four weeks. In acute tropical sprue enterobacterial colonization of the jejunal mucosa has been described and treatment with tetracycline produced elimination of the organisms and improvement in absorption (Tomkins et al., 1975). Patients who received metronidazole were advised to avoid alcohol for the duration of treatment because of its reported disulfiram-like actions. *Giardiasis lamblia* was the only parasitic pathogen found in these patients and no bacterial pathogens were isolated by stool culture. The parasitological diagnosis was made on stool examination in 34 patients (85 per cent of the whole group). In 6 patients the parasitological diagnosis was made only on examination of mucosal impression smears of jejunal aspirate. Three of these patients had severe diarrhoea and marked malabsorption.

Malabsorption was present in 29 of 40 symptomatic patients with giardiasis. Twenty-three had impaired D-xylose absorption, in 20 vitamin B_{12} absorption was low, and 15 patients had steatorrhoea. More severe malabsorption was associated with more marked histological abnormalities. Improvements in absorption and jejunal morphology followed anti-giardial treatment. Though the pathogenicity of *G. lamblia* in man has been disputed, there is a substantial body of evidence which supports the role of the parasite in causing symptomatic disease in man. Diarrhoea is the most common symptom. A persisting bowel upset that continues for weeks or months is typical of giardiasis, but this is not a feature of acute undifferentiated diarrhoea of the tropics. Malabsorption in giardiasis has been reported from a variety of geographical locations, and has a wider geographical distribution than tropical sprue. Though there is no specific feature which distinguishes tropical sprue, it usually improves in response to a prolonged course of antibiotics, often with folate or vitamin B_{12} supplements.

In any subject who has a bowel upset which persists for weeks or months after an initial acute onset the possibility of giardiasis should be considered, even in subjects whose travels have been limited to Europe. Single negative stool examinations are insufficient to exclude the diagnosis and small intestinal aspiration and biopsy may be necessary to demonstrate the parasite.

REFERENCES

Tomkins A. M., Drasar B. S. and James W. P. T. (1975) Bacterial colonisation of jejunal mucosa in acute tropical sprue. *Lancet* **1**, 59.

Wright S. G., Tomkins A. M. and Ridley D. S. (1977) Giardiasis: clinical and therapeutic aspects. *Gut* **18**, 343.

PRODUCTION OF ALCOHOL IN THE SMALL INTESTINE BY FERMENTATION

Hiroshi Kaji and his colleagues (1976) describe the 'auto-brewery syndrome'—repeated attacks of alcoholic intoxication due to overgrowth of *Candida (albicans)* in the gastrointestinal tract. The auto-brewery syndrome or so-called 'drunkenness disease' is gastrointestinal moniliasis, the patient becoming inebriated after taking foods of carbohydrate nature. It is caused by alcohol produced by the fermentation of carbohydrates due to the action of yeast, chiefly those belonging to the *Candida* group, abnormally proliferated in the gastrointestinal tract. Thirty-two cases have been reported in Japan, but they have not been reported in other countries. The most frequent have followed operations of the stomach, duodenum and gallbladder. The use of antibacterial compounds seems to be another important factor. It is easily treated by the administration of antifungal agents.

[Perhaps it does occur elsewhere in other countries.—F. A. J.]

REFERENCE

Kaji H., Asanuma Y., Ide H., Saito N., Hisamura M., Murao M., Yoshida T. and Takahashi K. (1976) The auto-brewery syndrome—the repeated attacks of alcoholic intoxication due to the overgrowth of *Candida (albicans)* in the gastrointestinal tract. *Materia Med. Polona* **4** (29), 429.

PRACTOLOL PERITONITIS

Marshall et al. (1977) report 16 patients with practolol peritonitis from the University Departments of Medicine and Pathology, University of Bristol, and the Departments of Medicine and Diagnostic Radiology, Bristol Health District. Peritonitis caused by the beta-adrenoreceptor blocking drug, practolol, had been first recognized in this department in 1974. This resulted in restricted availability and now withdrawal of the drug. A disturbing feature is the development of symptoms of peritonitis in some cases up to 18 months after cessation of treatment. It is necessary to remain alert to the possibility of more cases presenting in the future.

Practolol peritonitis has now been shown to have characteristic features which should make diagnosis possible and differentiate the conditions from other peritoneal disorders. The duration of practolol therapy has usually been prolonged. All the patients had taken the drug for longer than one year. A possible delay in the development of symptoms after cessation of treatment is also firmly established. Abdominal pain, vomiting, loss of weight and an abdominal mass are the predominant clinical features. Although the abdominal mass has caused considerable diagnostic confusion, these presenting symptoms in a patient who is taking or has taken practolol should make the diagnosis clear. Laparotomy with dissection and removal of the thickened peritoneum is considered the treatment of choice for practolol peritonitis. The condition has worsened in the one patient in the study not yet subjected to surgery and this progression has also been seen in others awaiting laparotomy. There are considerable risks to operating on ill, usually wasted patients with underlying cardiovascular disease, but alternative treatments with both corticosteroids and azathioprine have been ineffective. Drugs rarely produce a reaction affecting the peritoneal cavity. Although involvement of the retroperitoneal tissues in patients treated with serotonin antagonists is well recognized, practolol produces changes only in the peritoneum around the small intestine. The process usually stops at the ileal caecal valve.

The mechanism by which the drug induces the change is unknown. It is possible that this is either a drug allergy or a pharmacological action of practolol. If a pharmacological effect of beta-adrenoreceptor blockade is responsible for practolol peritonitis and the practolol syndrome, it would be difficult to explain why this beta-blocking agent only is implicated. An ocular reaction to propranolol and skin lesions in patients taking both propranolol and oxprenolol have been reported. No case of peritonitis alone has been described in patients treated with propranolol or oxprenolol only. One patient presented with the disease while taking oxprenolol, and lesions similar to those induced by practolol were reported in a patient taking propranolol. Definite radiological changes occur in patients on both propranolol and oxprenolol. These worsen when treatment is continued but, in every case, regress within four weeks of stopping the beta blocker.

The authors conclude that practolol peritonitis is a serious and life-threatening disease. If the patient is well enough when symptoms develop the treatment of choice is surgical. Some patients on beta-blocking drugs other than practolol develop bowel changes whilst on treatment. It is not yet known whether these are similar to practolol peritonitis.

REFERENCE
Marshall A. J., Baddeley H., Barritt D. W., Davies J. D., Lee R. E. J., Low-Beer T. S. and Read A. E. (1977) Practolol peritonitis. A study of 16 cases and a survey of small bowel function in patients taking β-adrenergic blockers. *Q. J. Med.* New Series, XLVI, No. 181, 135.

Oesophagus, stomach and small intestine: surgical

SIR JAMES FRASER Bt, BA, CM (Edin), FRCS

RECURRENCE OF DUODENAL ULCERATION AFTER PROXIMAL GASTRIC VAGOTOMY WITHOUT DRAINAGE

In spite of the encouraging results that have been reported on the medical treatment of duodenal ulcer following the introduction of cimetidine, it is apparent that a proportion of the patients with this pathology will continue to require operation. Of all the different procedures that have been used for this condition proximal gastric vagotomy without drainage undoubtedly causes the least disturbance to the physiology of the stomach and duodenum, and so far appears to provide at least an equal possibility of a successful outcome when compared with the traditional methods. Since the operation was first introduced by Amdrup and Jensen (1970) and Johnston and Wilkinson (1970), there have been many reports describing early experiences and the results in terms of functional status have been promising and apparently fully justify the early expectations. As the follow-up period has lengthened, however, special attention has been drawn to the possibility of recurrent ulceration, not least because of the observation that there is undoubtedly a very wide variation in the incidence reported from centre to centre.

Table 1. FOLLOW-UP AT 3 – 6 YEARS AFTER THE OPERATION

Total number undergoing operation	99
Operative deaths	0
Late unrelated deaths	4
Loss to follow-up	2
Cases traced 3 – 6 years after operation	93

Table 2. DIAGNOSIS OF RECURRENT ULCERATION

Certainty of diagnosis	No. of cases	%
Proved at laparotomy	3	4·3
Proved at X-ray	1	
Strongly suspected	2	2·1

In one of the most recent reports de Miguel (1977) presents his personal results based on a series of 99 patients with duodenal ulceration operated upon between December 1970 and August 1973, and on whom there is now a 3 – 6 year follow-up. The series which unfortunately is sequential rather than comparative includes 84 males and 15 females and is restricted to ulceration of the duodenum, patients with an associated gastric ulcer being excluded. Follow-up was possible in 93 of the 99 patients, a rate of 94 per cent, 2 patients were lost to the survey and 4 died from unrelated causes. 51 patients were submitted to radiological studies, this including all who complained of major or minor gastric symptoms. The composition of the survey and the diagnosis of recurrent ulceration is shown in *Tables* 1 and 2.

It is of interest that the 6 patients with recurrent duodenal ulceration — an overall rate of 6·4 per cent — were all males and generally presented between 12 and 18 months after the operation, there being one exception who took 3½ years to appear. Three of the patients with recurrence were subjected to further operation in the form of a partial gastrectomy with reported good results, three were treated medically.

In discussing his results de Miguel makes two observations. First, in respect of the operative procedure, there appeared to be no difference between his earlier technique in which the residual innervated antral segment was 5 – 6 cm and the later development in which the segment was 8 cm, the latter affording an improvement in early postoperative gastric emptying. Second, that the recurrence rate of established duodenal ulceration was 4·3 per cent and of suspected ulceration was 2 per cent, a rate that is very comparable to the anticipated rate of 6 per cent following selective vagotomy with drainage and reported by Amdrup (1973) and de Miguel (1974), but is at variance with many of the proximal vagotomy series that have so far appeared in the literature. It is interesting, however, that the incidence in these reports varies widely from 1 per cent by Grassier (1973), 4 per cent by Wastell and Wilson (1974) to 22 per cent by Kronberg and Madsen (1975). It may also be significant that most do not include a medium or a long term follow-up. The importance of this factor is not yet fully apparent and will obviously take some years to resolve. However, although 5 out of the 6 recurrent ulcers reported by de Miguel appeared within eighteen months of operation 1 was a late developer. Johnston and Goligher (1976) have also reported an incidence with time and Amdrup et al. (1974), whose early results from the Aarhus series were excellent with no cases of recurrent ulceration, later found a rate of 8 per cent. It must also be accepted that there may be an increasing incidence of postoperative gastric ulcer and that provided proximal gastric vagotomy follows the pattern associated with other types of vagotomy with and without a drainage procedure, this may not become apparent until much later, the average lapse with the older operations being 5 years or more.

In spite of these complications this report adds further to the evidence confirming the effectiveness of proximal vagotomy as the likely preferred method of treating duodenal ulceration. However, it does remind us that it is not totally without problems and a long term follow-up will be required before its true worth is confirmed. Unfortunately, it does not add to the evidence concerning the relative merits of the various available procedures. For this the results from several randomized trials currently in progress will have to be awaited.

REFERENCES

Amdrup E. (1973) In: Sirgus W. (ed), *Clinics in Gastroenterology,* Vol. 2. Philadelphia, Saunders, pp. 387 – 412.

Amdrup E. and Jensen H. E. (1970) Selective vagotomy of the parietal cell mass preserving innervation of the undrained antrum. *Gastroenterology* **59**, 522 – 527.

Amdrup E., Jensen H. E., Johnston D. et al (1974) Clinical results of parietal cell vagotomy (highly selective vagotomy) two to four years after the operation. *Ann. Surg.* **180**, 279 – 284.

Grassier G., Orecchia M. D., Sbuelz M. D. et al (1973) Early results of the treatment of duodenal ulcer by ultraselective vagotomy without drainage. *Surg. Gynecol. Obstet.* **136**, 726 – 728.

Johnston D. and Goligher J. C. (1976) Selective? highly selective? or truncal vagotomy in 1976: A clinical appraisal. *Surg. Clin. North Am.* **56**, 1313 – 1334.
Johnston D. and Wilkinson A. R. (1970) Highly selective vagotomy without a drainage procedure in the treatment of duodenal ulcer. *Br. J. Surg.* **57**, 289 – 295.
Kronberg O. and Madsen P. (1975) A controlled randomized trial of highly selective vagotomy versus selective vagotomy and pyloroplasty in the treatment of duodenal ulcer. *Gut* **16**, 261 – 271.
De Miguel J. (1974) Late results of bilateral selective vagotomy and pyloroplasty for duodenal ulcer: 5 – 9 years follow-up. *Br. J. Surg.* **61**, 264 – 269.
De Miguel J. (1977) Recurrence after proximal gastric vagotomy without drainage for duodenal ulcer: a 3 – 6 year follow-up. *Br. J. Surg.* **64**, 473 – 476.
Wastell C. and Wilson T. (1974) Proximal gastric vagotomy. *Proc. R. Soc. Med.* **67**, 41 – 43.

INCISIONAL HERNIATION IN APPENDICECTOMY WOUNDS

Most modern literature and all surgical textbooks describe incisional herniation through the anterior abdominal wall but the great majority restrict their descriptions and comments to defects occurring in the various vertical incisions usually with a discussion about the methods of repair and the suture materials used. Appendicectomy incisions are dismissed as resulting in neither dehiscence nor hernias. This is unfortunately a misconception. In 1920 Bancroft reported an incidence of such postoperative herniation of up to 15 per cent and Wolff and Hindman in 1952 an incidence of 11 per cent, but in both series it was pointed out that sepsis, wound drainage and the age of the patient were all highly relevant to the outcome.

Table 1. INCIDENCE OF HERNIATION AFTER APPENDICECTOMY ACCORDING TO AGE AND SEX

Age group	Total Incidence	Herniation %	Men Incidence	Men Herniation	Women Incidence	Women Herniation
10 – 89 yrs	10/7316	0·16	3/3777	0·079	7/3539	0·19
40 – 49 yrs	2/363	0·65	1/250	0·40	1/113	0·88
60 – 69 yrs	5/524	1·19	1/260	0·38	4/246	1·51
70 – 79 yrs	2/196	0·79	1/120	0·83	1/66	1·51
80 – 89 yrs	1/70	1·43	0/50	—	1/20	5·0

Recently Pollet has reported on 10 patients with incisional herniation through an appendicectomy wound admitted for repair to the Aberdeen Hospitals between 1971 and 1974, and he has therefore provided us with the facts about the contemporary situation. A total of 7316 patients underwent appendicectomy between 1961 and 1974 and the incidence of herniation by sex and age is given in *Table* 1.

The interval between appendicectomy and the patients' arrival in hospital with herniation either for elective repair or as an emergency ranged from less than one to ten years. The average age of the patients with hernia was 61·6 years with a range of 40 – 84; 7 were females of whom 5 were described as obese. The appendix at the time of the original operation was described as gangrenous in 7, suppurative in 2 and inflamed in 1. Six patients had wound drains and 4 drains into the peritoneal cavity. Postoperative wound sepsis was recorded in 7 cases. The incidence of gangrenous appendicitis is shown for 10 year age groups in *Table* 2.

The incidence is higher in males but remains constant in each sex except in the 40 – 49 age groups and in females over 70 years of age.

This retrospective survey is by no means comprehensive since it deals only with those patients admitted to hospital. However, it does confirm that although appendicectomy is a common operation its long term complications are rarely discussed and that incisional herniation is undoubtedly a problem. The risk may be small in young males with early appendicitis but it becomes increasingly significant after operations for gangrenous appendicitis where there has been wound sepsis, in obesity and in female patients over 40 years. It also points out that the operative repair is not without risk especially when performed as an emergency and that there may be a case for a long term follow-up of the high risk groups particularly in the case of the obese elderly female in whom strangulation must, if at all possible, be avoided.

Table 2. INCIDENCE OF GANGRENOUS APPENDICITIS IN MALES AND FEMALES 1961 – 74 INCLUSIVE

	Men			Women		
Age	No. of appendectomies	Gangrenous appendicitis		No. of appendectomies	Gangrenous appendicitis	
		No.	%		No.	%
10 – 19	1162	77	6·6	1148	44	3·8
20 – 29	665	56	8·4	854	15	1·7
30 – 39	329	35	10·6	357	16	4·5
40 – 49	322	41	13·8	289	28	9·7
50 – 59	175	15	8·6	175	7	4·0
60 – 69	140	13	9·3	203	8	3·9
70 – 79	77	9	12·3	112	37	33·1
80 – 89	49	5	10·2	74	13	17·5

REFERENCES

Bancroft F. W. (1920) Acute appendicitis. *J.A.M.A.* **130**, 1635.
Pollet J. (1977) Appendicectomy wounds do herniate. *J. R. Coll. Surg. Edinb.* **22**, 274 – 276.
Wolff W. I. and Hindman R. (1952) Acute appendicitis in the aged. *Surg. Gynecol. Obstet.* **94**, 239.

BURST ABDOMEN

The preceding article illustrates one area in which there has been a dearth of information concerning one relatively small aspect of surgical practice and goes so far as to suggest that surgical opinion and attitudes have as a result been adversely affected. It is probable that a similar situation exists in the attitudes within the profession to the problems of the burst abdominal wound, though in this case the information is too much rather than too little and is sometimes conflicting.

In an excellent reading Leading Article in the *Lancet* (1977) the topic is again presented in full and the evidence put into a proper perspective. The author points out that as a consequence usually of the retrospective evaluation of heterogenous series of patients, surgeons have been persuaded that a low but steady rate of abdominal wound disruption in the order of 5 – 7 per cent is inevitable and it matters not at all what suture materials or techniques are used. This inference is almost certainly untrue, the small but undoubted effect of materials or method often being obscured by other factors which occur often enough, such as sepsis, malnutrition, obesity or the effect of acute haemorrhage. Alternatively all the methods which are known to have a high disruptive rate may have a common factor possibly related to the technical procedure and which increases the likelihood of disruption if some other unfavourable circumstance exists. Such an explanation might explain the undoubted ability of some surgeons to achieve long series of laparotomies with exceedingly small rates of disruption. It is suggested that the feature of surgical practice common to these surgeons is the use of heavy non-absorbable sutures inserted with large bites, not dissimilar to that which would be used to close a burst wound.

In developing this theme the article discusses in detail the relation between the mechanical forces acting within a sutured wound and its subsequent disruption. It quotes the work of Dudley (1970), who pointed out that a large bite with heavy material obviously distributes stresses on a longer suture/tissue interface and thus reduces the force per unit area more than does a fine neat stitch. It continues by referring to the more recent report from Jenkins (1976), who has taken the mathematical analysis approach a stage further by pointing out that in the first few days after an abdominal operation increases in abdominal girth from gaseous distension may lengthen a vertical wound by as much as 30 per cent. When a continuous suture has been used and inserted tightly the tension at the suture/tissue junction must rise proportionately and when interrupted sutures are used the distance between the bites must increase. Furthermore, with continuous suturing the tension rises exponentially, the smaller the initial bite the greater the consequence of both, the shorter the total length of suture material relative to that of the wound.

Wound closure with big bites very loosely inserted may appear to be coarse and to challenge the accepted tenets of surgical practice, but Jenkins' experience with this technique now extends to 1500 consecutive vertical abdominal incisions all repaired with monofilament nylon and he admits to only one burst abdomen. Surgeons must appreciate that if wound disruption is indeed at the 5 per cent level throughout the country it must constitute a substantial surgical burden and a significant extra commitment on the Health Service. Jenkins' analysis points to the view that the burst abdomen is nearly always mechanical in origin; that it can be prevented and that if surgeons think mechanically while they sew and suppress their prejudices it will be prevented.

REFERENCES

Dudley H. (1970) Layered and mass closure of the abdominal wall: a theoretical and experimental analysis. *Br. J. Surg.* **57**, 664 – 668.

Jenkins T. P. N. (1976) The burst abdominal wound — a mechanical approach. *Br. J. Surg.* **63**, 873 – 876.

Leading Article (1977) Burst abdomen. *Lancet* **1**, 28.

PHOTOCOAGULATION IN THE CONTROL OF BLEEDING EXPERIMENTAL GASTRIC ULCERATION

In company with many new agents the laser is being applied to an increasing range of medical problems. As an example of this, endoscopic laser photocoagulation is one of several techniques which are now being investigated for the control of upper gastrointestinal haemorrhage. Several systems are available, some of which are capable of delivering laser energy through a flexible endoscope and thereby providing a means of introducing the coagulative properties of the laser to the inside of the stomach. Also because the laser beam is carried in a quartz fibre wave guide passed down the biopsy channel of a standard fibre-optic endoscope and is, accurately focused, it can be manipulated under direct vision and directed to any point accessible to the endoscope. Three types of lasers have been used, carbon dioxide, argon and Nd:YAG, and of these the argon source appears to be the most suitable in that it has the best depth of penetration and therefore is effective without the dange of perforation; it is also visible.

However, at its present stage of development much has to be done to investigate the destructive effects of laser photocoagulation on the gastric wall and its mucosa both in respect of the properties of the laser itself and the local histological changes that result from it. Amongst these are the variables which determine the energy delivered such as the power of the beam, the time of exposure and the area of mucosal involvement, while the histological changes include the depth of penetration and the rate of healing after the initial coagulation.

At this stage it is claimed that argon laser photocoagulation is a practical technique for the management of gastointestinal haemorrhage, and that with suitable equipment bleeding can be safety controlled, in the majority of cases with complete healing of the ulceration. However, the investigations on which the claim is based are for the most part restricted to animal experiments and the most recent report comes from Silverstein et al. (1977), at the University of Washington. They describe an experimental model in which acute bleeding gastric ulcers were produced at gastrotomy, the ulcer being then coagulated by a high powered (6·5±1·0 W) endoscopic argon laser. Bleeding was controlled in 13 out of 16 animals, there were no perforations of the stomach wall and each ulcer was completely healed within fourteen days. Although it is accepted that this work is in its early stages, the authors claim that the results are eminently satisfactory and should stimulate further and more extensive evaluation, hopefully with an eventual clinical application in hospital patients. This report is one of many that have recently appeared in the literature and the majority are most encouraging as to the ultimate potential of photocoagulation in surgical practice, and in particular in the management of the bleeding peptic ulcer. It may be some time before it is universally available to the clinician but it does raise hopes of a valuable alternative to a major operation in the management of what is often a most hazardous surgical situation.

REFERENCE

Silverstein F. E., Protell R. L., Piercey J., Rubin C. E., Auth D. C. and Dennis M. (1977) Endoscopic laser treatment. *Gastroenterology* 73, 481 – 486.

Colon, rectum and anus: surgical

J. C. GOLIGHER ChM, FRCS

CARCINOMA OF THE COLON AND RECTUM

Suture technique for anterior resection of the rectum

Anastomotic dehiscence is a well recognized complication of anterior resection, though estimates of its frequency vary greatly (Goligher, 1975, Goligher et al., 1970; Wilson and Beahrs, 1976). In part these variations reflect differences in the assiduity with which the complication is sought, and, in particular, whether radiological studies after a small opaque enema and possible a gently conducted digital and sigmoidoscopic examination are used in the postoperative period to test the integrity of the suture line (Goligher et al., 1970). But other factors, such as the type of patient and the height of the anastomosis are significant in this connection, and, perhaps most important of all from the practical point of view, is the possible influence of the actual technique of anastomosis employed. There has been much discussion recently on the relative merits of one-and two-layer methods of suture. In the last two or three years there have been several publications providing good objective information on this question.

As mentioned in the *Medical Annual* 1976 (p. 51), Everett (1975) reported the results of a well controlled trial of one- or two-layer methods of suture for anterior resection. This confirmed the findings of an earlier controlled study of Irvin et al. (1973) that, so far as *high* anterior resection is concerned, there was virtually no difference in the incidence of anastomotic leakage according to whether a one- or two-layer technique of suture has been employed. But with *low* anterior resection, there was a significant difference in favour of one-layer suture, with a dehiscence rate of $18\cdot2$ per cent for this technique as contrasted with 50 per cent for the two-layer technique, most of the dehiscences after either method being detected only on radiological study. At about the same time Matheson and Irving (1975) recorded their uncontrolled experience of a one-layer technique of anastomosis in 52 consecutive cases of anterior resection, using radiological assessment of the results, with a dehiscence rate of only $5-7$ per cent.

But still more recently Goligher et al. (1977) have published the results of their controlled trial of one- and two-layer techniques for high and low colorectal anastomoses (*Tables* 1 and 2). It will be seen that a slight advantage emerges for the two-layer technique for both high and low anastomoses, and this achieves statistical significance with the high anastomoses, but, because of the relatively smaller numbers of cases involved, not with the low anastomoses. Why there should be a conflict in the findings of this study and Everett's (1975) is difficult to understand, but, on the evidence available, it would seem reasonable for the average surgeon to adopt either one- or two-layer anastomosis for anterior resection according to this personal preference.

When a two-layer technique is chosen, many surgeons favour a continuous inner all-coats suture of catgut and an outer row of interrupted nonabsorbable stitches, such as silk or Ethiflex. But in this connection a recent controlled trial by Clark et al. (1977) is of interest. They compared catgut and Dexon for the inner layer of the anastomosis in 194 patients undergoing resection for colorectal cancer, the integrity of anastomoses in the rectum or left colon being ascertained by postoperative X-ray studies as described above. The patients having Dexon did better than those sutured with catgut. Of 52 patients having low or high anterior resection and left hemicolectomies in the Dexon group, 13·5 per cent developed anastomotic dehiscence, but of 52 patients having the same operations in the catgut group, 36·5 per cent had dehiscence. There would thus seem to be a good argument for using Dexon (or Vicryl) instead of catgut for the inner layer of a two-layer suture technique for rectal anastomoses.

Table 1. ANASTOMOTIC DEHISCENCE AFTER HIGH ANTERIOR RESECTION
(From Goligher et al., 1977)

Type of anastomosis	No. of cases treated	Anastomotic dehiscence		
		Evident clinically	Detected only radiologically	Total
Two-layer	41	0	7	7 = 17.2%
One-layer	43	1	15	16 = 37·.%
All operations	84	1 = 1·2%	22 = 26·2%	23 = 27·4%

Table 2. ANASTOMOTIC DEHISCENCE AFTER LOW ANTERIOR RESECTION
(From Goligher et al., 1977)

Type of anastomosis	No. of cases treated	Anastomotic dehiscence		
		Evident clinically	Detected only radiologically	Total
Two-layer	25	4	6	10 = 40%
One-layer	26	4	11	15 = 58%
All operations	51	8 = 16%	17 = 33%	25 = 49%

Use of an omental wrap to protect colorectal anastomoses

A debatable issue in abdominal surgery is the value of wrapping round intestinal anastomoses a piece of greater omentum, either in the form of a free graft without blood supply or as a pedicle graft with an intact arterial supply. Carter et al. (1972) were unimpressed by the effect of reinforcing intestinal anastomoses with omentum in the rabbit—a free graft seemed to increase the chances of anastomotic leakage, and a pedicled omental graft did not improve the survival rate of the animals. In further experimental work on dogs, McLachlin and Denton (1973) confirmed the uselessness of a free omental graft, but found that a pedicle graft of omentum wrapped round a devascularized anastomosis of small bowel considerably lessened the incidence of leakage. Subsequently, McLachlin et al. (1976) were able to demonstrate in the dog that wrapping a pedicle graft of omentum round a devascularized anastomosis after anterior resection in the dog was similarly beneficial.

[Of course, the conditions produced by McLachlin in his experiments are distinctly artificial in that the blood supply to the bowel taking part in the anastomosis has been deliberately impaired, whilst in clinical practice every effort is made to ensure that the supply to the end of bowel being joined in the anastomosis is adequate. But it would be reasonable to suppose that, if an omental pedicle graft can help in one situation it might be helpful in avoiding or restraining leakage in the other situation.—J. C. G.]

Despite the conflict in the experimental evidence, a number of surgeons have strongly advocated the use of a pedicle graft of omentum to wrap round suture lines in clinical practice, and particularly those resulting from anterior resection of the rectum, oesophagectomy and certain urological conditions (Turner-Warwick et al., 1967; Turner-Warwick, 1976; Silen, 1975; Localio, 1975; Goldsmith, 1977). In certain patients with an abundant greater omentum it is a relatively simple matter to wrap a portion of this structure round even somewhat inaccessible anastomoses, such as those resulting from anterior resection: but in other cases, if omentum is to be used for this purpose, it is necessary to detach it from the transverse colon and most of the greater curve of the stomach to make a long omental tail deriving its blood supply from the right gastroepiploic artery (*Fig.* 1). The omentum can as a rule most conveniently be passed down to the pelvis in the right paracolic gutter.

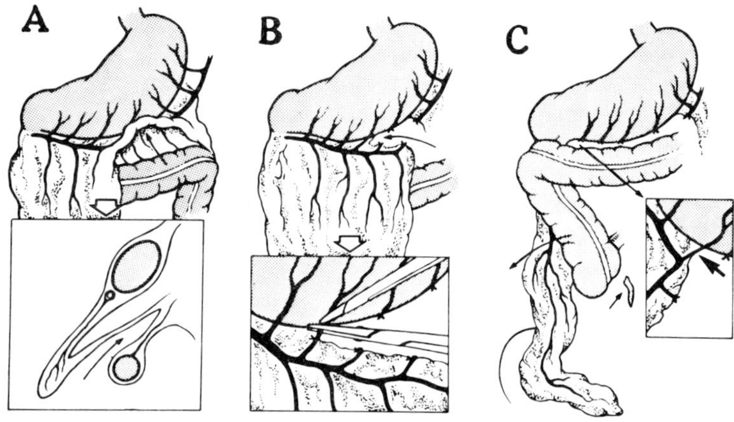

Fig. 1. Mobilization of the omentum. (Reproduced from the *Journal of Urology.*)

[Your Reviewer is not aware of any really objective clinical information that establishes beyond doubt the protective value of omental wrapping, but, for an outlay of 10 – 12 minutes of operative time to prepare the graft, it is perhaps worth adopting this relatively simple and innocuous practice. —J. C. G.]

Alternative sphincter-saving resections to anterior resection for rectal cancer

For most surgeons during the past couple of decades, the radical surgical treatment of rectal cancer has resolved itself into the use of two types of operation—abdominoperineal excision with permanent iliac colostomy, the method used for most cases, and anterior resection with colorectal anastomosis, the operation employed for growths of the upper third or half of the rectum, depending mainly on the sex and obesity of the patient and the expertise of the surgeon. Other forms of sphincter-saving excision than anterior resection have also been available for many years, but, because of technical difficulties and uncertainties of result, especially as regards anorectal continence, these alternative procedures have not hitherto found lasting favour, at any rate in this country. However, more recently there has been a fresh upsurge of interest in these other types of conservative surgery for rectal cancer, as a substitute not so much for anterior resection as for abdomino-perineal excision in patients with growths which are pathologically acceptable for excision with sphincter conservation, but are technically unsuited for anterior resection. It may be helpful to summarize some of the published work on these methods and to attempt a relative appraisal in the light of your Reviewer's own experience:

1. Abdomino-anal pull-through excision

As its name implies, this operation involves resection through the abdomen and then restoration of continuity by pulling the colon stump through the anal canal. Several different techniques exist for performing it. In one, before the colon stump is drawn through the anus, the lining of the anal canal is excised (Bacon, 1945, 1960; Waugh et al., 1955): in another the anal sphincters are divided (Babcock, 1947): and in yet another the anorectal remnant is left intact and in situ, whilst the colon is pulled through it (Black, 1952). A further variant is for the small anorectal stump to be everted through the anus for an *immediate* colo-anal anastomosis from below (Maunsell, 1892; Weir, 1901; Lloyd-Davies, 1950), as in the Swenson operation for Hirschsprung's disease, or for a *delayed* anastomosis after 10 – 14 days (Turnbull and Cuthbertson, 1961; Cutait and Figlioni, 1961). There are various postoperative complications peculiar to the abdomino-anal operation, but the overall immediate mortality seems to be roughly similar to that of low anterior resection. As regards ultimate cure of the disease, it is difficult from the published data to obtain a reliable assessment of the curative value of the method relative to that of ordinary abdominoperineal excision, but several highly respected surgeons such as Waugh et al. (1955) convinced themselves that the abdomino-anal pull-through technique was satisfactory from this point of view. One aspect of the operation about which there are very considerable differences of opinion is the quality of anorectal function preserved by it. No doubt the functional results are considerably influenced by the precise technique employed, which may partly explain why they have been variously rated as, in general, excellent (Bacon, 1960; Black and Botham, 1958), indifferent (Waugh and Turner, 1958; Kratzer, 1967; Kennedy et al., 1970), or poor (Goligher et al., 1965). Certainly, as Bennett et al. (1972) have stressed, there is a tendency for function to improve in time.

2. Abdomino-transanal excision with sutured colo-anal anastomosis

For this operation, devised by Parks (1972, 1977 a and b), the patient is placed in the lithotomy – Trendelenburg position, and the resection is carried out through the abdomen, leaving a small anorectal remnant 4 – 5 cm long, as measured from the anal verge. The splenic flexure is mobilized to make sure that the stump of lower descending or upper sigmoid colon will be able to stretch easily to the anal region leaving slack bowel in the pelvis. The surgeon now moves to the perineal end for the colo-anal anastomosis which is done from below through the anus, stretched widely open by means of a bivalve or trivalve speculum. In the original technique the cut edge of the colon stump, passed down by an assistant, was united to the cut upper edge of the anorectal stump by a circumferential series of interrupted catgut or Dexon sutures, the speculum being progressively rotated to expose each sector of bowel wall in turn. More recently it has been found that a more secure anastomosis is obtained, if, as a preliminary to the colo-anal suture, the mucosa of the anorectal remnant is excised from below, starting at a point $0 \cdot 5 - 1$ cm above the pectinate line and proceeding to the upper cut edge of the stump. This manoeuvre is facilitated by first of all injecting saline into the submucosa. The actual dissection is best done with sharp-pointed slightly curved scissors, each sector of the bowel circumference being exposed in turn by rotation of the anal speculum. The end of the colon is then sutured to the cut edge of anal mucosa just above the pectinate line, the sutures also taking a good bite of the internal sphincter. It is an advantage to pass 3 or 4 sutures between the cut upper edge of the muscle coat of the anorectal stump and the outer aspect of the colon stump; this is done either from below, before the colo-anal mucosal suturing begins, or from above after the anastomosis is complete.

Though the conduct of the colo-anal anastomosis can, at times, be rather difficult, it is surprising how well it usually heals. But leaks do sometimes occur, with resulting infection, which may considerably prolong convalescence and lead to stenosis or a poor functional result (Parks, 1977a; Lane and Parks, 1977; your Reviewer's personal experience). What is sadly lacking at the moment is a detailed comprehensive analysis of the complication rate and state of postoperative anorectal function with this method in a really large series of cases. It is already clear, however, from Lane and Parks' (1977) report and from your Reviewer's experience that function can in some cases be perfect, or nearly so, though often only after a tiresome period of frequent bowel actions and partial incontinence for several weeks after closure of the covering transverse colostomy (which should always be employed in connection with this operation). It is still too soon for any attempt at appraisal of the operation in terms of cure of the carcinoma.

3. *Abdomino-sacral resection*

In this operation the growth is resected together with most of the rectum and sigmoid colon, first by an abdominal phase (with the patient in the ordinary supine head-down position), and then by a sacral phase (with the patient turned on to his right side and the coccyx removed through a transverse or oblique post-anal incision) and a low colorectal anastomosis is constructed through the posterior wound. The method has recently been revived in America by Localio (Localio and Baron, 1973), who actually does the whole operation without moving the patient but having him on his right side throughout. He has reported challenging results with this procedure in a large series of patients with an operative mortality of 2 per cent and with anastomotic dehiscence in only 14 per cent, even though he does not usually employ a covering colostomy. Though the anastomoses lie as a rule $4 - 5$ cm from the anal verge and the patients do have severe diarrhoea and often some incontinence during the early weeks after the operation, eventually most of them are fully continent and do not wear anal pads. Localio and Eng (1975) do not seem to have had much trouble with the sacral wound [but your Reviewer found that infection and some degree of breakdown were not uncommon in 20 patients submitted to this operation, and a persistent faecal fistula developed in one of them.—J. C. G.]. The long term results recorded by Localio and Eng (1975) as regards cure of the carcinoma are difficult to evaluate, but are certainly not discouraging.

4. Abdomino-transsphincteric resection

Mason (1976a, 1977a and b) has developed a modification of the abdomino-sacral resection in which the patient is put in a prone jack-knife position for the posterior phase, and the classic sacral approach with excision of the coccyx is replaced by the posterior transsphincteric approach that he has advocated for dealing with villous papillomas of the rectum (Mason, 1970). One slight difference from this latter approach is that only the external anal sphincter and levator muscles are divided, the internal sphincter and mucosal lining of the anal canal are preserved intact. Mason (1977a and b) maintains that this form of posterior incision gives better access than the ordinary sacral incision with coccygectomy, and that through it the rectum, previously mobilized during the abdominal phase, can be divided just above the top of the internal sphincter and a colo-anal anastomosis easily performed. The levator and external sphincter are reconstituted by suture and the wound closed with suction drainage.

Though Mason (1976b, 1977a and b) has strongly championed this technique for low rectal carcinomas and claimed excellent function after it, it is difficult to find in his writings any detailed account of his series of patients so treated in regard to complications and functional results in individual cases.

[In choosing from amongst these alternative methods it seems to your Reviewer that an important consideration for British surgeons is the fact that abdominoperineal excision in this country is now almost invariably done by the synchronous combined technique with the patient in the litho-Trendelenburg position. This position is also very convenient for anterior resection or abdomino-anal resection, but is quite unsuited for abdomino-sacral or abdomino-transsphincteric excision, for either of which a side or prone position is needed for proper access for the posterior phase, and the abdominal phase is usually done with the patient in an ordinary supine head-down position. As a consequence, if, as sometimes happens, the lesion is found at laparotomy to be unsuitable for a sphincter-saving resection and to require abdominoperineal excision, this procedure has to be carried out by the classic Miles technique, for which the average surgeon is ill-equipped by training. Probably, therefore, the best policy for him is to have his patients with rectal cancer come to operation in the lithotomy – Trendelenburg position, and, if he finds a need for an alternative procedure to abdomino-perineal excision or anterior resection, to use some variant of the abdomino-anal theme.

Another alternative to be considered is an extension downwards of the range of anterior resection by the use of the new Russian SPTU suture gun—mentioned in *Medical Annual* 1976 (p. 49)—with which it is sometimes possible to achieve anastomoses as low as 4·0 and 4·5 cm from the anal verge with little morbidity. Also to be borne in mind for small, well differentiated, low lying frank rectal carcinomas, particularly in poor risk subjects, is the possibility of local destruction by diathermy (Madden and Kandalaft, 1971) or contact irradiation (Papillon, 1973), or removal by snaring or by local excision per anum (Parks, 1977b) or through a posterior transsphincteric approach

(Mason, 1977a). These methods can certainly be curative in appropriate patients, the difficulty being to select suitable cases, and surgical opinion on this matter is divided.—J. C. G.]

Surgical treatment of hepatic metastases from colorectal carcinoma

Wilson and Adson (1976) give a very interesting report from the Mayo Clinic of 60 patients with colorectal cancer and associated hepatic metastases who, during the years 1949—72 inclusive, underwent excision of metastases in addition to removal of the bowel lesion itself. In 40 of the cases the liver deposits were solitary, in 20 multiple. They varied in size from 1 to 15 cm in diameter, but in three-quarters they were 5 cm or less. In 39 patients the metastases were amenable to removal by wedge excision, in 10 cases segmental excision was necessary, and in 11 the lesions were so large as to require standard hepatic lobectomy. Approximately 80 per cent of the causal colorectal cancers were well differentiated, and just over 50 per cent had associated lymph node metastases.

Only 1 patient died in the immediate postoperative period, the cause of death being gastric stress ulceration. Follow-up data are available on all the survivors for periods of 2—3 years. No patient who had multiple hepatic metastases survived for 5 years, but 15 of the 36 with a single metastasis and eligible for 5-year follow-up lived for 5 years or more, and 8 patients were alive without evidence of recurrence 10 or more years after operation.

For comparison the authors have put together retrospectively a 'control' group of patients with colorectal cancer and associated metastases who, during the same period, due to differences in the attitude of various members of the surgical staff to the management of metastases, merely had colorectal resection without excision of the hepatic lesions. In making up this so-called 'control series', cases with very gross, obviously quite irremovable liver metastases were excluded, and only those with metastases roughly comparable to those in the operated series were chosen. Obviously such a concocted group is open to criticism as a control series, but for what it is worth, it is to be noted that none of the 'control' cases survived 5 years.

A final point is that most of Wilson and Adson's (1976) long survivors were patients who had had not formal hepatic lobectomy but a much more limited form of excision. [This paper will encourage many surgeons to reconsider their philosophy in regard to the management of hepatic metastases in cases of colorectal cancer and to adopt a more aggressive approach to single liver deposits. With the aid of computerized tomography it may be possible in the future to determine more accurately the solitary nature of an hepatic metastasis with a view to a direct attack at a second intervention, by which time Dukes' categorization of the primary lesion should also be available and might further influence the decision whether to proceed or not.—J.C.G.]

REFERENCES

Babcock W. W. (1947) *Surg. Gynecol. Obstet.* **85**, 1.
Bacon H. E. (1945) *Surg. Gynecol. Obstet.* **81**, 113.
Bacon H. E. (1960) *Dis. Colon Rectum* **3**, 393.
Black B. M. (1952) *Arch. Surg.* **65**, 406.
Black B. M. and Botham R. J. (1958) *Arch. Surg.* **76**, 688.
Bennett R. C., Hughes E. S. R. and Cuthbertson A. M. (1972) *Br. J. Surg.* **59**, 723.
Carter D. C., Jenkins D. H. R. and Whitfield H. N. (1972) *Br. J. Surg.* **59**, 129.
Clark C. G., Wyllie J. H., Haggie S. J. and Renton P. (1977) *World J. Surg.* **1**, 501—506.

Cutait D. E. and Figlioni F. J. (1961) *Dis. Colon Rectum* **4**, 335.
Everett W. G. (1975) *Br. J. Surg.* **62**, 135.
Goldsmith, H. S. (1977) *Surg. Gynecol. Obstet.* **144**, 584.
Goligher J. C. (1975) *Surgery of the Anus, Rectum and Colon,* 3rd ed. London, Baillière Tindall.
Goligher J. C., Graham N. G. and De Dombal F. T. (1970) *Br. J. Surg.* **57**, 109 – 118.
Goligher J. C., Duthie H. L., De Dombal F. T. and Watts J. McK. (1965) *Br. J. Surg.* **52**, 323.
Goligher J. C., Lee P. W. G., Simpkins K. C. and Lintott D. J. (1977) *Br. J. Surg.* **64**, 609.
Irvin T. T., Goligher J. C. and Johnston D. (1973) *Br. J. Surg.* **60**, 457.
Kennedy J. T., McOmish D., Bennett R. C., Hughes E. S. R. and Cuthbertson A. M. (1970) *Br. J. Surg.* **57**, 589.
Kratzer (1967).
Lane R. H. S. and Parks A. G. (1977) *Br. J. Surg.* **64**, 596.
Lloyd-Davies O. V. (1950) *Proc. R. Soc. Med.* **43**, 706.
Localio S. A. (1975) Personal communication.
Localio S. A. and Baron B. (1973) *Ann. Surg.* **178**, 540.
Localio S. A. and Eng K. (1975) *Curr. Probl. Surg.* **12**, 1.
McLachlin A. D. and Denton D. W. (1973) *Am. J. Surg.* **125**, 134 – 139.
McLachlin A. D., Olsson L. S. and Pitt D. F. (1976) *Surgery* **80**, 306 – 311.
Madden J. L. and Kandalaft S. (1971) *Am. J. Surg.* **122**, 347.
Mason A. Y. (1970) Personal communication.
Mason A. Y. (1976a) *Proc. R. Soc. Med., Med., Suppl. to Vol.* 65 1.
Mason A. Y. (1976b) *Proc. R. Soc. Med.* **69**, 237.
Mason A. Y. (1977a) In: *Surgical Techniques Illustrated* (ed. Malt R. and Robinson F.). Boston, Little Brown, Vol. 2, No. 2, pp. 71 – 89.
Mason A. Y. (1977b) Personal communication.
Matheson N. A. and Irving A. D. (1975) *Br. J. Surg.* **62**, 239.
Maunsell H. W. (1892) *Lancet* **2**, 473.
Papillon J. (1973) *Proc. R. Soc. Med.* **66**, 1179.
Parks A. G. (1972) *Proc. R. Soc. Med.* **65**, 975.
Parks A. G. (1977a) Personal communication.
Parks A. G. (1977b) In: *Surgical Techniques Illustrated* (ed. Malt R. and Robinson F.). Boston, Little Brown, Vol. 2, No. 2, p. 63.
Silen W. (1975) Personal communication.
Turnbull R. P. jun. and Cuthbertson A. M. (1961) *Cleve. Clin. Q.* **28**, 109.
Turner-Warwick R. T. (1976) *J. Urol.* **116**, 341.
Turner-Warwick R. T., Wynne E. J. C. and Handley-Ashken M. (1967) *Br. J. Surg.* **54**, 849.
Waugh J. M. and Turner J. C. jun. (1958) *Surg. Gynecol. Obstet.* **107**, 777.
Waugh J. M., Block M. A. and Gage R. P. (1955) *Am. Surg.* **142**, 752.
Weir R. F. (1901) *J. A. M. A.* **37**, 801.
Wilson S. M. and Beahrs O. H. (1976) *Am. Surg.* **183**, 556.
Wilson S. M. and Adson M. A. (1976) *Arch. Surg.* **111**, 330.

INFLAMMATORY BOWEL DISEASE

Sexual function after ileostomy and proctocolectomy

Patients who have to undergo ileostomy and proctocolectomy for ulcerative colitis or Crohn's disease are often relatively young and one of their main anxieties is that the presence of an ileostomy may render them sexually less attractive. In addition, their surgeon will allways be concerned about the possibility of trauma to the autonomic nerves in the pelvis during the rectal excision, which may result in interference with subsequent sexual (or bladder) function. A number of studies has shown that even in the best hands there is a small but definite risk of this complication after proctocolectomy (Stahlgren and Ferguson, 1958; May, 1966; Watts et al., 1966; Daly and Brooke, 1967; Burnham et al., 1977). A recent postal enquiry by Burnham et al. (1977) on behalf of the Ileostomy Association of Great Britain and Ireland has confirmed the findings of these earlier studies and thrown further light on the sexual problems of ileostomists.

Questionnaires were sent to 540 ileostomists and 376 replies were received, all but 13 of the respondents being married. Though between 30 and 50 per cent of the patients considered the ileostomy to be something of an embarrassment and felt that it rendered them sexually less attractive, this view was shared by only 6 – 9 per cent of the husbands and wives. Between 10 and 14 per cent found that sexual intercourse was more difficult because of the ileostomy, mainly because of a fear, usually unsubstantiated, that the bag might come off during the act.

As regards impotence in male patients, 5 per cent were completely impotent, and another 10 per cent were partially impotent, whilst 7·6 per cent noted failure of ejaculation. The age of the patient seemed to be an important factor in regard to the incidence of these complaints, for 5 of the instances of complete impotence occurred in the 35 patients over the age of 45 and none of the 61 patients under the age of 35, which suggests that there may be psychogenic as well as a neurogenic factor in the causation of the trouble. As for female patients, nearly a third of them had some new perineal or vaginal discomfort at intercourse after operation, but the proportion of women experiencing an orgasm increased slightly following the proctocolectomy.

It has been suggested by Lytle and Parks (1976) that if the dissection for removing the rectum for inflammatory bowel disease is kept specially close to the rectal wall, and in particular if the plane of dissection from the perineal aspect is taken between the internal and external anal sphincters instead of through the ischiorectal fossae, the incidence of sexual dysfunction may be lessened. But good evidence to support this contention has not yet been provided.

REFERENCES
Burnham W. R., Lennard-Jones J. E. and Brooke B. N. (1977) *Gut* **18**, 673.
Daly D. W. and Brooke B. N. (1967) *Lancet* **2**, 62.
Lytle J. A. and Parks A. G. (1976) *Gut* **17**, 392.
May R. E. (1966) *Br. J. Surg.* **53**, 29.
Stahlgren L. H. and Ferguson L. K. (1958) *New Engl. J. Med.* **259**, 873.
Watts J. McK., De Dombal F. J. and Goligher J. C. (1966) *Br. J. Surg.* **53**, 1014.

Liver and pancreas: medical

SHEILA SHERLOCK MD, FRCP, FRCP(Edin), FRCCP(Hon), FACP(Hon)

NON-A, NON-B VIRAL HEPATITIS

The last 10 years have seen considerable advances in our knowledge concerning the aetiology of acute viral hepatitis. The discovery by Blumberg of an antigen originally called 'Australia antigen' and now termed 'Hepatitis B surface antigen (HB$_s$Ag)' allowed diagnosis of type B, the form usually transmitted parenterally and having a relatively long incubation period. This type can develop without an apparent prior exposure and about 50 per cent of sporadic adult cases of acute hepatitis in urban areas of the United States may be of this type. Those attacks of acute viral hepatitis which are HB$_s$Ag negative could be explained in different ways. They might still be patients with acute type B hepatitis in whom the HB_sAg has become negative by the time of serological testing. Antibody to hepatitis B core antigen appears during the acute phase identifying type B hepatitis, even if HB_sAg is not detected. Type B hepatitis therefore can now be reliably identified.

The patient might be suffering from type A hepatitis. Antibodies to this virus can now be detected, permitting specific diagnosis of this aetiological form. Some patients may have hepatitis related to the Epstein-Barr virus or to cytomegalovirus, but these can also be excluded by specific laboratory tests. When all this has been done, there remains a residual group which has been diagnosed by exclusion and which has been designated 'non-A, non-B hepatitis'. Dienstag and colleagues (1977), from Bethesda, Maryland, and from Los Angeles, have identified 20 such patients. Clinical characteristics resemble those of type A hepatitis. Serum transaminase levels were similar and the duration of hospital stay in both was 11 days. One patient had a fulminant course and died. There was a striking predominance of women, most of them more than 35 years old. Eight of the non-A, non-B patients had exposures traditionally associated with type B hepatitis, including blood transfusions (4 cases), plasmapheresis (1 case) and occupational contact with sick or convalescent patients with hepatitis (3 cases). In the 4 transfusion-associated cases, the incubation periods were 19, 28, 49 and 96 days.

Re-checks of the sera taken in the 1950s from asymptomatic blood donors implicated in the transmission of viral hepatitis in volunteers have revealed that some of these were carrying non-A, non-B infection (Hoofnagle et al, 1977). The incubation period was 18 – 89 days. One of the donors was a chronic carrier. Two recipients developed mild chronic liver disease with fatigue, liver enlargement and abnormal flocculation tests. The bromsulphthalein test was normal. This suggests that non-A, non-B viral hepatitis appears to be associated with a chronic carrier state and with chronic liver disease.

REFERENCES
Dienstag J. L., Alaama A., Mosley J. W., Redeker A. G. and Purcell R. H. (1977) Etiology of sporadic hepatitis B surface antigen-negative hepatitis. *Ann. Intern. Med.* **87**, 1.
Hoofnagle J. H., Gerety R. J., Tabor E., Feinstone S. M., Barker L. F. and Purcell R. H. (1977) Transmission of non-A, non-B hepatitis. *Ann. Intern. Med.* **87**, 14.

TREATMENT OF PRIMARY BILIARY CIRRHOSIS WITH D-PENICILLAMINE

Primary biliary cirrhosis is a disease of unknown aetiology in which non-suppurative destruction of intrahepatic bile ducts leads to progressive cholestasis (obstructive jaundice). Death ensues a variable period of time after diagnosis, usually with bleeding oesophageal varices, liver failure and infection. Treatment is largely symptomatic. In primary biliary cirrhosis, the liver copper concentrations are raised, often into the range found in Wilson's disease. This is presumably the result of long-standing failure of biliary copper excretion, since 80 per cent of absorbed copper is normally removed in the bile. Accumulation of hepatic copper in the later stages of primary biliary cirrhosis may damage hepatocytes and provoke collagen synthesis. D-penicillamine chelates copper, increasing its excretion in the urine and decreasing tissue copper concentrations. Two prospective controlled trials of

D-penicillamine treatment in primary biliary cirrhosis have now been reported. In the first trial from the Royal Free Hospital, London, Jain and co-workers (1977) report the use of 900 mg D-penicillamine daily to 19 primary biliary cirrhosis patients with 13 receiving placebo. After 3 months, patients taking D-penicillamine showed a significant reduction in serum aspartate transaminase concentrations compared with the placebo group, and this reduction seemed to be sustained. Liver biopsies showed that the mean liver copper concentration had fallen and histology demonstrated less cholestasis in the treated group. Side effects such as acute nausea, urticaria and proteinuria led to withdrawal of treatment in 5 patients. In the second trial, reported from the Mayo Clinic, Rochester, Minnesota, Deering and colleagues (1977) gave increasing doses up to a maintenance of 1 g D-penicillamine daily to patients with primary biliary cirrhosis. Other patients received a placebo. Significantly increased urinary copper excretion was noted in the treated cases and liver copper values decreased significantly over those taking placebo.

Because of the variable and often long natural history of PBC, many years must elapse before it is known whether or not cirrhosis, portal hypertension and liver failure are prevented by D-penicillamine and whether survival is prolonged. In the meantime, for an illness for which no other form of therapy seems to offer a prospect of halting or delaying progressive liver damage, treatment with D-penicillamine, preferably within control trials, is recommended despite the high incidence of toxicity. The maintenance dose should probably be about 600 mg daily when side effects will be reduced.

REFERENCES

Deering T. B., Dickson E. R., Fleming C. R., Geall M. G., McCall J. T. and Baggenstoss A. H. (1977) Effect of D-penicillamine on copper retention in patients with primary biliary cirrhosis. *Gastroenterology* **72**, 1208.
Jain S., Scheuer P. J., Samourian S., McGee J. O'D. and Sherlock S. (1977) A controlled trial of D-penicillamine therapy in primary biliary cirrhosis. *Lancet* **1**, 831.

NON-SURGICAL REMOVAL OF COMMON BILE DUCT STONES

This problem is reviewed by Classen and Ossenberg (1977), from Hamburg, West Germany. Despite routine intra-operative cholangiography, common bile duct stones are overlooked in up to 14 per cent of patients. Because of the high rate of complications (over 50 per cent) that can be expected in cases of untreated cholelithiasis, the need to remove the stones from the common bile duct is imperative. If a T-tube is still in position in the bile ducts, the stones may be approached through it. This may be done by introducing the controllable catheter of Burhenne which can be manipulated by remote control and the stone can be extracted (Burhenne et al., 1974). Small calibre fibrescopes have also been devised allowing the extraction of stones via a T-tube and direct visual control (Yamakawa et al., 1975). Attempts have also been made to dissolve the gallstones by infusion through the T-tube. Sodium cholate solutions have been used continuously over a maximum of 10 days at a flow rate of 30 ml per hour and have been successful (Way et al., 1972; Lansford et al., 1974). Diarrhoea is a complication. Continuous heparin infusions have also been employed, the principle being fragmentation of the stone. This was successful in 22 of 30 patients and has no undesirable side effects (Gardner, 1973).

The introduction of retrograde cannulation of the common bile duct via the sphincter of Oddi allows removal of common bile duct stones with the aid of endoscopic papillotomy (Classen and Safrany, 1975). The papillotomy is done with a wire snare and a high frequency diathermy current. The stone is then removed with Dormia catheters. Eleven-hundred-and-seven endoscopic papillotomies have been performed, mainly in Western Europe. In 63 per cent of patients the stones spontaneously disappeared some days after. In a further 26 per cent of patients, stones could be extracted by means of the Dormia basket. Thus, in 89 per cent of cases, endoscopic papillotomy succeeded in removing common duct stones (Classen and Ossenberg, 1977). The complication rate was 1·08 per cent, mainly septic cholangitis, pancreatitis and bleeding. The indications are isolated papillary stenosis, common bile duct stones overlooked at surgical operations on the biliary tract, common bile duct stones causing obstruction in patients who have a high surgical risk. Younger patients, i.e. those less than 50 years old, presenting with an intact papilla of Vater, should probably have a surgical choledochotomy so that the function of the papilla is preserved.

REFERENCES

Burhenne H. J., Richards V., Mathewson C. and Westdahl P. R. (1974) Non-operative extraction of retained biliary tract stones requiring multiple sessions. *Am. J. Surg.* **128**, 288.
Classen M. and Ossenberg F. W. (1977) Non-surgical removal of common bile duct stones. *Gut* **18**, 760.
Classen M. and Safrany L. (1975) Endoscopic papillotomy and removal of gallstones. *Br. Med. J.* **4**, 371.
Gardner B. (1973) Heparin for common duct stones. *N. Engl. J. Med.* **289**, 592.
Lansford C., Mehta S. and Kern F. Jr. (1974). The treatment of retained stones in the common bile duct with sodium cholate infusion. *Gut* **15**, 48.
Way L. W., Admirand W. H. and Dunphy J. E. (1972) Management of choledocholithiasis. *Ann. Surg.* **176**, 347.
Yamakawa T., Mieno K. and Shikata J. (1975) Improved choledochofiberscopes and non-surgical removal of retained biliary calculi under direct visual control. *Gastroenterology* **68**, 1051.

RATIONAL SEQUENCE OF TESTS FOR PANCREATIC FUNCTION

The investigation of patients with suspected pancreatic disease still presents considerable practical problems to the clinician. Symptoms may be attributed to other abdominal diseases and the results of tests such as the detection of steatorrhoea are not specific. Biochemical investigation of the duodenal aspirate, after pancreatic stimulation (Lundh test), is of definite value in detecting pancreatic insufficiency but can be normal in the presence of pancreatic disease. ^{75}Se-selenomethionine scanning rarely misses pancreatic abnormality but carries a high incidence of falsely abnormal results and does not distinguish between causes of pancreatic disease. More recently, endoscopic retrograde pancreatography has permitted direct visualization of the pancreatic ducts. This technique may provide an accurate pathological diagnosis, but is more invasive and hazardous than other tests of pancreatic function. Mitchell and his colleagues (1976), from the Royal Free Hospital, London, have therefore attempted to evaluate scanning and endoscopic pancreatography in relation to other tests in order to determine the most efficient combination for the routine clinical diagnosis of pancreatic disease. The final diagnosis was known in 100 patients studied and was compared with the scan and endoscopic pancreatographic findings.

The first step is the radioisotope scan. A normal scan precludes the necessity for further investigation since it is a reliable indicator of a normal pancreas. If abnormal, the scan should be followed by endoscopic pancreatography, which when abnormal, has a high chance of producing a definite diagnosis. This leaves a small group with an abnormal scan, but a normal retrograde pancreatogram—a diagnostically unhelpful combination—with a mixture of false positive scans and false negative pancreatograms. The final stage in these patients should be a Lundh test which, if abnormal, reliably indicates pancreatic disease. The proposed sequence of tests would have correctly diagnosed 78 of the 81 patients, although one with carcinoma would have been missed.

REFERENCE
Mitchell C. J., Elias E., Agnew J. E., Summerfield J. and Dick R. (1976) Rational sequence of tests for pancreatic function. *Br. Med. J.* **2**, 1307 – 1309.

Gallbladder and pancreas: surgical

J. E. TRAPNELL MA, MD, FRCS

THE MANAGEMENT OF BLEEDING OESOPHAGEAL VARICES

Over the past four or five years there have been a number of useful contributions on the management of haemorrhage from oesophageal varices and the subject has recently been well reviewed by Johnston (1977a). Control of haemorrhage may be achieved either by reducing pressure within the portal system by some form of shunt, or by direct attack on the varices themselves. The value of a properly constructed portacaval shunt is now well established, for this operation will almost eliminate the risk of recurrent bleeding; however, particularly with the end-to-side shunt portal systemic encephalopathy becomes an increasing problem. In addition, a number of individual trials have failed to demonstrate that either a prophylactic or therapeutic portacaval shunt significantly prolongs life, for in those with progressive liver disease the underlying condition continues to advance, while those with a non-progressive disease may bleed again intermittently but are unlikely to die from the haemorrhage alone. The shunting operation is a major procedure carrying a fairly formidable mortality, particularly in those where the liver disease is severe, and the question has therefore been asked as to whether any alternative method of control of haemorrhage is available. It has also become apparent that the selection of patients for shunting is critical, as is the timing of the operation. Only Orloff et al. (1977) still appear to favour a policy of immediate shunting of patients who are bleeding.

In the majority of centres, when varices are diagnosed as the cause of haematemesis, control is first achieved by conservative measures; the value of transfusion with fresh blood, the infusion of pitressin and the use of oesophageal tamponade with the Sengstaken – Blakemore tube is well documented and at the same time oral antibiotics are given and the colon is washed out to reduce the risk of encephalopathy. With these measures 24 – 48 hours of time can be bought so that the patient's general condition can be improved. This allows a more thorough assessment as to what form of further treatment is best for him individually. Patients will probably fall into one of four categories (Johnston, 1977a).

1. Clearly if the patient is in coma it is pointless to attempt surgery and in this group conservative measures should be continued in the hope that the patient's general condition will improve and then one of the subsequent three alternative forms of management can be reconsidered.

2. Patients with serious jaundice or marked ascites do poorly with surgery and in this group of cases it has been suggested that injection sclerotherapy is the best form of management. The details of this technique have been well described by Johnson (1977). He prefers the use of a rigid oesophagoscope to the flexible fibre-optic instruments. The Negus oesophagoscope gives a good view, allows the use of a wide bore sucker and the tip of the instrument can be rotated to compress the varix that has just been injected. Finally, this instrument obstructs the flow above the point of injection thus keeping the sclerosant solution in the vein. Johnson uses 5 per cent ethanolamine in preference to sodium tetradecyl sulphate, as the latter is more irritant if it should be extravasted. Following injection the oesophagoscope is left in place, compressing the veins which have been injected for three minutes, and a Sengstaken tube is then passed and inflated in the usual way to a transmitted pressure of 40 cm of water. A Levine's tube is passed through the lumen into the stomach so that the oesophageal tube can be left in place for 24 – 36 hours. The stomach can be aspirated and drugs such as lactulose and magnesium sulphate can also be put down into the stomach. Johnson reports that the results of this form of treatment have been satisfactory with control of 25 bleeding episodes by one or, at the most, two injections. There were no significant complications.

3. Direct surgical attack on the varices and ligation, whether by the Borema – Crile or Walker methods, requires a thoracotomy and carries an operative mortality of 40 per cent. Johnston (1977b) has now reported his experiences with the SPTU gun, which is easy to use and effective. In order to employ this instrument the abdomen is opened through a midline incision, the diagnosis of varices is confirmed, the pre-oesophageal peritoneum is divided transversely and the oesophagus is mobilized with preservation of the vagi. A small gastrostomy is then made in the anterior wall of the stomach about 6 cm below the cardia. The nozzle of the gun is introduced into the lower oesophagus and the gap between the conical head and the cylindrical body of the instrument is opened. A stout linen thread is now passed around the oesophagus and tied so that a flange of oesophageal wall is introduced between the two sections of the gun. The head and the body of the instrument are then approximated and with the pulling of the trigger there is both a simultaneous resection of a disc of full thickness oesophageal wall and a re-anastomosis with 12 metal staples. With release of the head of the gun it is now a simple matter to withdraw the instrument from the stomach and the gastrostomy is closed. It is Johnston's practice to ligate the left gastric vein routinely in all these cases, and, where indicated, splenectomy or splenic artery ligation may also be carried out. Postoperatively nasogastric aspiration and intravenous therapy are continued for 5 days and during this time no oral fluids are allowed. A Gastrografin swallow on the fifth day is performed to confirm that the anastomosis is watertight. Johnston has used the technique on 12 patients in all of whom a portal-systemic shunt was contraindicated.

One patient died postoperatively from respiratory failure while in hospital and another died six weeks later, but he had, in addition, a primary hepatoma. There was no instance of anastomotic leak but 4 cases developed an oesophageal stricture requiring dilatation on two or three occasions each. Only 1 patient bled postoperatively and this took the form of a persistent ooze for about a week after operation. There was no late bleeding up to seven months on follow-up. Clearly this is an interesting development which, because it is simple may well find a place in the general management of bleeding varices.

4. A small number of patients with good liver function stop bleeding with conservative measures only. It is this group which may be selected for shunting but it is preferable to wait for some weeks after the acute haemorrhage before surgery is undertaken. From a review of the literature and as a result of a personal series of 58 patients Johnston has concluded that it is unwise to perform a conventional shunt in patients with acute variceal bleeding; in those with Child's Grade C liver disease; in patients with diabetes mellitus; in cases where the liver biopsy is unfavourable; in those with inadequate veins and in patients over 50 years of age.

The most exciting new development in the field of shunt surgery is Warren's concept of selective decompression of the oesophageal varices while maintaining the hepatic blood flow (Warren et al., 1969). This operation, by disconnecting the splenic vein and joining the *distal* end to the renal vein, gives a decompression of the oesophago-gastric varicele bed, while at the same time preserving the normal portal blood supply to the liver. It thus lowers the incidence of encephalopathy markedly. The operation is technically difficult and is contraindicated in the presence of ascites and in the absence of a good portal blood flow. Reports are now beginning to appear of the effectiveness of this type of selective shunt (Britton, 1977; Mosimann and Loup, 1977) and on follow-up the incidence of re-bleeding is very low. This is perhaps because thrombosis of the shunt appears to be rare and, most important of all, the frequency of postshunt encephalopathy is minimal with this type of operation. It is hoped that the value of selective spleno-renal shunts will be further established when the results of ongoing trials are published, and these are keenly awaited.

REFERENCES

Britton R. C. (1977) The clinical effectiveness of selective portal shunts. *Am. J. Surg.* **133**, 506–511.

Johnson A. G. (1977) Injection sclerotherapy in the emergency and elective treatment of oesophageal varices. *Ann. R. Coll. Surg. Engl.* **59**, 497–502.

Johnston G. W. (1977a) British Society of Gastroenterology. Annual Meeting, York.

Johnston G. W. (1977b) Treatment of bleeding varices by oesophageal transection with the SPTU Gun. *Ann. R. Coll. Surg. Engl.* **59**, 404–408.

Mosimann R. and Loup P. (1977) Efficacy and risks of the distal splenorenal shunt in the treatment of bleeding oesophageal varices. *Am. J. Surg.* **133**, 163–168.

Orloff M. J., Duguay L. R. and Kosta L. D. (1977) Criteria for selection of patients for emergency portacaval shunt. *Am. J. Surg.* **134**, 146–152.

Warren W. D., Fomon J. J. and Zeppa R. (1969) Further evaluation of selective decompression of varices by distal splenorenal shunt. *Ann. Surg.* **169**, 652.

MANAGEMENT OF JAUNDICE

The risks of surgery in a jaundiced patient with extrahepatic bile duct obstruction are well recognized. It is also generally accepted that mortality may be reduced by establishing drainage of the biliary system—hence the advocacy of a two-stage procedure for resection of a carcinoma of the head of the pancreas. The disadvantage of this technique has always been, however, that at the second laparotomy adhesions caused by a previous cholecyst-enterostomy impede and complicate the dissection. Also if there are complications following the initial drainage this may delay definitive surgery.

A report from Japan is therefore of interest. Mori et al. (1977) have described a technique of percutaneous transhepatic catheterization of the biliary system. Briefly they have combined the technique of percutaneous transhepatic cholangiography with the Seldinger technique. They first insert a cannula, and confirm its presence in the bile duct by injection of dye and cholangiography. This also allows the site of blockage to be identified. A guide-needle is then passed down through this needle, the needle is withdrawn and a catheter is passed over the guide-wire into the bile duct in the usual fashion. Mori et al. have performed this technique in 13 patients with very satisfactory results. The complications have been few although there was bleeding through the catheter on two occasions. From this experience they conclude that when such bleeding occurs the patient should be explored at once and an operative drainage should be performed. The 1 death in their series occurred when they did not follow this policy.

It would seem that this technique merits further evaluation for it would certainly be useful to be able to drain the biliary tract in this fashion. The Japanese workers were able to maintain this form of drainage for up to 5 weeks. The bilirubin and alkaline phosphatase levels fell very rapidly in the first 2 weeks and were approaching normal levels by 3 weeks in the majority of cases. Although slight leakage of contrast medium into the abdominal cavity along the catheter was occasionally observed, local or generalized peritonitis did not develop and emergency laparotomy was not required for this reason in any patient.

REFERENCE
Mori K., Misumi A., Sugiyama N., Okale N., Natsuoka T., Ishii J. and Akagi M. (1977) Percutaneous transhepatic bile drainage. *Ann. Surg.* **185**, 111 – 115.

WHITHER TRASYLOL AND GLUCAGON?

The value of Trasylol (aprotinin) and glucagon in the treatment of acute pancreatitis has always been controversial, for there have been strong proponents for and against each of these treatments.

Trasylol was first introduced in Germany in 1958, but early enthusiasm was based on short, often anecdotal reports, and it was not until 1974 that the first full, controlled trial was reported (Trapnell et al., 1974). This study examined the effect of Trasylol and placebo in 105 patients undergoing their first attack of either gallstone or idiopathic pancreatitis. The two groups were comparable for age, for apparent severity of onset and for the duration between the onset of the illness and administration of the drug. When the code was broken it was found that there was a significant difference between the treated group of 52 cases with 4 deaths (7·5 per cent) and the control group of 53 patients of whom 13 (25 per cent) had died. When patients over the age of 50 were considered the difference between the two groups was even more significant. This report caused some interest and Trasylol began to be used more widely, although it was pointed out at that time (*Medical Annual,* 1974, p. 95) that the drug should not be fully accepted on the basis of one trial alone.

Now two further studies have been reported, although so far only one has been published, but both conclude that Trasylol was ineffective for neither showed any difference in mortality between the treated and the' control groups. In the Medical Research Council study (Cox et al., 1977) 257 cases were divided into three groups: placebo 123 cases with 13 deaths (11 per cent mortality), a Trasylol-treated group of 66 cases with 6 deaths (9 per cent) and 68 patients who received glucagon with 8 deaths (12 per cent mortality). From Glasgow there has been a report (Imrie, 1977) of 161 cases collected over almost 3 years with a total of 14 deaths equally divided between the treated and controlled groups, a mortality of 8·7 per cent.

So whither Trasylol? Each of these studies can be criticized in different ways. In the first there was a mortality of 25 per cent in the controlled group, and this has received much adverse comment. However, this is not really a valid criticism of the trial for two reasons. First, unfortunately all these cases are dead, so that the statistic is not open to observer variation. Then it must also be conceded that percentage case mortality is a factor, not just of the number of deaths, but of diagnostic input as well (Trapnell and Duncan, 1975). Percentage case mortality rates should not, therefore, be used as a basis for comparison between one series and another, whether they are separated by time or geography. The M.R.C. study may be criticized because the full spectrum of pancreatic disease was included and therefore cases of post-operative, alcoholic and steroid pancreatitis, as well as recurrent acute pancreatitis, were included in the trial with their varying mortalities. The Glasgow experience is more uniform, as one would expect from one centre, but the question must be asked, if the control group mortality is only 8 – 10 per cent, do 161 cases or even 257 patients, as in the M.R.C. study, provide sufficient material to achieve a significant difference in death rate, especially when a three-way split is made.

Apart from the statistical query, the results of these two reports are very uniform, in contrast to the first study reported, and therefore the value of Trasylol must once again be questioned. There is good evidence both that it is effective and that it is ineffective, so presumably the present situation will continue where each clinician will decide for himself whether or not to use the drug, more on the basis of personal prejudice and preference rather than on established scientific fact!

The case for glucagon has never been as strong as for Trasylol, and it was fully discussed in the 1974 *Medical Annual* (p. 94). The theoretical rationale for its use is questionable, and the original clinical report was based on a comparison of mortality rates between two series of cases which were quite dissimilar. The only controlled trial of glucagon to be published in Britain so far is that from the M.R.C. (Cox et al., 1977) and this gives no support to the suggestion that glucagon might be valuable. There is still a strong body of opinion that glucagon reduces the pain of acute pancreatitis and therefore the general analgesic requirement in this condition. However, pain must be regarded as a highly subjective symptom which is very difficult to assess in any individual patient and it is open to great variation in acute pancreatitis in any event. It therefore seems likely that glucagon will not find a place in the general management of patients with acute pancreatitis.

As a postscript it needs to be stressed that at the present time there is no form of treatment which has been shown to be unequivocably beneficial in the management of this condition and this must be a source of continuing concern to those who are involved in this particular field.

REFERENCES
Cox A. G. et al. (1977) Death from acute pancreatitis. *Lancet* **2**, 632 – 635.
Imrie C. W., Benjamin I. S., Ferguson J. C. et al. (1978) A single-centre double-blind
　trial of Trasylol therapy in primary acute pancreatitis. *Br. J. Surg.* **65**, 337 – 341.
Trapnell J. E. and Duncan E. H. L. (1975) Patterns of incidence in acute pancreatitis.
　Br. Med. J. **2**, 179 – 183.
Trapnell J. E., Rigby C. C., Talbot C. H. and Duncan E. H. L. (1974) A controlled
　trial of Trasylol in the treatment of acute pancreatitis. *Br. J. Surg.* **61**, 177 – 182.

THE DIAGNOSIS OF PANCREATIC CYSTS

Pancreatic cysts may complicate either acute or chronic relapsing pancreatitis. Their identification and diagnosis is important as a guide to treatment, but until recently a confident diagnosis could only be made either if the cyst was very large, and so was palpable, or at operation. In the last 5 years both endoscopic retrograde pancreatography (ERP) and ultrasonic scanning have become more widely available. The value of the scan in differentiating between a solid and a cystic mass of the pancreas is now well established. The place of ERP in the diagnosis of cysts is, however, controversial. Cotton (1977) considers that the presence of a pancreatic cyst is a contra-indication to the use of endoscopic pancreatography because of the risk that the procedure may introduce infection and so transform the cyst into an acute abscess with its attendant severe complications and the need for emergency surgical intervention.

In contrast Andersen et al. (1977) have reported a series of 14 patients from Copenhagen where ERP and ultrasonography were performed in each case: 11 cysts were verified surgically while 3 were verified by ultrasonically-guided puncture and aspiration. Comparison of the two methods reveals that the pancreatic duct was successfully cannulated in 12 of the 14 cases. In 4 patients communication between the cyst and the duct system was demonstrated. In a further 3 cases there was doubtful filling of the cyst but other abnormalities in the duct system were noted; while in 5 patients the diagnosis of the cyst was suggested because of a total obstruction of the main pancreatic duct. There were no clinically significant complications due to ERP.

Ultrasonic scanning again gave the correct diagnosis of the cyst in 12 patients. In 8 cases ultrasonic guided puncture of the cyst was carried out, and in 5 of these patients puncture was repeated several times so that a total of 19 punctures, all of which were successful at the first attempt are reported. Fluid was aspirated and dye was introduced to demonstrate the cyst on each occasion and the diameter of the cysts were measured. These varied from 2 cm to 19 cm. Andersen et al. report that 1 patient had been followed for 20 months without an ultrasoncially demonstrable recurrence of a cyst which when it was originally aspirated was 11 cm in diameter. Except for 1 patient with a small cyst 2 cm in diameter, who developed fever and slight epigastric tenderness for 2 days after a puncture, there were no complications due to percutaneous puncturing of these cysts.

From this report it would seem not only that ultrasonic scanning is a more reliable method of diagnosis of a pancreatic cyst, but that it can in addition be used as a method of introducing a needle, thus allowing aspiration of fluid. Open surgical drainage of pancreatic cysts carries a mortality of the order of 10 per cent and Andersen et al. therefore suggest that guided percutaneous puncture and repeated aspiration should be undertaken as a method of treatment in these cases.

REFERENCES

Anderson B. N., Hancke S., Nielsen S. A. D. and Schmidt A. (1977) The diagnosis of pancreatic cyst by endoscopic retrograde pancreatography and ultrasonic scanning. *Ann. Surg.* **185,** 286–289.
Cotton P. B. (1977) Progress Report: E.R.C.P. *Gut* **18,** 316–341.

ANAESTHESIA AND ANALGESIA

R. S. J. CLARKE BSc, MD, PhD,
FFA RCS

ADVERSE REACTIONS TO DRUGS USED IN ANAESTHESIA

It has become increasingly common to hear a description of an anaesthetic induction somewhat as follows. The patient, a young healthy woman, was given a typical dose of the intravenous agent plus suxamethonium 75 mg. She was intubated without difficulty but when an attempt was made to inflate the lungs the resistance was very high. She was then seen to be flushed and cyanosed and the pulse was weak. The tube and cuff were checked and she was re-intubated but the problem was clearly intractable bronchospasm. After 15 minutes of ventilation with oxygen, aminophylline, hydrocortisone and 1 litre of dextran 70 she was able to breathe and pressure was returning to normal. At this stage the face and especially the eyelids were puffy and swollen but the swelling gradually subsided over 24 hours. The operation was postponed, to be performed a week later under neurolept anaesthesia. The problem still remained, however, as to what to advise the patient about future anaesthetics.

This type of episode has been described many times in print since the first such reaction to thiopentone was reported (Hayward and Kiester, 1957). However, since the great majority of patients recover with only symptomatic treatment most cases remain unreported but are simply discussed among colleagues.

The topic was mentioned in the 1972 *Medical Annual* (p. 74) in connection with thiopentone and propanidid and indeed the latter drug has virtually passed out of use because of the severe histaminoid reactions that were reported. Further reviews of published reactions to these two drugs appear in the comprehensive survey of *Intravenous Anaesthesia* by Dundee and Wyant (1974). In the light of these reports reactions to Althesin (alphaxalone) were observed critically soon after it came into widespread clinical use and reports began to appear in print (Avery and Evans, 1973; Healy, 1973; Mehta, 1973). A prospective survey was started and case reports invited from anaesthetists who had experienced such anaphylactoid reactions. The report on the first 100 of these (Clarke et al., 1975) is summarized in *Table* 1, omitting those not clearly anaphylactoid and those probably due to the muscle relaxant or poor

**Table 1. CLASSIFICATION OF 81 HYPERSENSITIVITY REACTIONS
FOLLOWING INTRAVENOUS ANAESTHESIA
(From Clarke et al., 1975)**

Type of reaction	Intravenous anaesthetic used			
	Althesin	Thiopentone	Epontol	Total
Histaminoid	17	2	—	19
Histaminoid with bronchospasm	25	8	—	33
Bronchospasm only	10	2	—	12
Cardiovascular collapse	7	—	4	11
Delayed histaminoid	6	—	—	6

health. The method of reporting (to the Department of Anaesthetics of The Queen's University of Belfast or Glaxo Laboratories or the CSM) and background to the study inevitably resulted in an emphasis on reactions to Althesin. It is clear also that there may well have been reactions not reported or erroneously attributed to the anaesthetic rather than the muscle relaxant. Nevertheless, the survey gives some idea of the type of reaction seen, the importance of the patient's history, the treatment and the prognosis.

The descriptive terms were used in the hope that some pattern would emerge either with one drug having a particular type of reaction or reactions to a second dose being different from those after a primary exposure. However, no clear pattern can be seen. The histaminoid reactions with flushing, oedema and hypotension can have additional bronchospasm and the latter can occur on its own. There are all degrees of the reactions though, in fact, none of the patients having Althesin died (except in one instance which was considered to be due to the poor health of the patient). Four died after histaminoid and bronchospasm reactions to thiopentone. Erratic reporting and variable treatment may well explain this apparent discrepancy.

As judged by these reports and manufacturers' estimates of doses of drug given, the incidence of reactions to Althesin appeared to be about 1 in 11 000 administrations. Figures for propanidid are in the range of 1 in 2 000 to 1 in 1 000 (Dannemann and Lubke, 1970; Kay, 1972) and for methohexitone 1 in 7 000 (Driggs and O'Day, 1972). The incidence for thiopentone is probably less than for any of these drugs (Dundee and Wyant, 1974).

Since the first 100 cases were collected reports have continued to flow in, though most are as yet unpublished. The same agents are still implicated, with the addition of methohexitone, and the proportion following Althesin remains high. Furthermore, some reports (Watt, 1975; Fisher, 1976; Evans and Keogh, 1977) indicate an incidence of reactions to Althesin of about 1 in 1 000 administrations which, if universally true, would be dangerously high. Much depends on the definition of a reaction but the fact that these three publications come from different areas makes it difficult to explain them by local sensitivity. A broader picture of the problem was given at a symposium on 'Allergy and Anaesthesia' in Nancy, in 1975. Almost every drug the anaesthetist uses, from atropine to antibiotics, was shown to be associated with reactions, some truly anaphylactic, others merely non-specific histamine liberation (Vignon et al., 1976; Moneret-Vautrin et al., 1976).

The role of Cremophor EL, the organic solvent in Epontol and Althesin, has been suspect since Althesin was found to cause similar reactions to Epontol. However, it has not been found to liberate histamine when given intravenously to volunteers (Doenicke et al., 1973) and in addition Althesin has not caused cutaneous reactions in anaesthetists sensitive to Epontol (Sneddon and Glew, 1973; Dundee et al., 1974). On the other hand, because of its surface activity, it could present the anaesthetic molecules or their antigenic grouping to the receptor in a particular way. Alternatively it could block inhibitors of complement activation which would explain the involvement of complement by the so-called 'alternate pathway' in so many of these reactions (Watkins et al., 1976). Some involvement is supported by the fact that diazepam, which is sparingly soluble in water, causes scarcely any adverse reactions when injected as Valium, dissolved in propylene glycol and benzoic acid; but in Scandinavia it is also available in Cremophor EL as Stesolid and many reactions have been reported to this mixture during the last two years. It must, however, be remembered that drugs in organic solvents have a bad record of venous thrombosis, going back to hydroxydione in the nineteen-fifties, and intravenous diazepam has recently been shown to cause thrombophlebitis in up to 39 per cent of patients (Hegarty and Dundee, 1978).

It might be supposed that patients who have hypersensitivity reactions to intravenous anaesthetics would be more likely to have a history of asthma, hay fever or eczema than the general population. However, Clarke and his colleagues found an incidence of only 15 per cent of such histories in the patients followed-up. A similar figure was found in a survey by Sigiel, but Moneret-Vautrin et al. (1976) have found that while this holds true for minor reactions the percentage of patients with an atopic history in those with *severe* anaesthetic reactions was as much as 41 per cent. To interpret these figures one must know the frequency of atopy in the general population and in various studies 14 – 15 per cent seems to be the general level. A more detailed study has recently been carried out questioning 10 000 patients throughout the British Isles before surgery and an $8 \cdot 5$ per cent incidence of atopy was found. It has therefore not been possible yet to show a statistical relationship between atopy and reactions, though evidence is suggestive (Clarke et al., 1977; Clarke, 1979).

In the broader field of patients with a history of drug or food allergies, there does seem to be a significant correlation. The same survey of 10 000 preoperative patients recorded a general incidence of allergy of $13 \cdot 5$ per cent (most commonly to penicillin), whereas in patients who have had adverse reactions 29 per cent have an allergic history. There is, as one would expect, a strong cross-relationship between atopy and allergy so it does seem likely that they are both predisposing factors. The other factor investigated is previous exposure to the same anaesthetic. This is difficult to evaluate because as many as 66 per cent of the surgical population have had an anaesthetic previously, thiopentone being used in the majority of cases (Clarke et al., 1977). All one can say is that at least one-third of patients reacting have not had the same drugs previously and it seems likely that two different types of reaction are involved between those already sensitized and those receiving the drug for the first time.

In the last three years a wide variety of rections has been analysed for complement and immunoglobulin changes (Watkins et al., 1976; Watkins et al., 1978). One of the first considerations was to distinguish between anaesthetic disasters due to overdosage, aspiration of gastric contents etc. and true hypersensitivity reactions. This is now clearly possible by measurement of plasma complement C 3 consumption and conversion in sequential blood samples over 24 hours. Furthermore, the barbiturate reactions are usually of the immune-mediated type involving IgE, whereas Althesin reactions more often involve direct activation of C 3 and the 'alternate pathway'.

Histamine liberation following administration of muscle relaxants (particularly tubocurarine) has been known for many years but a true hypersensitivity reaction was thought to be rare. However, in the survey by Clarke and his colleagues, skin testing showed that 2 of the 100 reported reactions were probably due to suxamethonium and 2 to pancuronium. Other reports (Clark, 1973; Heath, 1973; Tweedie and Ordish, 1974) have revealed reactions to most of the muscle relaxants, the French workers laying particular stress on suxamethonium (Vignon et al., 1976). These drugs are often given about the same time as the induction agent and it will probably never be possible to attribute the blame in all instances. Skin testing, though widely carried out, probably gives too many false positive reactions to be reliable.

The management of severe histaminoid reactions is now well standardized and even after collapse complete recovery is to be expected. Bronchospasm was usually treated with aminophylline 250 – 500 mg and hydrocortisone 500 – 1000 mg. Arterial hypotension was treated with a rapid intravenous infusion of fluid, generally 500 – 2000 ml sodium lactate injection compound BP. Antihistamine drugs are of some value both in prophylaxis of anticipated reactions and in treatment of obvious histamine release, but the symptomatic treatment is probably more valuable. Administration of adrenaline is clearly useful but most anaesthetists are reluctant to use this drug without an ECG and clear knowledge of the cause. Since these reactions often occur in circumstances where no resuscitation provision is available the simple safe measures are more often employed. The mortality is probably about 5 per cent of reported reactions but should undoubtedly be less if correct measures were taken rapidly. There appears to be very little justification for using intravenous anaesthetics in isolated dental surgeries whether the reaction rate is 1 in 1 000 or 1 in 10 000 and it will never be possible for such places to be provided with adequate resuscitation equipment.

REFERENCES

Avery A. F. and Evans A. (1973) Reactions to Althesin. *Br. J. Anaesth.* **45**, 301 – 302.

Clark R. M. (1973) Reactions to pancuronium. *Br. J. Anaesth.* **45**, 997.

Clarke R. S. J. (1979) Hypersensitivity reactions to intravenous anaesthetics. In: Dundee J. W. (ed.), *Current Topics in Anaesthesia: New Intravenous Drugs in Anaesthesia*. London, Arnold.

Clarke R. S. J., Dundee J. W., Garrett R. T., McArdle G. K. and Sutton J. A. (1975) Adverse reactions to intravenous anaesthetics: a survey of 100 reports. *Br. J. Anaesth.* **47**, 575 – 585.

Clarke R. S. J., Fee J. P. H. and Dundee J. W. (1977) Factors predisposing to hypersensitivity reactions to intravenous anaesthetics. *Proc. R. Soc. Med.* **70**, 782 – 784.

Dannemann H. and Lubke P. (1970) Complications during anaesthesia with Epontol. *Z. Prakt. Anaesth. Wiederbeleb.* **5**, 273.

Doenicke A., Lorenz W., Beigl R., Bezecny H., Uhlig G., Kalmar L., Praetorius B. and Mann G. (1973) Histamine release after intravenous application of short-acting hypnotics: a comparison of etomidate, Althesin (CT 1341) and propanidid. *Br. J. Anaesth.* **45**, 1097 – 1104.

Driggs R. L. and O'Day R. A. (1972) Acute allergic reaction associated with methohexital anaesthesia: report of 6 cases. *J. Oral Surg.* **30**, 906 – 909.

Dundee J. W., Assem E. S. K., Gaston J. H., Keilty S. R., Sutton J. A., Clarke R. S. J. and Grainger D. (1974) Sensitivity to intravenous anaesthetics: report of 3 cases. *Br. Med. J.* **1**, 63 – 65.

Dundee J. W. and Wyant G. M. (1974) *Intravenous Anaesthesia*. Edinburgh, Churchill Livingstone.

Evans J. M. and Keogh J. A. M. (1977) Adverse reactions to intravenous anaesthetic induction agents. *Br. Med. J.* **2**, 735 – 736.

Fee J. P. H., McDonald J. R., Clarke R. S. J., Dundee J. W. and Pal P. K. (1978) The incidence of atopy and allergy in 10 000 preanaesthetic patients. *Br. J. Anaesth.* **50**, 74.

Fisher M. M. (1976) Severe histamine mediated reactions to Althesin. *Anaesth. Intensive Care* **4**, 33 – 35.

Hayward J. R. and Kiester G. L. (1957) Severe allergic reactions during thiopental sodium anaesthesia. *J. Oral Surg.* **15**, 61 – 63.

Healy T. E. J. (1973) Bronchospasm following Althesin induction. *Lancet* **2**, 975.

Heath M. L. (1973) Bronchospasm in an asthmatic patient following pancuronium. *Anaesthesia* **28**, 437 – 440.

Hegarty J. E. and Dundee J. W. (1978) Local sequelae following the i.v. injection of three benzodiazepines. *Br. J. Anaesth.* **50,** 78.
Kay B. (1972) Brietal sodium in children's surgery. In: Lehmann C. (ed.), *Das Ultrakurznarkoticum Methohexital,* pp. 149 – 158. Berlin, Springer-Verlag.
Mehta S. (1973) Anaphylactic reaction to Althesin. *Anaesthesia* **28,** 669 – 672.
Moneret-Vautrin D. A., Duc M. and Sigiel M. (1976) Étude de différents facteurs de risque du déclenchement d'accidents aux anesthésiques et myorelaxants. *Ann. Anesth. Franc.* **17,** 165 – 174.
Sneddon I. B. and Glew R. C. (1973) Contact dermatitis due to propanidid in an anaesthetist. *Practitioner* **211,** 321 – 323.
Tweedie D. G. and Ordish P. M. (1974) Reactions to intravenous agents (Althesin and pancuronium). *Br. J. Anaesth.* **46,** 244.
Vignon H., Gay R. and Laxenaire M. C. (1976) Observations cliniques d'accidents anaphylactoids per et post anesthésiques. Resultat d'enquêtes a posteriori. *Ann. Anesth. Franc.* **17,** 117 – 121.
Watkins J., Udnoon S., Appleyard T. N. and Thornton J. W. (1976) Identification and quantitation of hypersensitivity reactions to intravenous anaesthetic agents. *Br. J. Anaesth.* **48,** 457 – 461.
Watkins J., Udnoon S. and Taussig P. E. (1978) Complement activation pathways and adverse (anaphylactoid) responses to i.v. anaesthetic agents. *Br. J. Anaesth.* **50,** 73.
Watt J. M. (1975) Anaphylactic reactions after use of CT 1341 (Althesin). *Br. Med. J.* **3,** 205 – 206.

EMERGENCY REPLACEMENT OF BLOOD LOSS

Views on the best fluid for emergency blood volume replacement change with place and time and there are many who rigidly maintain the principle that, if a patient has lost blood, it is blood and nothing else that should be transfused. There are, however, many objections to this view. The most obvious is that cross-matched blood is not available initially and that even Group O Rh negative blood may produce minor incompatibilities leading to haemolysis and predisposing to renal failure. In addition, any stored blood is acidotic with a high plasma potassium level and low erythrocyte 2 – 3 DPG. This latter biochemical abnormality results in a shift to the left of the oxygen dissociation curve and reduces its value for transporting oxygen to the tissues. A quite separate aspect is that by dilution of the blood with 'clear fluids' the viscosity is reduced and low molecular weight dextrans in particular improve capillary circulation. The oxygen-carrying capacity of the blood is reduced but this is less important to the tissues than the arterial oxygen tension and capillary blood flow.

There is therefore much to be said in favour of using crystalloids as the initial transfusion fluid. The ideal crystalloid solution for infusion should resemble the extracellular fluid since its main role is to prevent its depletion rather than to replace blood lost. It cannot be regarded as a plasma expander and probably only remains in the vascular compartment for 30 – 60 minutes. Only by giving many times the volume of blood lost can Ringer-lactate solution be used as a true plasma expander and then only at the risk of pulmonary and peripheral oedema.

The accepted safe limit is therefore about 3 litres or 40 per cent of the blood volume. The safe level of haemodilution is probably to a haematocrit of 28 per cent, but this includes dilution with colloids.

There can be no doubt that if purified human plasma and its fractions were readily available and cheaper, foreign colloids would pass out of use. Since, however, we will need them for many years their properties should be understood (Doenicke et al., 1977). In general, the higher the molecular weight (MW) the longer the molecule will be retained in the bloodstream.

Thus, dextran 140 (MW = 140 000) acts as a plasma expander for 1 – 2 days, dextran 70 for about 5 hours and dextran 40 for about 2 hours, the latter causing an osmotic diuresis as it is excreted. The proportion not excreted is slowly oxidized over several weeks. On the other hand, the larger the molecule the less effective, weight for weight, the maintenance of the colloid osmotic pressure (cf. MW of albumin 70 000; globulin 140 000). The higher MW dextrans cause some aggregation of erythrocytes in vitro and interfere with cross-matching of blood. Samples for blood typing should therefore always be taken before the infusion is started. The smaller molecules appear to have the reverse action in vivo and prevent the tendency of cells to sludge in capillaries where tissue perfusion is poor.

Dextrans are produced by the bacterium *Leuconostoc mesenteroides* B 512 from an agar-sugar-yeast mixture. They are available as 6 or 10 per cent solutions in 5 per cent dextrose or normal saline. There are 150 000 and 110 000 MW solutions (Dextraven), dextran 70 (Lomodex, Macrodex, Gentran 70) and dextran 40 (Lomodex, Rheomacrodex and Gentran 40). There do not appear to be any harmful effects from the dextrans on hepatic or renal function.

Gelatin is derived from hydrolysis of animal collagen tissue such as bone and the product can be cross-linked to give a stable molecule of MW 35 000. They have a half life in the bloodstream of 2 – 3 hours. The most commonly used of gelatins in the UK is Haemaccel which is cross-linked with hexamethylene di-iso-cyanate. The incidence of adverse reactions with gelatins is somewhat higher than with the dextrans but with both it is between 1 in 1 000 and 1 in 10 000 administrations. In general, reactions resemble those with intravenous anaesthetics, varying from a bright flush to life-threatening bronchospasm or hypotension. They are commoner on the European continent, where these substances are more widely used, than in the UK, but if fatalities are to be avoided, everyone involved should be aware of them (Fanous et al., 1977; Ring and Messmer, 1977). It must always be remembered that the incidence of reactions to transfused blood is even higher.

Blood-component therapy is greatly increasing in use as the transfusion centres are able to make these fractions more generally available. The old dried plasma contained fragments of broken down cells, a high level of potassium and a risk of serum hepatitis. Purification has avoided these problems and Plasma Protein Fraction, apart from its cost, would be the ideal colloid plasma expander. It consists of about 83 per cent albumin with 17 per cent of α and β globulins so that it is practically equivalent to plasma — except for the absence of the labile clotting factors. These can best be supplied by interspersing Fresh Frozen Plasma or cryoprecipitate in which the plasma has been separated from the cells soon after donation and stored deep frozen. Platelets should also be given intermittently to maintain adequate haemostasis. The usual regime consists in maintaining the blood volume (judged by central venous pressure) with Ringer-lactate and PPF, the haematocrit above 80 with packed red cells and the clotting properties with FFP and platelets in the ratio of 1 unit of each for every 5 units of packed red cells.

Blood warmers have greatly improved in safety and convenience so it seems best to give any large transfusion at body temperature. Blood filters still cause considerable irritation if transfusion is urgent but unless fresh blood or platelets are being given they are certainly desirable to remove cell aggregates and foreign materials (Dunbar et al., 1974). The speed of infusion can then be maintained with a pressure bag.

REFERENCES

Doenicke A., Grote B. and Lorenz W. (1977) Blood and blood substitutes. *Br. J. Anaesth.* **49**, 681 – 688.

Dunbar R. W., Price K. A. and Cannarella C. F. (1974) Microaggregate blood filters: effect on filtration time, plasma haemoglobin and fresh blood platelet counts. *Anesth. Analg. (Cleve.)* **53**, 577 – 583.

Fanous L. H., Gray A. and Felmingham J. (1977) Severe anaphylactoid reactions to dextran 70. *Br. Med. J.* **2**, 1189 – 1190.

Ring J. and Messmer K. (1977) Incidence and severity of anaphylactoid reactions to colloid volume substitues. *Lancet* **1**, 466 – 469.

RECENT ADVANCES IN HAEMATOLOGY

A. S. DOUGLAS DSc, MD, FRCP,
FRCP Edin, FRCP Glas, FRCPath and
A. A. DAWSON MD, FRCP (Edin),
MRCPath

APLASTIC ANAEMIA

There now seems to be some light at the end of the tunnel for patients developing severe aplastic anaemia in adult life. For several years, conventional therapy has consisted of corticosteroids, to try to protect the patient from the haemorrhagic manifestations, plus synthetic androgens, especially high-dose oxymetholone; the latter, though stimulant to the marrow of some children with hypoplastic anaemias, was never of certain value in adults. In addition to these drugs, all-important has been supportive management, with RBC concentrates, platelet concentrates, and the use of a cell separator for white blood cells, with appropriate careful reverse barrier nursing and also prompt treatment of infections. However, the mortality with conventional treatment has remained at 80 – 90 per cent, most patients dying within 6 months of diagnosis.

Bone marrow transplantation

The place of transplantation of bone marrow from HLA-identical siblings is becoming established. The work on patients with aplastic anaemia began in Seattle around 1970, since when a bone marrow transplant registry has been formed in America, and there have been major improvements in the technique. Now 45 per cent of patients who have a transplant survive for 1 to more than 5 years with complete haematological normality, and a prospective study of early marrow transplantation has demonstrated its superior efficacy over conventional therapy (Camitta et al., 1976).

Apart from such careful prospective trials, it is easy to obtain too optimistic an outlook, since not all the failures are reported. More than half the patients do not have a compatible sibling. The finding of identical tissue-type (HLA) status between donor and patient should be followed by evidence of reciprocal non-stimulation of cells in vitro in mixed lymphocyte culture (MLC) tests. In this technique lymphocytes from donors and recipients are cultured together; when compatability is present there is no growth of the lymphocytes; when incompatible then the lymphocytes from recipient and donor both proliferate. The problem is marrow-graft rejection, and to prevent it, a large dose of cytotoxic drug (usually cyclophosphamide) to suppress the patient's immune mechanism is given. Of 73 patients in Seattle the graft was rejected in 21, and a second graft was rarely successful. In patients with rejection, death is from infection related to the pancytopenia (Storb et al., 1977).

Clinical and laboratory prognostic features

In a survey of 62 transplanted patients published as a report by the Advisory Committee of the Bone Marrow Transplant Registry (1976), clinical prognostic pointers emerge. The longer after diagnosis before transplantation, the lower was the survival rate; 55 per cent were alive when the transplant took place within 3 months of diagnosis compared with 13 per cent when the transplant was delayed more than 9 months from diagnosis. The greater the number of pre-transplant transfusions, the lower was the survival. Also, the younger the patient, the better; survival being significantly higher in the under-21s than the over-21s. Infection in the patient at the time of graft was not a contraindication to the graft nor did it affect survival.

Storb and his colleagues (1977) found that the two important prognostic factors which affected graft 'take' were (1) the MLC test and (2) the number of donor marrow cells obtained. Evidence of cross-reaction in the MLC test, or in another test of cell-mediated immunity—the ^{51}Cr release assay, suggests immunization of the patient against 'minor' histocompatibility antigens of the donor, presumably by preceding blood transfusion. If donor and patient have a positive MLC test then a more powerful (and therefore more toxic) conditioning regimen has to be used, which may include procarbazine, plus antithymocyte globulin, plus total body irradiation; these regimens are still at the investigational stage. It is important to harvest as many donor cells as possible. Failing a minimum of 3×10^8 marrow cells/kg body weight, Storb and his colleagues suggest giving donor haemopoietic stem cells from the buffy coat layer of the peripheral blood, so long as post-grafting methotrexate is given to prevent early graft *v*. host disease.

Immunosuppressive therapy alone

The fact that successful marrow engraftment from a sibling can occur at all in aplastic anaemia is in favour of the belief that the patient's basic lesion is a defect of the pluripotential haemopoietic stem cell, either as an intrinsic defect, or due to adverse circumstances. There have been reports of remission after HLA-incompatible transplants where the transplant appears to have been destroyed (Jeannet et al., 1976; Territo, 1977), and this has led workers to consider the effects on the disease of massive immunosuppressive therapy alone. In a single case report, the patient was given high-dose intravenous cyclophosphamide for 4 days, then supported throughout subsequent severe pancytopenia to relative normality, apart from a moderately low platelet count, a frequent finding in patients in remission after aplastic anaemia (Baran et al., 1976). The possible reason for this success may be that the lymphocytes in aplastic anaemia have some inhibitory effect on the patient's stem cell.

Possible immunological pathogenesis of aplastic anaemia

Some confirmation of this has been provided by Hoffman and colleagues (1977), who demonstrated in tissue culture that peripheral blood lymphocytes from aplastic patients inhibit the erythroid colony formation of marrow from normal subjects, while serum from the patients had no effect. This demonstrated the same cell-mediated inhibition as they had found previously in congenital hypoplastic anaemia. That the granulocyte series is also inhibited was demonstrated by an increase in the number of granulocytic colonies in tissue culture by adding antilymphocyte globulin to aplastic marrow (Ascensão et al., 1976). The finding is of practical importance in explaining the failure of some grafts of HLA-compatible cells, if some of the patient's lymphocytes capable of suppressing haematopoiesis persist; it explains the success of immunosuppressive therapy alone; and it suggests a fundamental effect of suppressor lymphocytes in the aetiology of aplastic anaemia.

Good (1977) provides evidence of this effect of lymphocytes from the marrow (but not the peripheral blood) of some patients with aplastic anaemia. He indicates that suppressor lymphocytes may suppress the proliferative responses of T lymphocytes, the synthesis and secretion of immunoglobulin by B lymphocytes, and plasma-cell differentiation, and may thus act as important controls of lymphoid cell population and function. He believes that in aplastic anaemia, the suppressor T cells are a secondary phenomenon, just as these same cells, found in common variable hypogammaglobulinaemia, are usually secondary to the immunodeficient state, and not the cause of it.

REFERENCES

Advisory Committee of Bone Marrow Transplant Registry (1976) Bone marrow from donors with aplastic anaemia. *J.A.M.A.* **236,** 1131 – 1135.

Ascensão J., Kagan W., Moore M., Pahwa R., Hansen J. and Good R. (1976) Aplastic anaemia: evidence for an immunological mechanism. *Lancet* **1,** 669 – 671.

Baran D. T., Griner P. F. and Klemperer M. R. (1976) Recovery from aplastic anaemia after treatment with cyclophosphamide. *N. Engl. J. Med.* **295,** 1522 – 1523.

Camitta B. M., Thomas E. D., Nathan D. G., Santos G., Gordon-Smith E. C., Gale R. P., Rappaport J. M. and Storb R. (1976) Severe aplastic anaemia: a prospective study of the effect of early marrow transplantation on acute mortality. *Blood* **48,** 63 – 70.

Good R. A. (1977) Aplastic anaemia—suppressor lymphocytes and haematopoiesis. Editorial. *N. Engl. J. Med.* **296,** 41 – 42.

Hoffman R., Zanjani E. D., Lutton J. D., Zalusky R. and Wasserman L. R. (1977) Suppression of erythroid-colony formation by lymphocytes from patients with aplastic anaemia. *N. Engl. J. Med.* **296,** 10 – 13.

Jeannet M., Speck B., Rubinstein A., Pelet B., Wyss M. and Kummer H. (1976) Autologous marrow reconstitutions in severe aplastic anaemia after ALG pre-treatment and HL-A semi-incompatible bone marrow cell transfusion. *Acta Haematol. (Basel)* **55,** 129 – 139.

Storb R., Prentice R. L. and Thomas E. D. (1977) Marrow transplantation for treatment of aplastic anaemia. *N. Engl. J. Med.* **296,** 61 – 66.

Territo M. C. For UCLA Bone Marrow Tansplantation Team (1977) Autologous bone marrow repopulation following high dose cyclophosphamide and allogenetic marrow transplantation in aplastic anaemia. *Br. J. Haematol.* **36,** 305 – 312.

PENICILLIN-RELATED BLEEDING

McClure and associates (1970) observed purpuric bleeding in patients receiving carbenicillin in high dosage and found that the administration of the drug caused a prolonged bleeding time and impaired ADP-induced platelet aggregation. This finding has been repeatedly confirmed and several other penicillins have been shown to have the same effect, including penicillin G and ampicillin. Cazenave et al. (1973) showed that penicillin G in high concentration in vitro inhibited platelet adhesion to collagen and the release reaction, as well as ADP-induced aggregation; they suggested that the penicillins might act by coating the platelets and blocking their receptor sites to aggregating agents.

When frank bleeding occurs in patients it is usually when the antibiotic has been given in very high dosage, particularly in patients with renal fanure, whose platelet function may already be defective, and in whom very high blood concentration may be reached.

REFERENCES
Cazenave J. P., Packman M. A., Guccione M. A. and Mustard J. F. (1973) Effects of
    penicillin G on platelet aggregation, release, and adherence to collagen[1] (36980).
    Proc. Soc. Exp. Biol. Med. **142**, 159 – 166.
McClure P. D., Casserly J. G., Monsier C. and Crozier D. (1970) Carbenicillin-induced
    bleeding disorder. *Lancet* **2**, 1307 – 1308.

THROMBOCYTOPENIA DURING HEPARIN THERAPY

Thrombocytopenia has recently been observed in a surprising number of
patients during treatment with heparin (Bell, 1976). A further 5 patients were
reported by Babcock and associates (1976). The patients were receiving
heparin for conventional reasons and in none was there any clinical evidence
of haemostatic failure during heparin administration; the thrombocytopenia
was often profound ($10 - 35 \times 10^9$/litre). During $1974 - 5$ a prospective
study was conducted at the Johns Hopkins Hospital (Bell et al., 1976). In 16
out of 52 patients who were treated for 5 or more days with continuous
intravenous infusions of beef lung heparin, severe thrombocytopenia
developed. This usually occurred $2 - 10$ days after starting heparin therapy, in
contrast to the immediate fall in platelet count noted in earlier reports.

The mechanism of the thrombocytopenia is obscure. Heparin is not
available as a chemically pure substance, and is contaminated with the animal
tissue from which it is derived. Bell and his colleagues noted a fall in platelet
count in patients treated with heparin derived both from beef lung and from
intestinal mucosa, and no single batch of heparin was responsible. Whether
the thrombocytopenia is a manifestation of hypersensitivity to the heparin
itself or to a tissue contaminant is not known. Neither the time lag to
development of thrombocytopenia, nor the finding that only one third of the
52 patients were affected, favours an immunological mechanism. Half of the
16 patients with thrombocytopenia had collateral evidence of disseminated
intravascular coagulation, not a surprising finding when a product derived
from animal sources is used. Zucker (1974) reports that heparin enhances
primary aggregation, induces aggregation by causing the release reaction, and,
as a result, may reduce the release reaction subsequently provoked by in
vivo stimuli normally leading to effective haemostasis.

As a next stage, it is important for other investigators to follow the platelet
count in patients treated routinely with heparin.

REFERENCES
Babcock R. B., Dumper C. W. and Scharfinan W. B. (1976) Heparin-induced immune
    thrombocytopenia. *N. Engl. J. Med.* **295**, 237.
Bell W. R. (1976) Thrombocytopenia occurring during heparin therapy. *N. Engl. J.
    Med.* **295**, 276.
Bell W. R., Tomasulo P. A., Alving B. M. and Duffy T. P. (1976) Thrombocytopenia
    occurring during the administration of heparin in a prospective study of 52 patients.
    Ann. Intern. Med. **85**, 155.
Zucker M. B. (1974) Effect of heparin on platelet function. *Thromb. Diath. Haemorrh.*
    33, 63.

BLOOD VISCOSITY

Viscosity is the resistance offered by a liquid attempting to change its shape.
Until recently in studies on blood flow there has been emphasis on the

importance of the driving pressure and the calibre of the vessels rather than on the physiology and pathology of blood viscosity (Dormandy, 1970). Determinations of viscosity involve not just plasma but whole blood, and there are many unresolved issues because of the difficulties of measurement.

Factors influencing whole blood viscosity

HAEMATOCRIT

With an increasing haematocrit the greater is the blood viscosity. Rapid administration of intravenous fluid produces haemodilution with a rapid lowering of blood viscosity. This is the rationale in the use of various intravenous solutions, including low molecular weight dextran, in the treatment of conditions giving rise to haemoconcentration. Dormandy (1970) showed that a reduction of haematocrit from 50 per cent to 45 per cent produced a 12 per cent fall in viscosity; this simultaneously reduced the haemoglobin by 10 per cent (1·4 g/dl). The oxygen carrying capacity per unit of blood was reduced, but this was more than compensated by the increase in blood flow.

RED CELL AGGREGATION

At rest red cells form three-dimensional continuous networks of rouleaux. With the application of increasing shear stress these continuous networks are broken down, first into smaller formations of rouleaux, which then disperse into discrete cells. Aggregation of red cells at low and very low rates of shear has been considered of great importance in accounting for the high viscosities found with these conditions of flow (Copley et al., 1975).

RED CELL INTERNAL VISCOSITY

At flow velocities close to zero human blood may have a viscosity of 100 – 10 000 times greater than water. At high flow velocities it may only be 2 – 10 times that of water (Dintenfass, 1965, 1966). If red cells were replaced by rigid spheres of the same dimension, the resultant 'fluid' would be solid at a haematocrit of 65 per cent. Blood remains fluid at a haematocrit of 95 per cent because the internal viscosity of the red cell is probably remarkably low.

RED CELL FLEXIBILITY OR DEFORMABILITY

Filming of the microcirculation in experimental animals shows the extraordinary ability of red cells to deform. Red cell flexibility can be measured by centrifugation filtration techniques using membranes with pores of standard diameter (Reid et al., 1975). There is a gross reduction in red cell deformability in patients with peripheral vascular disease of the lower limbs. It is possible that the effect on blood viscosity of β-blockers (Dintenfass and Lake, 1976) is mediated by the changes in red cell deformability. Mayer (1976) reported that the administration of oral anticoagulants reduced blood viscosity, and ascribed this to a fall of haematocrit value — possibly as a result of occult bleeding from the gastrointestinal and urinary tracts.

PLASMA FIBRINOGEN

Plasma fibrinogen levels have been shown to influence whole blood viscosity (Weaver et al., 1969). Dormandy and his colleagues have studied a large group of patients with peripheral arterial disease and intermittent claudication. The high blood viscosity in such patients was associated with abnormally raised plasma fibrinogen; lowering of the fibrinogen concentration with clofibrate resulted in a lowering of blood viscosity with accompanying symptomatic and objective improvement (Dormandy and Edelman, 1973; Dormandy et al., 1973, 1974).

Retinopathy in diabetics is due to small vessel disease; these patients have raised blood viscosity, but this is not correlated with the fibrinogen level (Hoare et al., 1976).

Clinical application

Phillips and Harkness (1976), in an excellent review of plasma and blood viscosity, agree that the clinical applications are not yet clear. However, the concepts of red cell deformability (which can be measured) and red cell internal viscosity (which cannot) are important to our understanding of blood flow through small vessels. In the aetiology of deep venous thrombosis the low shear rate in the calf veins with red cell aggregation, and raised fibrinogen concentration may be relevant. The role of fibrinogen in viscosity can be altered by defibrination with ancrod derived from the Malayan pit viper. The beta-blocking drugs require to be assessed as antithrombotic agents; in the present context this is because of their action on viscosity, but they are also antiplatelet drugs.

At a practical level, the measurement of plasma viscosity affords a useful non-specific index of disease, which closely parallels the findings of the ESR; it can be readily standardized and is not affected by age, sex, or by anaemia. It does require a more complex and expensive apparatus than does the ESR, however. In the future, measurement of blood viscosity could emerge as of sufficient immediate clinical importance to become a routine service responsibility of haematology departments.

REFERENCES

Copley A. L., King R. G., Chien S., Usami S., Skalak R. and Huang C. R. (1975) Microscopic observations of visco-elasticity of human blood in steady and oscillatory shear. *Biorheology* **12**, 257.

Dintenfass L. (1965) Viscosity of the packed red and white blood cells. *Exp. Mol. Pathol.* **4**, 597.

Dintenfass L. (1966) Viscometry of human blood for shear rates of $0 - 100\,000\ \mathrm{sec}^{-1}$. *Nature (Lond.)* **211**, 632.

Dintenfass L. and Lake B. (1976) Beta-blockers and blood viscosity. *Lancet* **1**, 1026.

Dormandy J. A. (1970) Clinical significance of blood viscosity. *Ann. R. Coll. Surg. Engl.* **47**, 211.

Dormandy J. A. and Edelman J. (1973) A new aetiological factor in deep venous thrombosis. *Br. J. Surg.* **60**, 187.

Dormandy J. A., Hoare E. M., Colley I., Arrowsmith D. E. and Dormandy T. L. (1973) Clinical, haemodynamic, rheological and biochemical findings in 126 patients with intermittent claudication. *Br. Med. J.* **4**, 576.

Dormandy J. A., Hoare E. M. and Dormandy T. L. (1974) Effect of clofibrate on blood viscosity in intermittent claudication. *Br. Med. J.* **4**, 259.

Hoare E. M., Barnes A. J. and Dormandy J. A. (1976) Abnormal blood viscosity in diabetes mellitus and retinopathy. *Biorheology* **13**, 21.

Mayer G. A. (1976) Blood viscosity and oral anticoagulant therapy. *Am. J. Clin. Pathol.* **65**, 402.

Phillips M. J. and Harkness J. (1976) Plasma and whole blood viscosity. *Br. J. Haematol.* **34**, 347.

Reid H. L., Dormandy J. A., Barnes A. J., Lock P. M. and Dormandy T. L. (1975) Impaired red cell deformability in peripheral vascular disease. *Lancet* **1**, 666.
Weaver J. P. A., Evans A. and Walder D. N. (1969) The effect of increased fibrinogen content on the viscosity of the blood. *Clin. Sci.* **36**, 1.

HAEMOGLOBIN AI LEVELS IN DIABETES MELLITUS

There are three minor components of normal haemoglobin—HbAIa, HbAIb and HbAIc—which are fast-moving components in a chromatographic system utilizing a particular ion-exchange resin (Allen et al., 1958). These three haemoglobins account for about 7 per cent of total haemoglobin, with HbAIc as the major component representing 5 – 6 per cent of total haemoglobin. HbAIc differs chemically from the major adult haemoglobin HbA ($\alpha_2\beta_2$). The β chains have an added hexose (glucose and mannose), and the consequence of this is a high affinity for oxygen.

An increased HbAI in diabetics was first observed by Huisman and Dozy (1962) and confirmed by Paulsen and Koury (1976); these high levels of HbAI are present in states of relative or absolute insulinopenia, including steroid-induced diabetes. In ketoacidosis in diabetics the levels rise even higher, and it requires at least a month for a return to that individual's baseline, or preketotic but elevated value. This decline occurs only as new red cells form under conditions less favourable to HbAI synthesis.

Abnormal amounts of HbA and HbAI resisted removal from diabetic red cell membranes by low ionic buffers, but yielded to hypotonic tris buffers. The elution of the HbAI resulted also in removal of integral membrane proteins. Such tight binding might well alter membrane elasticity and cell deformability—characteristics of possible relevance to cell movement through the microvasculature (Paulsen and Koury, 1976). The consequence of loss of red cell deformability on whole blood viscosity has been discussed above in the section on blood viscosity.

REFERENCES

Allen D. W., Schroeder W. A. and Balog J. (1958) Observations on the chromatographic heterogeneity of normal adult and foetal haemoglobin. A study of the effects of crystalization and chromatography on the heterogeneity and isoleucine content. *J. Am. Chem. Soc.* **80**, 1628.
Huisman T. H. and Dozy A. M. (1962) Studies on the heterogeneity of haemoglobin. V. Binding of haemoglobin with oxidised glutathione. *J. Lab. Clin. Med.* **60**, 302.
Paulsen E. P. and Koury M. (1976) Haemoglobin AIc levels in insulin-dependent and independent diabetes mellitus. *Diabetes* **25** (suppl. 2), 890.

BLEEDING TIME

The bleeding time test

With careful standardization of site, length, and depth of the incision much more precise information has recently been obtained from this test (Hirsh et al., 1976). The skin bleeding time test measures primary haemostasis in capillaries, precapillary arteries, and postcapillary venules. The test is sensitive to quantitative and qualitative platelet disorders, but is relatively insensitive both to coagulation disorders and vascular disorders (allergic purpura, Cushing's disease, and scurvy). Careful correlation was made with the platelet count. Prolongation of bleeding time starts when the platelet count falls to 100×10^9/litre. The time lengthens progressively until the count is

20×10^9/litre; below this, the time is infinite. The bleeding time tends to be shorter for any given platelet count in this range in chronic immune thrombocytopenia. As has long been accepted by the clinician, it has been confirmed that the bleeding time in thrombocytopenia is shortened by hydrocortisone.

The bleeding time is longer in normal women as compared with normal men. Administration of aspirin prolongs the bleeding time.

The haemostatic efficiency of stored human platelets has been measured. Storage at 4 °C for 24 hours caused loss of effectiveness. The haemostatic efficiency of the stored platelets could be sustained by manipulation of the pH. Platelets maintained frozen also retain their haemostatic properties.

REFERENCE
Hirsh J., Blajchman M. and Kaege A. (1976) The bleeding time test. *Workshop on Platelets,* Philadelphia, 1976 (Abstract).

FIBRINOLYSIS

The precise role of the fibrinolytic enzyme system in human physiology and pathology is uncertain. It seems likely, however, that it is concerned with wound healing and the restoration of vascular patency when there is partial or complete vessel occlusion by thrombus. Despite much endeavour over the last 15 years there is no clear definition of the therapeutic role of thrombolytic agents in human disease, but there have been advances in our knowledge of the fibrinolytic mechanism.

Circadian rhythm

The circadian periodicity of fibrinolysis has recently been confirmed by Cepelak and Cepelakova (1976); fibrinolysis is most marked at 4·00 p.m. and least at 4·00 a.m. This is not related to physical activity and is present in bedridden patients.

Fibrin removal by leucocytes

At least two recent investigators have produced evidence that the blood leucocytes are responsible for removing fibrin, probably independently of the conventional fibrinolytic (plasminogen – plasmin) system. Haverkate et al. (1976) reported on the leucocytes in normal subjects and in others suffering from rheumatoid disease. This property was related to granulocytes and not to lymphocytes or monocytes. Kwaan and Hatem (1976) have demonstrated similar properties of the white cells, emphasizing in particular the role of eosinophils. Fibrin is acted on at the surface of the cell, usually in shallow invaginations of the cell membrane. It has long been known that leucocytes are always intimately associated with thrombus. These authors suggest that eosinophils and neutrophils are concerned with the transformation of early fibrin and platelet depositions; the neutrophil leucocytes are of particular importance in the phagocytosis of platelets.

Cycloallin

Previous work on the onion has established its power to enhance natural fibrinolysis. The active principle appears to reside in the essential oil, which is rich in sulphur-containing compounds. Unfortunately, these last are also responsible for the particular taste and odour of onion and these limit its clinical application. Cycloallin, a sulphur-containing amino-acid and a normal constituent of onion, is free from these features and was known previously to have a property for enhancing fibrinolysis (Augusti et al., 1975). This material has now been synthesized and given in a dose of 0·25 g to human volunteers. Blood tested 1½ hours after ingestion showed a doubling of the fibrinolytic activity (Agarwal et al., 1977). This material is likely to be more acceptable for clinical testing than the anabolic steroids and phenformin, the other known orally effective pharmacological activators of fibrinolysis.

REFERENCES

Agarwal R. K., Dewar H. A., Newell D. J. and Das B. (1977) Controlled trial of the effect of cycloallin on the fibrinolytic activity of venous blood. *Atherosclerosis* **27**, 347.
Augusti K. T., Benaim M. E., Dewar H. A. and Virden R. (1975) Partial identification of the fibrinolytic activators in onion. *Atherosclerosis* **21**, 409.
Cepelak V. and Cepelakova H. (1976) Circadian periodicity of fibrinolysis and clinical trials. *Third Int. Conf. on Synthetic Fibrinolytic Thromolytic Agents—Progress in Fibrinolysis,* Glasgow (Abstact).
Haverkate F., Hegt V. N., Putte L. B. A. and Ginkel C. J. W. (1976) Fibrinolytic activity of human leucocytes. *Third Int. Conf. on Synthetic Fibrinolytic (Thrombolytic Agents—Progress in Fibrinolysis,* Glasgow (Abstract).
Kwaan H. C. and Hatem A. A. (1976) The lysis of early fibrin by eosinophils. *Third Int. Conf. on Synthetic Fibrinolytic Thrombolytic Agents—Progress in Fibrinolysis,* Glasgow (Abstract).

CLUSTERING OF EPSTEIN – BARR VIRUS (EBV)-ASSOCIATED AMERICAN BURKITT'S LYMPHOMA

Burkitt's lymphoma is the most frequent neoplasm in African children and in endemic areas has an incidence as high as 10 per 100 000 per year, with a peak occurrence between the ages of 6 and 8 years. The African tumour is almost invariably associated with the Epstein – Barr virus. The patients have a broader spectrum and higher titres of antibodies to EBV-determined antigens than controls. EB viral DNA is detectable in nearly all the tumours, and the tumour cells contain the EBV-associated nuclear antigen.

Sporadic cases of Burkitt's lymphoma have been found in the USA and Europe, and these are not usually EBV positive. Judson and colleagues (1977) investigated 4 patients with histologically confirmed Burkitt's lymphoma presenting during a 1-year period. These were young adults living within 50 km of each other in a rural area of Pennsylvania; 2 were related by marriage but there had been no contact with or between the other 2. All 4 patients showed spectra and titres of antibodies to antigens related to that virus characteristic of the disease as found in Africa.

Clustering has been demonstrated previously with other lymphomas, notably Hodgkin's disease (Vianna et al., 1971). Burkitt's lymphoma has the scientific and epidemiological advantage of having the EBV 'marker', so that careful follow-up of this and other groups might add considerably to current knowledge of aetiology.

REFERENCES

Judson S. C., Henle W. and Henle G. (1977) A cluster of Epstein-Barr-Virus-associated American Burkitt's lymphoma. *N. Engl. J. Med.* **297**, 465.

Vianna N. J., Greenwald P. and Davies J. N. P. (1971) Extended epidemic of Hodgkin's disease in high-school students. *Lancet* **1**, 1209.

'MYELOPROLIFERATIVE' SYNDROMES

The myeloproliferative diseases have always been resistant to precise definition; this is especially so with myelofibrosis, where diagnostic criteria are difficult to achieve, and where transitional states with other myeloproliferative disorders, especially polycythaemia vera, exist. Mulder and his colleagues (1977), using the name 'myelofibrosis with myeloid metaplasia', included in the group only patients with (1) an increase in fibrous tissue, collagen and/or reticulin in the marrow (2) proved extramedullary haemopoiesis on biopsy or histology of the spleen; (3) leucoerythroblastosis of the peripheral blood film; and (4) splenic enlargement.

Ferrokinetic studies

USING ^{59}Fe

These have proved of some value both in diagnosis and in therapeutic decision in myelofibrosis; the common finding is a faster plasma iron half-clearance time ($T\frac{1}{2}\,^{59}$Fe) and reduced red cell iron incorporation (Szur and Lewis, 1975). Surface counting shows extramedullary erythropoiesis in the spleen and, less constantly, in the liver.

USING ^{52}Fe SPLENIC UPTAKE

The short-lived ^{52}Fe, made in the cyclotron, has a half-life of 8·2 hours. With this isotope it is possible to use a sufficient dose for scanning techniques to identify the sites of RBC production, and to do serial studies at short intervals (Pettit et al., 1976). These workers demonstrated that the *splenic uptake* of ^{52}Fe in myelofibrosis represented movement of iron into developing erythroblasts, and not mere removal of iron by splenic reticuloendothelial cells. They found a high splenic uptake in myelofibrosis and a low or absent one in polycythaemia; there was a variable uptake in patients with 'transitional' myeloproliferative disorders, i.e. those with high RBC mass, hypercellular marrow, and leucoerythroblastosis in the blood film. In the future this technique could be applied to patients with polycythaemia vera to establish which are developing myelofibrosis. The test could also have therapeutic implications in deciding on splenectomy in those cases of myelofibrosis where red cells destruction after sequestration exceeds the splenic contribution to total erythropoiesis.

Development of leukaemia

Some patients who have progressed from polycythaemia vera to myelofibrosis terminate with acute leukaemia (myeloid or myelomonocytic). Polycythaemia vera has been treated with radioactive phosphorus (^{32}P) for over 20 years. The role of ^{32}P in the transition of polycythaemia vera to myelofibrosis and of the subsequent development of acute leukaemia once myelofibrosis has supervened are uncertain. In a large series of 306 patients with myeloproliferative disorders Rosenthal and Maloney (1977) had 18 cases of acute leukaemia, developing from 6 months to 20 years after initial diagnosis (of polycythaemia vera, myelofibrosis, and essential thrombocythaemia); and, because of their strict criteria in diagnosing the acute leukaemia, which is often difficult in these circumstances, they believe that the incidence is higher. (In other series the incidence has varied from 5 to 25 per cent of cases of myeloproliferative disorders.) There was an equal occurrence of leukaemia in both polycythaemia and myelofibrosis (the numbers of cases of essential thrombocythaemia were too small to compare). There was a higher male risk of developing acute leukaemia. The preleukaemic state lasted longer in polycythaemia than in myelofibrosis, and once leukaemia supervened survival was poor, with no remissions in these elderly patients. Using ^{59}Fe ferrokinetics an attempt has been made to define which patients with myelofibrosis will go on to develop acute leukaemia. Bentley and associates (1977) provided some evidence that it is those with a hypoplastic marrow pattern on ^{59}Fe ferrokinetic studies, who go on to blastic transformation.

Role of splenectomy

In patients with these myeloproliferative syndromes various therapies have been used, including ^{32}P, cytotoxic drugs, and splenic radiotherapy. In some patients splenectomy seemed to be followed rapidly by a blastic crisis, but this operation is not considered to be a predisposing factor (Silverstein and ReMine, 1974).

Until recent years splenectomy was contraindicated in the management of myelofibrosis; with limited supportive therapy and a decision to operate late in the course of the disease (by which time the spleen was enormous) the operative mortality was high. Crosby (1972) proposed early splenectomy in myelofibrosis, before splenomegaly produces functional or mechanical problems. It is well known that the iron overload produced by repeated transfusions carries a high mortality. Mulder and his colleagues (1977) described the effect of elective splenectomy in 19 patients, often referred to their centre rather late, and enumerated severe postoperative complications of bleeding, thrombosis, and hepatitis B. They still demonstrated that all but 2 patients (who died within 3 months of surgery) had a better quality of life, with improvement in white cell count and platelet count, and virtual disappearance of the leucoerythroblastosis. Survival was generally longer than in patients not so treated, so that with improved methods of monitoring splenic function, possibly by radioactive iron (^{59}Fe or [52]Fe), a further trial of early splenectomy in myelofibrosis seems timely.

REFERENCES

Bentley S. A., Murray K. H., Lewis S. M. and Roberts P. D. (1977) Erythroid hypoplasia in myelofibrosis: a feature associated with blastic transformation. *Br. J. Haematol.* **36**, 41 – 47.

Crosby W. H. (1972) Splenectomy in haematologic disorders. *N. Engl. J. Med.* **286**, 1252 – 1254.

Mulder H., Steenbergen J. and Haanen C. (1977) Clinical course and survival after elective splenectomy in 19 patients with primary myelofibrosis. *Br. J. Haematol.* **35**, 419 – 427.

Pettit J. E., Lewis S. M., Williams E. D., Grafton C. S., Bowring C. S. and Glass H. I. (1976) Quantitative studies of splenic erythropoiesis in polycythaemia vera and myelofibrosis. *Br. J. Haematol.* **34**, 465 – 475.

Rosenthal D. A. and Maloney W. C. (1977) Occurrence of acute leukaemia in myeloproliferative disorders. *Br. J. Haematol.* **36**, 373 – 382.

Silverstein M. N. and ReMine W. H. (1974) Sex, splenectomy and myeloid metaplasia. *J.A.M.A.* **227**, 424 – 425.
Szur L. and Lewis S. M. (1975) Iron kinetics. *Clin. Haematol.* **4** (2), 407 – 425.

HERPES ZOSTER IN THE IMMUNOSUPPRESSED

Herpes zoster is a common infection in immuno-compromised patients, in whom it is acutely debilitating, and may be life-threatening if it involves the viscera by dissemination. Methods of therapeutic attack have included the antiviral agent, idoxuridine, and the purine analogue, cytarabine (cytosine arabinoside), both of which have considerable toxicity in dosage suitable for systemic therapy. The related purine nucleoside, adenine arabinoside, is an antiviral agent which showed clinical usefulness in controlled trials of human herpes infection. In a controlled study in herpes zoster infection in immunosuppressed patients Whitley and his collaborators (1976) in the USA have reached some conclusions about the value of this material. The material itself is highly insoluble, so it has to be administered slowly by intravenous infusion, and is only available by special arrangement. However, unlike its relation, cytarabine, it has no obvious bone marrow or immunological toxicity, nor any other notable side-effect. It hastened cutaneous healing of herpetic lesions and significantly improved acute neuritic pain, but the trial did not allow an answer as to whether it prevented dissemination or reduced mortality.

Of immunosuppressed patients, those with the slowest rate of healing and at greatest risk of dissemination are those with reticuloendothelial tumours. In the normal population herpes zoster heals more rapidly in the younger than in the older.

The standard treatment should be the use of hyperimmune globulin; the latter is now more plentiful, being obtained from subjects convalescent from or immunized against varicella/zoster. In addition, the use of adenine arabinoside should be considered; while the results from controlled clinical trials are not at present available, the evidence is that adenine arabinoside is of value and equally effective in the younger as well as the older patient.

REFERENCE
Whitley R. J., Chien L. T., Dolin R., G-Alasso G. J., Alford C. A. and the Collaborative Study Group (1976) Adenine arabinoside therapy of herpes zoster in the immunosuppressed. *N. Engl. J. Med.* **294**, 1193 – 1199.

CARDIOVASCULAR DISEASE

B. L. PENTECOST MD, FRCP
J. L. MONRO FRCS
H. H. G. EASTCOTT MS, FRCS

Heart and major vessels: medical

B. L. PENTECOST MD, FRCP

VASODILATOR THERAPY IN CARDIAC FAILURE

The standard drug treatment of cardiac failure involves a combination of diuretics and a glycoside. The purpose of the diuretic is to reduce congestive symptoms such as peripheral or pulmonary oedema, and the glycoside, usually digoxin, theoretically increases myocardial contractility. Oedema may not always respond to diuretics, however, and the reduction in circulating volume which they produce may accentuate the problem of 'forward failure' or low stroke volume, with consequent under-perfusion of vital tissues. There is also some doubt about the value of digitalis in both the long term management of congestive failure in the absence of atrial fibrillation, and in some acute situations such as pump failure manifested as cardiogenic shock in myocardial infarction. A new pharmacological approach to the problem is centred around the possible therapeutic role of vasodilators in the management of cardiac failure.

In the presence of severe cardiac failure, the Starling curve, relating stroke volume or work to ventricular end diastolic pressure, is flattened. The function of the ventricle is further impaired by an apparently high degree of peripheral vascular resistance or arterial impedance which is partly due to an increased sympathetic neural stimulus. A reduction of arterial impedance in this situation tends to restore the normal curvilinear relationship between stroke volume and end diastolic pressure, or put another way shifts the Starling curve upwards and to the left, as a result of which the end diastolic pressure falls and the stroke volume rises (Cohn and Franciosa, 1977). Among the drugs influencing arterial impedance are hydrallazine, prazosin, minoxidil, and phenoxybenzamine, which are orally active, and phentolamine and sodium nitroprusside, which require to be given intravenously. Drugs dilating the venous circulation result in peripheral pooling of blood and may be expected to ameliorate congestive features of heart failure. Glyceryl trinitrate and isosorbide dinitrate act primarily in this way. It is important to note that in the presence of failure the systemic hypotension and tachycardia, which would normally tend to result from these drugs, are rarely observed but continue to be one potential hazard of such therapy.

One application of this approach has been in the management of severe pump failure complicating myocardial infarction. Chatterjee and his colleagues (1976) treated 40 such patients with intravenous nitroprusside by continuous infusion. Initial doses were low (16µg/min) and were gradually increased until the stroke volume rose and left ventricular end diastolic pressure fell. The therapeutic dose varied between 25 and 425µg/min and the regime was continued for between 4 hours and 27 days. In this group of patients, in whom the authors' previous experience would suggest an expected mortality rate of 80 per cent, some 56 per cent survived hospital admission, although there was a high mortality over the first six months after discharge. Hypotension is a potential hazard of this treatment and could further reduce myocardial blood flow. It was encountered occasionally but responded briskly to cessation of drug therapy and elevation of the legs. Thiocyanate poisoning was apparently not a problem but has been recorded in other studies in which medication has been continued for several days, making blood level estimations of thiocyanate an important precaution. In chronic congestive cardiac failure similar improvement in cardiac performance has been achieved with parenteral nitroprusside, but perhaps of greater interest to the clinician is the beneficial effect of oral treatment with isosorbide and phenoxybenzamine (Kovick et al., 1976). Among 12 patients responding favourably to parenteral therapy with nitroprusside, oral isosorbide was started in a dose of $2 \cdot 5 - 10$ mg every 2 hours of the waking day, and phenoxybenzamine (10 mg capsules) every $8 - 12$ hours. The dose of the latter drug was carefully titrated against any hypotensive effect before discharge from hospital. Over a period ranging from 3 to 21 months all survivors were subjectively improved and showed objective evidence of enhanced cardiac performance. A beneficial effect of oral isosorbide in a single dose of 20 mg in patients with congestive failure has been confirmed, mainly in the relief of congestive symptoms and signs, although patients with severely elevated left ventricular end diastolic pressure do show some increase in stroke volume (Williams et al., 1977).

Several other oral drugs have been evaluated in the management of congestive cardiac failure including the antihypertensive drug prazosin (Miller et al., 1977). In patients with long-standing severe left ventricular failure due to coronary artery disease, oral prazosin in a dose of $2 - 7$ mg produced a slight fall in arterial pressure together with a reduction in left ventricular end diastolic pressure and elevation in stroke volume. The effects persisted for at least 6 hours and constitute an encouraging finding for long term administration. In a similar manner, a single dose of from 50 to 100 mg hydrallazine has been shown to produce a substantial improvement in stroke volume among a group of patients with left ventricular failure due to severe myocardial disease (Franciosa et al., 1977). This beneficial effect was maintained for 4 hours, and was accompanied by a relatively slight increase in heart failure and fall in systolic blood pressure.

The eventual place of vasodilators in the management of cardiac failure remains to be established. When parenteral therapy with nitroprusside is indicated, particularly in the presence of myocardial infarction, haemo-dynamic monitoring is essential in order to avoid potentially dangerous systemic hypotension and to judge the dose at which haemodynamic improvement occurs. For long term medication in chronic failure with such drugs as oral hydrallazine, prazosin and isosorbide, clinical observations are probably adequate, but it is advisable to start therapy under careful supervision in order to avoid the potential hazard of tachycardia and hypotension which, according to published experience, appear to be rare. Doubts may also be felt over non-selective reduction in arterial impedance in that inappropriate redistribution of blood flow might follow. So far there has been no evidence of this problem, particularly within the coronary circulation itself, and indeed the haemodynamic effects of reducing the left ventricular after-load should result in a reduction of myocardial oxygen requirement, unlike the increase provoked by positive inotropic agents.

REFERENCES

Chatterjee K., Swan H. J. C., Kaushik V. S., Jobin G., Magnusson P. and Forrester J. S. (1976) Effects of vasodilator therapy for severe pump failure in acute myocardial infarction on short-term and late prognosis. *Circulation* **53**, 797.

Cohn J. N. and Franciosa J. A. (1977) Vasodilator therapy of cardiac failure. *N. Engl. J. Med.* **297**, 27.

Franciosa J. A., Pierpont G. and Cohn J. N. (1977) Hemodynamic improvement after oral hydrallazine in left ventricular failure. *Ann. Int. Med.* **86**, 388.

Kovick R. B., Tillisch J. H., Bereus S. C., Bramowitz, A. D. and Shine K. I. (1976) Vasodilator therapy for chronic left ventricular failure. *Circulation* **53**, 322.

Miller R. R., Awan N. A., Maxwell K. S. and Mason D. T. (1977) Sustained reduction of cardiac impedance and preload in congestive heart failure with the anti-hypertensive vasodilator prazosin. *N. Engl. J. Med.* **297**, 303.

Williams D. O., Bommer W. J., Miller R. R., Amsterdam E. A. and Mason D. T. (1977) Haemodynamic assessment of oral peripheral vasodilator therapy in chronic congestive heart failure: Prolonged effectiveness of isosorbide dinitrate. *Am. J. Cardiol.* **39**, 84.

MYOCARDIAL INFARCTION—SUDDEN DEATH AFTER HOSPITAL DISCHARGE

Several studies in the past have shown that the majority of deaths among patients discharged from hospital after acute myocardial infarction happen within the first few months. As with any acute coronary episode many such deaths occur suddenly and without warning, presumably as a result of ventricular fibrillation. It would clearly be of value if those convalescent patients at high risk from sudden death could be identified during their hospital admission, in order that some attempt be made to prevent the subsequent development of serious arrhythmias. Effective anti-arrhythmic drugs exist including oral procainamide, mexiletene, disopyramide and the beta-adrenoceptor blocking agents, but all have unwanted effects, including some depression of myocardial contractility, rendering their widespread use potentially hazardous. It is important for drug studies to concentrate on the high-risk subgroups: if this is not done there may be a failure to detect beneficial anti-arrhythmic effects as a result of dilution with low risk patients. In the last year observations on patients experiencing sudden death after hospital discharge have provided some clues as to the identification of this high risk sub-group and its possible treatment.

In one study among a group of 81 hospital patients recovering from myocardial infarction a careful assessment was made of both myocardial performance and cardiac rhythm approximately two weeks after admission (Schulze et al., 1977). Left ventricular ejection fraction, i.e. the ratio of stroke volume to end diastolic volume, was estimated by an isotopic technique measuring left ventricular blood volume, and a 24-hour electrocardiographic tape-recording was made with the patient fully active about the ward. The tape was subsequently analysed for rhythm disturbance. During a period of follow-up which varied from 2 to 16 months, 8 patients were judged to have died suddenly, i.e. within an hour, or from documented ventricular fibrillation in hospital. All 8 were found to have belonged to a sub-group comprising 26 of the original 81 patients each of whom showed a depressed left ventricular ejection fraction (less than 0·40), and complicated ventricular ectopic activity.

Ventricular ectopic activity in this study was defined according to Lown's criteria, and in the particular sub-group under consideration ventricular ectopic beats were either multifocal, coupled or bigeminal, or occurred in salvoes, i.e. short bursts of ventricular tachycardia, or exhibited the R on T appearance.

It was argued that this severe form of ventricular ectopic activity was the result of impaired myocardial function due to relatively extensive myocardial damage, and that a search for evidence of both left ventricular dysfunction and serious ventricular ectopic activity in the convalescent phase could identify a high risk sub-group of patients. An important aspect of the study was the emphasis placed upon arrhythmias occurring late in the hospital admission rather than in the acute stage, a point which was elaborated upon by Vismara and his colleagues (1977). They showed that the presence or absence of serious ventricular ectopic activity within the first few days of admission after myocardial infarction bore little or no relevance to the rhythm situation two weeks later. Again, late arrhythmias were found to occur more commonly among patients in whom the acute illness had been complicated by haemo-dynamic evidence of left ventricular failure, such as the appearance of a high pulmonary artery wedge pressure as measured by right heart catheterization. Vismara also demonstrated the futility of attempts at arrhythmia detection in the later stages of hospital admission by conventional 12 lead electrocardio-graphy, and emphasized the need for some form of ambulatory electrocardio-graphic tape monitoring. There was a significant correlation between ventricular ectopic activity during the late period of hospital admission and sudden death after discharge in this study, but not between sudden death and arrhythmias witnessed in the early acute stages of the admission.

Moss et al. (1977) also found that the majority of sudden deaths occurring after discharge from hospital occurred during the first few months. Among their own group of 759 patients, 42 deaths occurred within 6 months (the great majority within 2 months of discharge), and of these 62 per cent were judged to have been sudden, i.e. they were either unwitnessed or death occurred within 12 hours of the onset of symptoms. One particularly interesting aspect of this work was the observation that a high proportion of the sudden death patients had recently been treated with digitalis (70 per cent) and diuretics (49 per cent), but relatively few had been prescribed either anti-arrhythmic drugs or propranolol. It is therefore tempting to speculate that these patients represented a group with relatively more severe myocardial damage similar to the patients exhibiting a low ejection fraction in the study of Schulze et al. The lack of antiarrhythmic drug prescription may have been explained by a true absence of arrhythmias, or quite possibly by a failure to detect even serious ectopic activity by conventional physical examination.

The final results of the International Multicentre Practolol Study (1977) may throw some further light on this problem. Routine beta blockade with practolol beginning approximately two weeks after myocardial infarction was shown to reduce the incidence of sudden death in a large controlled study involving more than 3 000 post-infarction patients. These were highly selected and the study excluded anyone over the age of 70, those with congestive cardiac failure, bradycardia, asthma, and those patients with greater than first degree atrioventricular block. Subsequent analysis revealed that the beneficial effect was demonstrated primarily in patients with a pre-trial anterior infarction who, at the time of admission to the trial, had a diastolic blood pressure of less than the average 78 mm Hg for all patients included in the study. It is possible that the presence of a low diastolic blood pressure after recovery from an anterior infarction is evidence of relatively severe myocardial injury, even in the absence of clinically obvious cardiac failure.

The present state of knowledge therefore suggests that the peak incidence of sudden death after discharge from hospital is within the first few weeks or months. Patients who are most at risk appear to be those who have suffered extensive myocardial injury at the time of infarction and who, presumably as a direct result of the impaired ventricular performance, are shown to have complicated ventricular activity during the later stages of admission. Techniques for recording and analysing 24 electrocardiographic tapes are now widely available, but the work involved in routine patient screening would be considerable and its value requires confirmation. The detection of impaired myocardial contractility, which is not obvious as cardiac failure, by non-invasive techniques is less easy. Reliance may need to be placed upon the careful recording of clinical and radiological evidence of left ventricular failure, or impending failure, in the acute stages of the illness in order to select those patients with more extensive myocardial damage. More studies are certainly required to identify the high risk sub-group with the object of further evaluation of anti-arrhythmic therapy.

REFERENCES

Moss A. J., de Camilla J. and Davis H. (1977) Cardiac death in the first six months after myocardial infarction; Potential for Mortality Reduction in the Early Post-Hospital Phase. *Am. J. Cardiol.* **39,** 816.
Multicentre International Study: Supplementary Report (1977) Reduction in mortality after Myocardial Infarction with long term beta adrenoceptor blockade. *Br. Med. J.* **2,** 419.
Schulze R. A., Strauss H. W. and Pitt B. (1977) Sudden death in the year following myocardial infarction. *Am. J. Med.* **62,** 192.
Vismara L. A., Vera Z., Foerster J. M., Amsterdam E. A. and Mason D. T. (1977) Identification of sudden death risk factors in acute and chronic coronary artery disease. *Am. J. Cardiol.* **39,** 821.

DIABETES AND THE MYOCARDIUM

The majority of patients suffering from diabetes mellitus die as a result of cardiovascular disease, perhaps as many as 20 per cent from myocardial infarction. Diabetic patients treated for myocardial infarction in hospital appear to have a higher mortality than non-diabetic patients although there is some disagreement as to the comparative prognosis. In three recent studies undertaken in Coronary Care Units hospital mortality ranged from 24 to 35 per cent for diabetic patients: in each series the mortality was significantly higher than among non-diabetic patients by a factor of from 1·26:1 to 2:1 (Soler et al., 1974; Harrower and Clarke, 1976; Tansey et al., 1977). The question is why do diabetics fare so badly? Several possibilities exist including increased atheroma production as a result of hyperlipidaemia, impaired glucose availability to the myocardium, a specific defect in myocardial function (diabetic cardiomyopathy), or some factor relating to previous drug therapy. Accumulated experience from the above studies and that of Soler et al. (1975) suggests that certain clinical features appear to identify patients with a high mortality after myocardial infarction. Females, particularly obese females, fared particularly badly, so too did patients with retinopathy or with poor biochemical control of diabetes either before or immediately after the onset of infarction. It seems unlikely that all the increased risk factors would act through a final common pathway and that diabetes mellitus diminishes the chance of patient survival after myocardial infarction by several mechanisms.

Interest has recently centred on the possibility of a specific defect in myocardial function which is independent of coronary artery disease amongst patients suffering from diabetes.

Seneviratne (1977) investigated a group of 28 insulin dependent diabetics with no clinical evidence of cardiovascular disease by measurement of the systolic time intervals. This technique involves simultaneous recording of the phonocardiogram, electrocardiogram and the carotid pulse. The left ventricular ejection time and pre-ejection time may then be measured, and the ratio of the two intervals provides an indication of myocardial contractility. This technique is not without its critics but when performed in the circumstances of these studies it provides a useful non-invasive measure of ventricular performance. Among all 14 patients with clinical evidence of microangiopathy, as judged by the presence of proliferative retinopathy or heavy proteinuria (more than 3 grams in 24 hours), there was evidence of impaired left ventricular function, whereas among the diabetics without obvious microangiopathy there was no such evidence. All patients were, of course, free from clinical signs or symptoms of cardiac disease, but it was concluded that impaired myocardial contractility as the result of microangiopathy could facilitate the development of cardiac failure in response to such cardiovascular problems as hypertension or myocardial infarction. The findings were subsequently confirmed by echocardiography in some of the patients. Such a finding would go some way towards explaining the 70 per cent mortality encountered in one study (Soler et al., 1975) one month after myocardial infarction among patients with evidence of retinopathy and treated with oral hypoglycaemic drugs. Using the same technique of systolic time interval measurement an earlier study (Ahmed et al., 1975) had also shown impaired left ventricular function among a group of 25 diabetic patients which appeared to be independent of age, sex, duration of diabetes or drug therapy. Data on the presence or absence of retinopathy and proteinuria was, however, not included. A group of patients with relatively mild diabetes, requiring treatment with diet alone or oral hypoglycaemic drugs, revealed no evidence of impaired myocardial contractility (Sykes et al., 1977). The cause of a diabetic cardiomyopathy remains unknown but changes in the wall of the myocardial capillary could be of fundamental importance (Yodaiken, 1976). Patients with evidence of retinopathy and renal disease have also been shown to exhibit increased blood viscosity which may lead to further impairment of myocardial perfusion (Barnes et al., 1977). Further research is required into the possibility of a diabetic cardiomyopathy together with an assessment of the influence of effective diabetic control of any disordered myocardial function.

The deficiency in myocardial performance so far described is not accompanied by symptoms and signs of failure, indeed the degree of abnormality demonstrated is well short of that seen in cardiac failure. The clinical picture of congestive cardiac failure may, however, result from coronary artery disease in the absence of such localized structural problems as left ventricular aneurysm or papillary muscle dysfunction, a condition often labelled ischaemic cardiomyopathy. In a detailed study based on coronary angiography Dash et al. (1977) set out to test the hypothesis that the cardiomyopathic syndrome due to coronary artery disease was more common among diabetics than non-diabetic patients. The syndrome was defined clinically as the presence of congestive cardiac failure and was associated with a reduced left ventricular ejection fraction determined angiographically. The incidence of the cardiomyopathic syndrome was indeed more frequent among the diabetic patients than among the age and sex matched non-diabetics, but its presence was associated with a similarly high number of major proximal arterial occlusions and stenoses in both groups. There was, however, a significantly greater tendency for the diabetic patients with a high incidence of proximal arterial lesions to develop the signs of congestive failure. The authors concluded that given a similar degree of arterial disease the diabetic myocardium may be more vulnerable to infarction. It is possible that this tendency to more extensive myocardial injury among the diabetic patients is another expression of an underlying myocardial fault.

REFERENCES

Ahmed S. S., Jaferi G. A., Narang R. M. and Regan T. J. (1975) Pre-clinical abnormality of left ventricular function in diabetes mellitus. *Am. Heart J.* **89**, 153.

Barnes A. J., Locke P., Scudder P. R., Dormandy T. L., Dormandy J. A. and Slack J. (1977) Is hyperviscosity a treatable component of diabetic microcirculatory disease. *Lancet* **2**, 789.

Dash H., Johnson R. A., Dinsmore R. E., Francis C. K. and Harthorne C.W. (1977) Cardiomyopathic syndrome due to coronary artery disease, II: increased prevalence in patients with diabetes mellitus: a matched pair analysis. *Brit. Heart J.* **39**, 740.

Harrower A. D. B. and Clarke B. F. (1976) Experience in coronary care in diabetics. *Br. Med. J.* **1**, 126.

Seneviratne B. I. B. (1977) Diabetic cardiomyopathy: the preclinical phase. *Br. Med. J.* **1**, 1444.

Soler N. G., Bennett M. A., Pentecost B. L., Fitzgerald M. G. and Malins J. M. (1975) Myocardial infarction in diabetes. *Q. J. Med.* **125**.

Soler N. G., Pentecost B. L., Bennett M. A., Fitzgerald M. G., Lamb P. and Malins J. M. (1974) Coronary care for myocardial infarction in diabetics. *Lancet* **1**, 475.

Sykes C. A., Wright A. D., Malins J. M. and Pentecost B. L. (1977) Changes in systolic time intervals during treatment of diabetes mellitus. *Br. Heart J.* **39**, 255.

Tansey M. J. B., Opie L. H. and Kennelly B. M. (1977) High mortality in obese women diabetics with acute myocardial infarction. *Br. Med. J.* **1**, 1625.

Yodaiken R. E. (1976) The relationship between diabetic capillaropathy and myocardial infarction: a hypothesis. *Diabetes* **25**, Suppl. 2, 928.

Heart and major vessels: surgical

J. L. MONRO FRCS

THE COST EFFECTIVENESS OF CARDIAC SURGERY

In these days of economic difficulty, the question is inevitably being asked whether we can afford some of the more expensive types of treatment provided by the N.H.S., and the finger of suspicion seems to fall fairly regularly on cardiac surgery. However, it is in fact easy to justify the continuance of an active cardiac surgical programme.

Despite the fact that the types of cardiac surgical procedure offered are continually becoming more daring, the operative mortality continues to fall, and this in turn increases the cost effectiveness. The number of people in the older age group being operated upon also continues to rise, and gratifyingly without significant increase in operative mortality (De Bono et al., 1977; Ross and Monro, 1977). However, there must be an upper age limit to what is an economic reality.

Bypass techniques have become more efficient and simplified, and this in turn has cut costs. Whereas it used to be commonplace to use more than eight or ten units of blood per case, now by using a fluid prime and returning all blood to the patient, some centres are averaging little more than two units of blood per case (Ross and Monro, 1977), and sometimes no homologous blood is used at all.

The length of time a patient undergoing cardiac surgery stays in hospital following operation is now usually ten or twelve days and this lessening of the hospital stay also reduces costs.

The exact cost of a cardiac surgical operation varies from one unit to another, and unfortunately the D.H.S.S. seems to have little up to date information about this. However, two recent and quite independent attempts have been made to cost a cardiac surgical operation, one at St Thomas's Hospital, London (Morgan et al., 1977) and the other at The Wessex Regional Cardiac and Thoracic Centre in Southampton (Monro et al., 1978). Both reports deal with a patient undergoing aortic valve replacement but excluded the capital cost of equipment already in the units and are therefore very comparable.

The group at St Thomas's Hospital found that the total cost for their patient was £2 755. This excluded the cost of cardiac catheterization, and the patient, who was in the intensive care unit for three days, spent a total of 20 days in hospital. The group in Southampton found that the total cost for their patient undergoing a similar operation was £2 037 and this included a 7-day stay for preoperative cardiac catheterization. The Southampton patient was 1 day in the intensive care unit, and the admission for valve replacement lasted 18 days. Perhaps more helpful would be to assess the cost of one of these patients undergoing cardiopulmonary bypass surgery alone and exclude the cost of the valve, which at approximately £300 for a Starr – Edwards and £400 for a Carpentier – Edwards xenograft could be added later. If a stay of 18 days is average, the cost at St Thomas's would be approximately £2 100 and, at Southampton, £1 450.

Both these estimates were prepared by meticulously costing the progress of one patient undergoing a similar procedure, which was thought to be representative of the unit's work. An alternative method is to add up the total cost of running a unit performing open heart surgery and to divide by the number of bypass procedures. This in fact has also been done at Southampton, and the two figures were very close.

One further interesting fact emerging from the St Thomas's investigation was that the cost of an oesophagectomy done at the same hospital, on a patient who stayed 24 days in hospital was £1 870. Whereas no one can deny the right of a patient with carcinoma of the oesophagus to have a chance of curative resection, if one thinks in cost effective terms the likely 5-year survival rate for these 2 patients undergoing aortic valve replacement and oesophagectomy is respectively 80 and 10 per cent. One can appreciate that when the cost of operation is respectively £2 755 and £1 870 in the same unit, cardiac surgery clearly comes out well on top.

If one allows for a 15 per cent per year increase in costs, in round figures the cost at 1977 prices for a representative open heart operation in a typical London teaching hospital is likely to be about £2 400 compared with £1 700 in a provincial teaching hospital regional cardiothoracic unit, exclusive of the cost of any valves or other hardware inserted.

It is important to know, not only the early and late mortality of various cardiac operations, but the quality of life to be expected, and the improvement to be gained by operation. A study has been undertaken at The Wessex Cardiac and Thoracic Centre in Southampton (Ross et al., 1977) to look into just this aspect of cardiac surgery. It was found that whereas only 33 per cent of males of working age were at work preoperatively 66 per cent had returned to work 8 months postoperatively. Apart from the fact that many would have died fairly soon without operation, this marked improvement in the quality of life, as demonstrated by the ability to work, makes operation seem well worth while. A similar increase in the ability in women to do housework etc. was noted, and in the elderly a marked reduction in the dependance on others was found.

In financial terms, the sickness benefit that such a patient with aortic stenosis would receive from the State, together with the loss of tax because the patient was not working, would together probably equal the cost of an operation for aortic valve replacement in about two years. So apart from prolonging the patient's life and relieving his symptoms, the high percentage of patients that return to work support the reasoning in favour of cardiac surgery despite its apparent relatively high cost.

Many patients will have been on drugs preoperatively that can be stopped following the operation, and this is also a saving. Those patients who have a prosthetic valve inserted will need to be on anticoagulants for life and the cost of the warfarin and the anticoagulant control must be added to the total cost. In this respect, a tissue valve such as a xenograft which does not need anticoagulants, though initially more expensive, probably pays for itself within two or three years.

Although there can be little argument about the cost effectiveness of cardiac surgery for the vast majority of patients, we are probably still feeling our way at either end of the age range. Despite considerable advances in infant and neonatal cardiac surgery there are still some conditions, such as the hypo-plastic left heart syndrome, which are considered inoperable. Furthermore with advances in techniques, improved results have been achieved with the treatment of many conditions in infancy, so that a one stage corrective procedure can now be performed rather than an initial palliative, and later corrective procedure. This, of course, in addition to improving the overall survival, saves money.

At the other end of the scale, although patients over 65 years of age can undergo cardiac surgery without an increased operative mortality (De Bono et al., 1977), there must be a limit, and probably only the fittest patients over 70 years of age will benefit.

The increasing frequency of operations being performed for coronary artery disease, while lagging well behind the U.S.A., is likely to pose a big financial problem for the N.H.S. The saphenous vein aorta-coronary artery bypass graft has been shown to be extremely effective in the relief of angina. The operation carries a very low mortality and the increased survival achieved which is now becoming more apparent in patients with the most severe disease, is responsible for the increasing popularity. However, coronary artery disease is extremely common, and if we follow the North American example, could be swamped by it. It is likely that we would in this country have to increase the number of coronary artery bypass operations by the total number of bypasses in this country per year, if we were to begin to cope with the disease on the same scale as it is being treated in the U.S.A., Australia and New Zealand. From all the evidence, this would indeed be cost effective, but would need a radical rethinking in the scale of services provided by the N.H.S.

In summary, a cardiac surgical operation costs in the region of £2 000, and while this may seem expensive relative to the cost of some other operations the benefit to the patient is enormous, and the cost to the State is in many cases paid back within two years by the patient's return to work.

REFERENCES
De Bono A. H. B., Milstein B. B. and English T. A. H. (1977) Valve replacement in the elderly. Reported at The Annual Meeting of The Society of Thoracic and Cardio-vascular Surgeons, London.
Monro J. L., Mollo S., Brookbanks S. and Ross J. K. (1978) The cost of cardiac surgery. *Br. Med. J.* In the press.
Morgan K., Didsbury F. and Braimbridge M. (1977) The cost of a cardiac surgical operation. Reported at The Annual Meeting of The Society of Thoracic and Cardiovascular Surgeons, London.
Ross J. K., Dowell A. E., Marsh J., Monro J. L. and Barker D. J. P. (1978) Wessex Cardiac Surgery Follow-Up Survey: the quality of life after operation. *Thorax* **33**, 3.
Ross J. K. and Monro J. L. (1977) Unpublished data.

FALLOT'S TETRALOGY

The combination of ventricular septal defect (VSD), pulmonary stenosis, overiding aorta and right ventricular hypertrophy, was first described by Fallot in 1888, and is known therefore as 'Fallot's tetralogy'. During development of the heart, the aorta is overiding and pushed forward to the right (dextroposed) (Becker et al., 1975) at the expense of the outflow tract of the right ventricle (infundibulum) which is therefore narrowed, giving rise to infundibular and often pulmonary valve stenosis. In the presence of this obstruction to the flow of blood to the lungs, the right ventricle finds it easier to push its desaturated blood through the coexistent large VSD, thus resulting in cyanosis of the patient. In turn the right ventricular muscle hypertrophies to withstand the increased pressure required to produce this right-to-left shunt. In order to effect correction of these defects, the VSD must be closed (with a patch) and the pulmonary infundibular and valvar stenosis removed. The right ventricular hypertrophy will therefore regress as the work required returns to normal and it is unnecessary and indeed impracticable to correct the overiding of the aorta. There is, of course, a considerable range of severity of the lesions found in Fallot's tetralogy, the main pulmonary artery and valve ring may be extremely narrow and one pulmonary artery may even be absent. Not surprisingly those patients with the more hypoplastic outflow tracts tend to be more severely affected, and therefore present earlier.

Well before correction was possible, Blalock performed the first palliative operation for Fallot's tetralogy (Blalock and Taussig, 1945). Using an idea of his colleague Helen Taussig, he anastomosed the subclavian artery to the pulmonary artery in a patient with Fallot's tetralogy. The increased flow of blood to the lungs resulted in an overall increase in arterial saturation, and the Blalock – Taussig shunt achieved considerable popularity. A more direct approach was popularized by Brock (1949) in which a blind infundibular resection and valvotomy was performed through the right ventricle and an increase in the flow of blood to the lungs was achieved.

Lillehei et al. (1955) first achieved correction of Fallot's tetralogy, using a cross circulation technique to enable the heart to be opened. However, with the use of cardiopulmonary bypass which had been introduced in 1953 (Gibbon, 1954), others also started to correct this challenging lesion. However, the initial operative mortality and morbidity was high due to poor knowledge of the anatomy of the bundle of His, rather primitive bypass apparatus then available and inadequate techniques for closing the VSD, but learning from their mistakes these early workers, such as Kirklin, developed the techniques which have now evolved for the safe correction of Fallot's tetralogy.

Despite improved results in older children, by the early 1960s (Malm et al., 1963) the operative mortality for correction in infancy was still prohibitive, and therefore most surgeons tended to use a two-stage approach in the management of this condition. In infants who developed severe cyanotic spells or progressive cyanosis, and would die without operation, a palliative procedure such as the Blalock – Taussig shunt, Brock procedure or latterly the aorta-to-right-pulmonary-artery anastomosis (Waterston et al., 1972) would be performed, and then, later, at perhaps the age of 5 years, a further operation for total correction would be undertaken.

The disadvantages of this two-stage approach are that there is a mortality for each operation and the intervening period between operations, when the child still has a right-to-left shunt and is therefore exposed to such dangers as the formation of a cerebral abscess and bacterial endocarditis.

In recent years, as a result of the improvement in techniques, and particularly that of deep hypothermia as popularized by Barratt-Boyes et al. (1971), corrective operations in infancy have become much safer. Several centres have reported excellent results with correction in infancy (Starr et al., 1973; Barrett-Boyes and Neutze, 1973), with a considerably lower mortality than the overall mortality of the two-stage approach. Obviously this early correction is preferable for patient, parents and surgeon, provided the mortality is less, as mentioned in an Editorial in the *Lancet* (1973).

Recently Castaneda et al. (1977) reported a series of 41 consecutive infants, in whom total correction of Fallot's tetralogy was performed and only 3 patients, all less than 3 months of age, died. In the experience of others palliation can carry a high operative mortality in this very young and desperately ill age group, in addition, of course, to later mortality. Therefore it would seem that in experienced units, total correction in infancy should be the approach of choice, the only possible exceptions being when there is extreme hypoplasia of the pulmonary arteries, or the presence of an anomalous left anterior descending coronary artery, across the outflow tract. It is also possible to delay the need for surgery in young infants with cyanotic spells, by the use of Inderal (propranolol).

When patients do not develop difficulties in infancy, the elective time for total correction should probably be about 3 or 4 years of age, and the operative mortality in this age group should certainly be less than 5 per cent.

One other factor that has been the subject of much discussion is the decision of whether or not to patch the outflow tract of the right ventricle, in order to obtain better relief of obstruction. It is more than 20 years since Lillehei first appreciated the need for this procedure (Lillehei et al., 1956) but still the incidence of patching varies from 5 per cent to more than 80 per cent, and there is still doubt as to whether the patch need be taken across the pulmonary valve ring. The decision to exchange pulmonary stenosis for probable regurgitation must inevitably be a compromise, and some degree of residual stenosis is often accepted in order to preserve a reasonably competent valve. It is difficult to know which patients will need an outflow patch, though a recent paper by Pacifico et al. (1977) has outlined the indication for patching across the valve ring as suggested by measuring the pulmonary valve ring at the time of surgery and patching if it is less than the diameter recommended in a carefully prepared table. Another approach (Monro, 1977) is to compare the size of the pulmonary artery and aorta on the preoperative angiogram, and if the former is less than 50 per cent of the latter patching across the valve ring is advised. The type of material used for the patch is probably unimportant, but the pericardium or Dacron cloth have been used for a long time. Recently good results have been reported using a segment of homograft aortic valve containing one cusp (unicusp homograft patch), in an attempt to preserve competence of the pulmonary valve, at least in the all important postoperative phase (Radley-Smith and Yacoub, 1977; Monro, 1977).

There have been few recent reports from centres in the United Kingdom. Whereas an operative mortality of 3 per cent for total correction for all patients referred has been reported (Monro, 1977), the overall operative mortality for the correction of Fallot's tetralogy in the United Kingdom, as reported in a general census for 1976 was as high as 15 per cent (English, 1977). Clearly this is unacceptable, and both emphasizes the fact that it is still a difficult condition to treat, and the fact that surgery for congenital heart disease should be concentrated into a few expert centres in this country, rather than spread thinly amongst all units.

Information is gradually accumulating about the long term follow-up of patients who have undergone total correction of Fallot's tetralogy. In general, the results are excellent, pulmonary regurgitation is tolerated well and provided the VSD has been securely closed, pulmonary stenosis adequately relieved and there are no conduction problems, the prognosis is extremely good. The longest follow-up reports are, of course, on patients who were operated upon when the corrective techniques were still developing and therefore can be expected to have somewhat less than perfect results. Poirier et al. (1977) in an excellent report from the Mayo Clinic reported on the follow-up of more than 300 patients up to 12 years postoperatively. The results were ideal in 80 per cent of patients, fair in 10 per cent, poor in 3 per cent and the late mortality rate was 4 per cent. Five per cent had a residual haemodynamic defect, and those patients with poor results had a higher incidence of inadequate relief of outflow tract obstruction.

Although in the early days of total correction, heart block was frequently encountered due to damage to the bundle of His which is in close proximity to the VSD, this is now rare as anatomical knowledge and techniques have improved. However, right bundle branch block is extremely common after total correction, but it remains to be seen whether this is of real importance.

In conclusion, it can be said that Fallot's tetralogy, which is the commonest type of cyanotic heart disease, can be successfully corrected with an operative mortality of less than 5 per cent and an extremely good long term prognosis. The argument still rages as to whether initial palliation or early correction should be offered when surgery becomes necessary in infancy. It would seem that the results achieved in good centres using the one-stage approach are consistently better than those achieved in the best centres using the two-stage approach. The choice will therefore depend on which centre the child can be sent to. However, as a result of the early corrective approach it is now becoming rare to operate on a child with Fallot's tetralogy over the age of 5 years, or indeed who has had previous palliation. Hopefully the horrific, polycythaemic older patients with Fallot's tetralogy will soon have gone for ever.

REFERENCES

Barratt-Boyes B. G. and Neutze J. M. (1973) Primary repair of tetralogy of Fallot in infancy using profound hypothermia with circulatory arrest and limited cardio-pulmonary bypass: a comparison with conventional two-stage management. *Ann. Surg.* **178**, 406.

Barratt-Boyes B. G., Simpson M. and Neutze J. M. (1971) Intracardiac surgery in neonates and infants using deep hypothermia with surface cooling and limited cardio-pulmonary bypass. *Circulation* **43** and **44**, Suppl. 1 – 25.

Becker A. E., Connor M. and Anderson R. H. (1975) Tetralogy of Fallot: A morphometric and Geometric study. *Am. J. Cardiol.* **35**, 402.

Blalock A. and Taussig H. (1945) The surgical treatment of malformations of the heart. *J.A.M.A.* **128**, 189.

Brock R. C. (1949) The surgery of pulmonary stenosis. *Br. Med. J.* **2**, 399.

Castaneda A. R., Freed M. D., Williams R. G. and Norwood W. I. (1977) Repair of tetralogy of Fallot in infancy: early and late results. *J. Thorac. Cardiovasc. Surg.* **74**, 372.

Editorial (1973) Management of Fallot's tetralogy. *Lancet* **2**, 306.

English T. A. H. (1977) United Kingdom Cardiac Surgical Register — report on pilot study. Annual meeting of The Society of Thoracic and Cardiovascular Surgeons, London.

Gibbon J. H. (1954) Application of a mechanised heart and lung apparatus to cardiac surgery. *Minn. Med.* **37**, 171.

Lillehei C. W., Cohen M., Warden H. E., Read R. C., Aust J. B., De Wall R. A. and Varco R. L. (1955) Direct vision intracardiac surgical correction of the tetralogy of Fallot, pentalogy of Fallot and pulmonary atresia defects: report of 10 cases. *Ann. Surg.* **142**, 41, 8.

Lillehei C. W., Cohen M., Warden H. and Varco R. (1956) Complete anatomic correction of the tetralogy of Fallot defect. *Arch. Surg.* **73**, 526.

Malm J. R., Bowman F. O., Jameson A. G., Ellis K., Griffiths S. P. and Blumenthal S. (1963) An evaluation of total correction of tetralogy of Fallot. *Circulation* **27**, 805.

Monro J. L. (1977) The surgery of Fallot's tetralogy — necessity for outflow patch. Second European symposium, London. June, 1977.

Pacifico A. D., Kirklin J. W. and Blackstone E. H. (1977) Surgical management of pulmonary stenosis in tetralogy of Fallot. *J. Thorac. Cardiovasc. Surg.* **74**, 382.

Poirier R. A., McGoon D. C., Danielson G. K., Wallace R. B., Ritter D. G., Moodie D. S. and Wiltse C. G. (1977) Late results after repair of tetralogy of Fallot. *J. Thorac. Cardiovasc. Surg.* **73**, 900.

Radley-Smith R. and Yacoub M. (1977) Clinical and haemodynamic results of primary total correction of Fallot's tetralogy in the first two years of life. *Br. Heart J.* **39**, 353.

Starr A., Bonchek, L. E. and Sunderland C. O. (1973) Total correction of tetralogy of Fallot in infancy. *J. Thorac. Cardiovasc. Surg.* **65**, 45.

Waterston D. J., Stark J. and Ashcraft K. W. (1972) Ascending aorta-to-right pulmonary artery shunts: Experience with 100 cases. *Surgery* **72**, 897.

Peripheral vascular diseases

H. H. G. EASTCOTT MS, FRCS

CORONARY ARTERY BY-PASS GRAFTING AND SUBSEQUENT SURGERY

Peripheral vascular surgeons and the physicians with whom they work are usually aware of the general risks and implications of arterial graft procedures in patients with evidence of ischaemic heart disease. Until recently all they could do was to try to ensure a smooth course through their ordeal and to limit the indications in such subjects to the more pressing ones, such as incipient limb loss, or the fear that an abdominal aortic aneurysm might rupture. Prospects are now improving with the advent of safe, routine surgery for myocardial ischaemia, which may now precede the correction of the peripheral vascular condition.

From Baylor University, Texas, McCollum (1977) reports favourably on his experience of coronary artery by-pass grafting (CABG) in 60 patients who were also known to require extracardiac surgery but were suffering from angina pectoris—indeed 25 had already experienced a myocardial infarct. After uneventful CABG 23 of the 60 were able to proceed to their other operation during the same hospital admission. The 37 remaining underwent secondary major surgery within an average of 8·9 months. Thirteen of the 60 had a further major procedure, and 4 had a third. There were no deaths and only 8 cardiovascular complications: 7 supraventricular arrhythmias and one pulmonary oedema. The author reminds us that in patients over 50 years of age major surgery in the presence of myocardial ischaemia carries a 6 per cent risk of infarction, so that when the need for multiple surgery arises the coronary grafting should be done first.

The number of conditions subsequently corrected in this series was as follows:

Resection of abdominal aortic aneurysm—16.
Aorto-iliac by-pass—12.
Femoro-popliteal by-pass—10.
Carotid endarterectomy—5.
Resection of thoraco-abdominal aneurysm—1.
Total peripheral arterial reconstruction operations—44.

The number of surgical procedures that were safely completed were:

Cholecystectomy—8.
Repair of hiatus hernia and operation for peptic ulcer—6.
Bowel resection—2.
Total non-vascular operations—16.

This development will allow vascular surgeons to extend their indications for the relief of less serious peripheral conditions, provided the CABG has been successful; indeed it could well be felt that a patient who had undergone heart surgery would be a particularly deserving case for lower-limb arterioplasty for intermittent claudication that was preventing his return to normal activities for his age. [At St Mary's Hospital, London we have already had experience of this kind. 10 patients underwent combined procedures with safe passage through two or more, and in one case five cardiovascular operations — a preliminary carotid endarterectomy, the CABG, a postoperative iliac embolectomy, and two femoropopliteal grafts for disabling claudication in early middle age. We feel that carotid stenosis should be attended to even before CABG, and that some symptomless cases should come to operation, particularly if the heart procedure is more than usually complex, or the carotid lesion is bilateral, or likely to affect the dominant hemisphere, or if the neck bruit is variable, suggesting activity and change in the thrombus—H. H. G. E.]

REFERENCE
McCollum C. (1977) Myocardial revascularisation before major surgery. *Surgery* **81,** 302.

HOW SAFE IS CAROTID ENDARTERECTOMY?

After more than 20 years of uncertain acceptance this operation is at last assuming a definable place in the prevention and treatment of stroke. Last year we considered the new non-invasive techniques that are helping to define the population at risk from neck artery obstruction, and also the medical and clinical neurological factors that bear upon the operative risk (*Medical Annual,* 1977/8, pp. 106 – 107). Now there is a thoughtful report from Boston on the hazards of carotid surgery and the safeguards that have been found to be useful for their avoidance (Matsumoto et al., 1977). No fewer than 130 consecutive carotid endarterectomy operations during the period 1974 – 1976 were available for study. There were 2 operative deaths, both from myocardial infarction, and 6 other non-fatal coronary occlusions. Neither of the deaths was stroke-related. There was one re-exploration for local bleeding. New neurological defects were surprisingly common for a series of this high quality, but almost all were peripheral nerve lesions of lower motor neuron type related to local operative damage. No fewer than 8·5 per cent had hypoglossal weakness. The vocal cord (2·3 per cent) and the cervical branch of the facial (1·5 per cent) were much less common. Upper motor neuron lesions (4·6 per cent) were all transient, though one of the coronary patients who died had weakness of one hand until his death later in the first day. These authors attribute their good results in respect of freedom from serious postoperative stroke less to the measurement of carotid stump pressure, which many others use as their guide to the need for an indwelling shunt, than to the close surveillance of the electroencephalogram.

[As this measurement is likely to be more relevant to incipient cerebral damage than the state of the pressure in one neck artery, they may well be correct. Now that simpler forms of EEG are becoming available as 'cerebral activity monitors' that do not impede the work of the surgeon or the anaesthetist, we may be seeing the wider use of the method in future. Our experience of it at St Mary's Hospital, London has been impressive in the few cases that we have so far had the opportunity of studying in this way—H. H. G. E.]

REFERENCE
Matsumoto G. H., Cossman D. and Callow A. D. (1977) Hazards and safeguards during carotid endarterectomy. *Am. J. Surg.* **133,** 458.

METHODS OF LUMBAR AORTOGRAPHY

Radiologists differ in their choice of access to the lumbar aorta; strong views are often expressed as to the relative advantages of the trans-femoral and the trans-lumbar routes. Statistics, however, are not so often presented. From Szilagyi and his colleagues in Detroit (Szilagyi et al., 1977) comes an analysis of their figures that supports the advocates of the trans-lumbar method. Among 14 550 examinations there were 2 deaths and 7 major complications. When these were compared with the previously published series collected from several sources with a total of 9438 examinations the latter results were less good in respect of fatalities, which number 10 (0·1 per cent, compared with 0·014 per cent in Detroit), though this higher figure was much influenced by 10 deaths from one large centre reported in 1964. Major complications were more nearly the same (0·16 per cent, compared with 0·05 per cent). The earlier literature was also reviewed for complication rates after trans-femoral catheterization for the purpose of lumbar aortography. Out of a total of 21 324 cases there were 15 fatalities and 265 major complications (0·07 per cent and 1·24 per cent respectively). Thus it seems that trans-femoral aortography is satisfactory on grounds of safety, with comparable death rates but a much higher incidence of complications.

This last finding is the one that surgeons are aware of; for it is they who are called in to repair the damage. Occlusion of the common femoral artery occurs too often in smaller centres where these examinations are only occasional. In particular the risk seems to be significantly higher in patients with occlusive arterial disease affecting the zone of catheterization, and also in women and in children whose arteries are small and therefore more vulnerable. Large haematoma at the groin is also familiar; it occurs in obese hypertensive subjects and may amount to actual false aneurysm. Yet it can be argued that with the femoral route at least it is possible to see the complications, whereas after leakage or mural arterial damage from trans-lumbar aortic puncture the effects are mostly hidden. Once again, it will be the surgeon who encounters the evidence when he exposes the abdominal aorta shortly after the diagnostic examination and finds fresh blood clot in the left flank and periaortic tissues. Many vascular surgeons will also have noticed that after trans-lumbar aortography the left foot becomes warmer and dry, indicating that the left sympathetic chain has been damaged. While no doubt this could explain some cases of hindquarter pain after the examination, it also accounts for the happier circumstance of a striking symptomatic improvement in left lower-limb ischaemia that was beginning to cause rest pain.

In summary, therefore, though trans-femoral aortography is clearly preferable when detailed examination of the abdominal aortic branches is required, allowing, as it does, the easy performance of lateral and repeated local views, it does carry real hazard for the patient with lower-limb arterio-sclerosis, especially in the hands of the less experienced operator. Moreover, he is the one most likely to select this procedure in the face of the real or imagined risks of trans-lumbar puncture, which, incidentally, is much disliked by many patients who undergo it without general anaesthesia.

REFERENCE
Szilagyi D. E., Smith R. F., Elliott J. P. and Hageman J. H. (1977) Translumbar aortography: a study of its safety and usefulness. *Arch. Surg.* **112,** 399.

THE SMALL ABDOMINAL AORTIC ANEURYSM
Opinion almost everwhere now favours the active, surgical approach to the

treatment of abdominal aortic aneurysm (AAA) in good-risk patients and nearly all those in whom the lesion is thought to be causing symptoms. Problems still arise, however, in cases of general medical unfitness and in asymptomatic, reluctant patients, particularly when the aneurysm is small.

Bernstein et al. (1976), reporting from La Jolla, a southern Californian retirement community, have used B-mode ultrasound scan (echography) to make serial measurements of the diameter of small AAAs in 49 poor-risk patients of mean age 68 years who were symptom-free on entry to the study. The examination was repeated at approximately 3-monthly intervals until either the measured increase in diameter during this time exceeded 0·4 cm, or the patient became symptomatic. *Fig.* 1 shows what happened to each of these

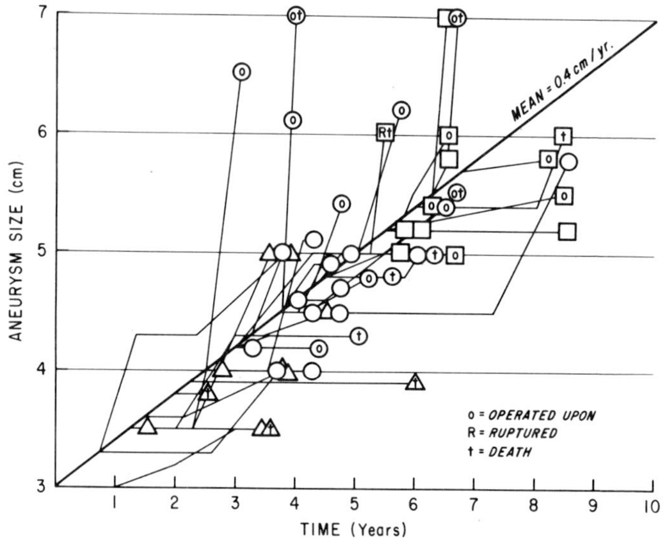

Fig. 1 Plot of the growth course of each of the 49 patients studied in which the aneurysm first is located at its initially diagnosed size on the mean growth line and then is traced to its present status. Triangles indicate the final observation of these aneurysms first diagnosed between 3·0 and 3·9 cm, circles indicate those first diagnosed between 4·0 and 4·9 cm, and the squares identify those 5·0 – 5·9 when first studied. (Reproduced from *Surgery.)*

49 patients, both clinically and as regards the growth rate of their aneurysms. It will at once be seen that there is wide variation of the individual cases from the mean growth line that they collectively form, marking the rate of 0·4 cm per year. Most of those removed from the series by operation were either greater than 5 cm in diameter or had been found on successive examinations to have undergone more rapid enlargement; in several instances this was dramatic and from a small starting size. In one case an expansion of nearly 2 cm in 2 months was found to be associated on echography with a posterior leak, which was asymptomatic but was confirmed at operation. One other patient ruptured his aneurysm during this conservative regimen and died after

an emergency operation. This sac had also expanded markedly, comparing the operative with the earlier ultrasound findings. There were 3 deaths after elective operation; all of these patients had shown a growth rate of 0·6 cm per year. From their study Bernstein et al. conclude that a small aneurysm of initial size 3 cm will take 7·5 years to reach 6·0 cm, at which stage they operate on all cases. Below this diameter, in high-risk patients they repeat echography at 3-monthly intervals. In favour of the conservative concept embodied in this interesting paper is the fact that 7 of the 49 patients who died of causes other than their aneurysm while under observation were spared a needless operation. There were 15 patients who showed no enlargement of the aneurysm during the study, including 5 in which the initial diameter was over 5 cm.

REFERENCE
Bernstein E. F., Dilley R. B., Goldberger L. E., Gosink B. B. and Leopold G. R. (1976) Growth rates of small abdominal aortic aneurysms. *Surgery* **80**, 765.

ULTRASOUND SCAN IN THE DIAGNOSIS OF PERIPHERAL ANEURYSMS

The difficulty often experienced in detecting, for example, a popliteal aneurysm and in estimating its size by clinical examination alone, is due, as with abdominal aortic aneurysm, most often either to the patient's obesity, or a tightness of the overlying tissues, or to both. In the popliteal fossa, with the knee at rest in extension, the fat and the deep fascia may transmit the arterial impulse in a manner highly suggestive of an aneurysm. Arteriography can be equally misleading, for even in quite a large aneurysm only the patent lumen through the thrombus may be shown.

Davis et al. (1977) have studied 34 selected patients with ultrasound scanning, including normal subjects, patients with abdominal aortic aneurysm and others with confirmed peripheral aneurysm. They concluded that the normal measurement of the femoral artery by this method is 1·1 cm (±0·3 cm) and the popliteal 0·9 cm (±0·2 cm). The 13 patients with peripheral aneurysm were readily confirmed as such with good clear images. These authors point out that other major deficiencies of arteriography in these cases can be overcome by the use of this simple, non-invasive method, including the common difficulty over slow arterial blood-flow rates that fail to reach or fill the aneurysm, and, even more important, with the thrombosed aneurysm that does not fill at all and may thus be missed completely. An easily reversible cause of limb damage may therefore be revealed only by ultrasound scan. Moreover, in patients with abdominal aortic aneurysm, in whom the suspicion of accompanying popliteal aneurysm is high and the tactics of aortic surgery may be involved, the ultrasound examination may exclude this likely cause of difficulty during aortic resection.

REFERENCE
Davis P. P., Neiman H. L., Yao J. S. T. and Bergan J. J. (1977) Ultrasound scan in diagnosis of peripheral aneurysms. *Arch. Surg.* **112**, 55.

AN UNSUSPECTED SOURCE OF AORTIC GRAFT INFECTION

Rejection of cloth polymer arterial prostheses due to infection is one of the most deadly and intractable complications in vascular surgery. Though it has been known for many years that abdominal aortic aneurysms can become infected through the bloodstream (Sommerville et al., 1959), little attention appears to have been paid to the possibility that pre-existing infection in such an aneurysm could explain some of the disastrous, haemorrhagic graft failures that all vascular surgeons know and fear. From Williams and Fisher (1977) comes a report on the results of bacteriological culture of 68 abdominal aortic aneurysms, swabs being taken from the thrombus content, fluid other than blood, and any necrotic or otherwise locally unhealthy-looking part of the aneurysm wall. Of these results 7 proved positive, and the organisms grown were all, except for a haemolytic streptococcus, insensitive to the prophylactic antibiotic that had already been administered. Massive antibiotic treatment appropriate to the culture findings was given as soon as the result was known. Three of the 7 patients died of causes unrelated to infection [but possibly indicative of the patients' poor general condition—H. H. G. E.]. Of the 4 who survived, none developed evidence of graft infection.

REFERENCES

Somerville R. L., Allen E. V. and Edwards J. E. (1959) Bland and infected arteriosclerotic abdominal aortic aneurysms: a clinicopathologic study. *Medicine (Baltimore)* **38**, 207.
Williams R. D. and Fisher F. W. (1977) Aneurysm contents as a source of graft infection. *Arch. Surg.* **112**, 415.

MYCOTIC ANEURYSMS REASSESSED

The literature of vascular disease contains many equivocal terms: for example, dissecting aneurysm when leaking abdominal aneurysm is meant, and the earlier confusion between Buerger's disease and arteriosclerotic gangrene. Mycotic aneurysm has long been another of these.

Patel and Johnston (1977) have put the record straight with a clear exclusion of pre-existing infected arteriosclerotic aneurysms and infected arterial prostheses. They examined the records of 14 patients at the Toronto General Hospital whose diagnosis was validated on these criteria. Of these patients 10 were shown to have developed their infection from intravascular sources (7 had bacterial endocarditis that had given rise to an infected embolus, and 1 showed a direct spread from the endocardium to the sinus of Valsalva). Identifiable sources of infection in the other 2 were found in the skin and in the urinary tract, and were the cause of septicaemia in both cases. In 4 patients the infection could be traced to a non-vascular origin: 2 from a surrounding inflammatory process and 2 from iatrogenically introduced infection via a trans-femoral catheter. Over the whole series the organisms responsible were many and varied. Blood culture was positive in 10 of the 14. Pain and fever were present in all cases. Among the 10 of intravascular origin 6 were palpable clinically and 5 had ruptured. In this group the results of operation were good. All 3 who received surgery survived; 2 unoperated patients both died. In the 4 erosive or extravascular cases, all operated, 2 died of secondary haemorrhage, and 2 survived. Over the whole series of 14 patients 10 were operated and 8 survived; 5 had ligation and excision only, with 2 deaths; and 4 had ligation, excision and vein grafting, with all surviving.

[This paper deals with a 32-year period; during that time the infective aspects of vascular disease have changed. Nevertheless, the authors give a clear account in modern terms of the true primary condition as Osler saw it, and as such it is a useful addition to a scanty and somewhat confused literature—H. H. G. E.]

REFERENCE
Patel S. and Johnston K. W. (1977) Classification and management of mycotic aneurysms. *Surg. Gynecol. Obstet.* **144,** 691.

CHILDREN'S DISEASES

BRIAN WEBB MD, FRCP, DCH
A. W. WILKINSON CHM (Edin),
FRCS ED, FRCS, FAAP (Hon)

Medical

BRIAN WEBB MD, FRCP, DCH

SODIUM CROMOGLYCATE FOR ECZEMA IN CHILDREN

It has now been shown that 10 per cent sodium cromoglycate ointment can be an effective and safe alternative to topical steroids in the treatment of atopic eczema in children (Haider, 1977). Sodium cromoglycate has been known to be effective in the treatment of asthma (Intal), rhinitis (Rynacrom, Lomusol), and vernal kerato-conjunctivitis (Opticrom). The drug acts by inhibiting the release of the chemical mediators of the immediate (type I) hypersentitivity reaction. Eczema is a skin disorder often associated with a high incidence of atopy.

In a randomized double blind trial, 42 children with chronic atopic eczema received either an ointment containing 10 per cent sodium cromoglycate in white soft paraffin or a placebo ointment consisting of the white soft paraffin base only. The ointments were to be applied twice daily for up to 12 weeks, but 16 of the 21 placebo-treated patients withdrew prematurely because treatment was ineffective compared with only 4 patients who withdrew among the sodium cromoglycate-treated children. Evaluation showed that 16 of the patients who used the 10 per cent cromoglycate ointment showed significant improvement in the signs of inflammation, lichenification and cracking and the symptoms of itching and sleep disturbance—the improvement being consistent week by week. At the end of the trial period 16 sodium cromoglycate-treated patients were judged to have benefited from treatment, compared to only 2 in the placebo group, the large majority having withdrawn from the trial on account of lack of progress. Not surprisingly, in the placebo group the benefit had been to the lichenification and cracking, presumably due to the ointment. No side-effects were observed during the trial period. It is worth noting that some earlier work using a weaker solution of 4 per cent sodium cromoglycate in cream had not shown any significant advantage to the patient.

Yaffe (1977) comments that even though adverse systemic effects should theoretically be minimal, since the drug is so poorly absorbed, we have to remember that the skin of infants is more absorbent than adults and remember the unexpected hexachlorophene absorption by infants and that eczematous/irritable skin is more absorbent than healthy skin.

It seems likely that this will prove to be a useful innovation in the treatment of infantile eczema, and a safe alternative to topical steroids in the treatment of atopic dermatoses.

REFERENCES
Haider S. A. (1977) Treatment of atopic eczema in children: clinical trial of 10 per cent
    sodium cromoglycate ointment. *Br. Med. J.* **1**, 1570.
Yaffe S. J. (1977) Cromoglycate for eczema. *Paediatric Alert* **2**, 56.

A FRESH LOOK AT RUBELLA VACCINATION IN BRITAIN

Of all the methods for prevention of handicap known at this time vaccination against rubella must be the most productive of good (MacKeith, 1977). The size of the problem can be understood when one considers that 30 000 children with congenital deformities, largely blindness, deafness and mental defect, resulted from the 1964 epidemic of rubella in the United States.

The practice in the United States since 1969 has been to immunize all children of both sexes between the ages of 1 and 12 years and for the present to undertake the *selective* immunization of women of child-bearing age.

In an excellent review of the present position in the United States Krugman (1977) shows that the use of more than seventy million doses of rubella vaccine there during the past seven years has had a profound effect on the epidemiology of rubella. Since the 1964 epidemic there has been a progressive decline in the number of reported cases of rubella for twelve successive years. The experience in New York City (illustrated in *Fig.* 1) shows the number of

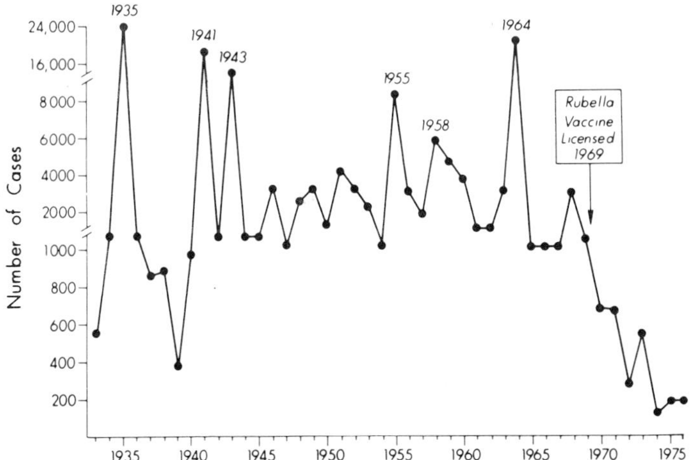

Fig. 1 Rubella in New York City (1933 – 1976): Note dramatic decrease in number of reported cases since licensure of vaccine in 1969. (Reproduced from the *Journal of Pediatrics.)*

reported cases which have declined to unprecedented low levels, less than 200 during each of the past three years. A corresponding decrease in the number of serologically confirmed cases of rubella in pregnant women has been reported by Cooper (1975), who reported that the number of cases of congenital rubella in New York City has also declined progressively since 1969.

The practice in the United Kingdom has been to immunize girls between the ages of 11 – 14 years but this does not, of course, much reduce the amount of rubella amongst pre-school and school-age children who can then bring the infection to a pregnant mother. Until rubella is conquered all women at high risk, such as nurses and school teachers of child-bearing age, should be offered serological testing and, if sero-negative, be offered vaccination against rubella. There are few complications to vaccination with rubella vaccine and even though the adult is more at risk of them than the child (Swartz et al., 1971) they are less likely to occur following immunization than following a natural rubella infection. Adverse reactions amongst children have been rare but perhaps about 20 per cent of young adults have minor joint pains lasting up to four or five days, which was half the incidence reported by Landrigan et al. (1974) in a carefully observed epidemic of rubella in adolescent males. There are fewer complications than with any other immunization apart from tetanus. All authorities are agreed that rubella vaccination during pregnancy is contraindicated, but at least Modlin et al. (1975) has produced evidence indicating that the risk of occurrence of a congenital malformation is much less following vaccination than with natural infection.

The success of the British policy of immunizing all the girls between 11 and 14 years (which some had reasoned would be more cost effective) is obviously dependent upon having a very high percentage of success, near 100 per cent, with this target group. Unfortunately Peckham et al. (1977) have found that only 71 per cent of the 16-year-old girls who were aged 12 when the rubella vaccine programme was implemented in 1970 had received rubella vaccine. This figure varied from 81 per cent for girls living in Scotland to 61 per cent for girls living in Wales. The lowest proportion of schoolgirls vaccinated had come from professional families and unskilled manual families; the former apparently because more attended independent schools where there was a lack of structure for administering vaccine, and the latter apparently accounted for by a missed opportunity of vaccination due to a higher number of school absences. If a selective rubella vaccination programme is to succeed then the vaccination of schoolgirls, who are a captive population, must be almost complete. If this were the case then vaccination of women of child-bearing age, which is complicated by the need to carry out a preliminary test to identify those who are susceptible to rubella, would then be only a temporary exercise aimed at protecting those who were over 14 when school vaccination was introduced. In 1969 Marshall had shown that before the introduction of rubella vaccine the number of women of child-bearing age who were susceptible to rubella was around 15 per cent.

If we are to prevent congenital rubella parents and schoolgirls will have to be told more about the severe complications that may result from getting rubella when pregnant. They must also be told that permission for vaccination should not be withheld on the grounds that the child is thought to have had clinical rubella because that fact correlates very poorly with the serological state.

In considering whether it is possible to make rubella immunization more acceptable to young girls, it is worth noting that Ganguly et al. (1974) have shown that rubella vaccine can be given as successfully by nose drop or by aerosol spray as by the subcutaneous route, and that this applies not only to the sero-conversion rate but also to the serum antibody titre levels obtained. Other information that may be helpful is that working with the measles vaccine which had been available for 13 years, as opposed to the rubella vaccine for only 7 years, Bass et al. (1976) came to the conclusion that unless the vaccine was given to an infant less than 1 year of age there would seem to be no need for re-vaccination with measles vaccine later. Ramos-Alvarez et al. (1975) have shown that measles and rubella vaccines were as safe and effective when given together as when given separately, the sero-conversion rate being over 98 per cent for both vaccines. Weibel et al. (1975) have shown that antibody persistence was the same for combined vaccines as for monovalent vaccines and indicated no alteration in the retention of immunity, the vaccines seeming to be just as protective as is recovery from the natural disease. It is possible that one day we may find that all that is necessary is the routine immunization of all 15-month-old infants with a combined measles and rubella vaccine.

The tragedy of lifelong damage to children from rubella can be prevented, but we shall either have to increase our efficiency in doing so within our present policy or, if that is not possible, re-evaluate our policy.

REFERENCES
Bass J. W., Halstead S. B., Fischer G. W. et al. (1976) Booster vaccination with further live attenuated measles vaccine. *J.A.M.A.* **235**, 31.
Cooper L. Z. (1975) Congenital rubella in the United States. *Prog. Clin. Biol. Res.* **3**, 1.
Ganguly R., Durrer B. and Waldman R. H. (1974) Rubella virus immunization of pre-school children via the respiratory tract. *Am. J. Dis. Child.* **128**, 821.
Krugman S. (1977) Present status of measles and rubella immunization in the United States: a medical progress report. *J. Pediatr.* **90**, 1.
Landrigan P. J., Stoffels M. A., Anderson E. and Witte J. J. (1974) Epidemic rubella in adolescent boys. *J.A.M.A.* **227**, 1283.
MacKeith R. (1977) Rubella vaccination. *Dev. Med. Child. Neurol.* **19**, 435.
Marshall W. C. (1969) Symposia Series in Immuno-biological Standardization, **2**, 68.
Modlin J. F., Brandling-Bennett A. D., Witte J. J. et al. (1975) A review of 5 years experience with rubella vaccine in the United States. *Pediatrics* **55**, 20.
Peckham C. S., Marshall W. C. and Dudgeon J. A. (1977) Rubella vaccination of schoolgirls; factors affecting vaccine uptake. *Br. Med. J.* **1**, 760.
Ramos-Alvarez M., Miller B. J., Jackson J. E., Schwarz A. J. and Bessudo L. (1975) Immunization of children with attenuated measles-rubella bivalent vaccine. *Am. J. Dis. Child.* **129**, 47.
Swartz T. A., Klingberg W., Goldwasser R. A. et al. (1971) Clinical manifestations, according to age, among females given HPV-77 duck rubella vaccine. *Am. J. Epidemiol.* **94**, 246.
Weibel R. E., Buynak E. B., McLean A. A. and Hilleman M. R. (1975) Long term follow-up for immunity after monovalent or combined live measles, mumps and rubella virus vaccines. *Pediatrics* **56**, 380.

COMPARISON OF INTAL AND THEOPHYLLINE IN CHRONIC ASTHMA IN CHILDHOOD

Intal (sodium cromoglycate) blocks the antigen-induced release of chemical mediators and when inhaled by sensitive individuals blocks antigen-induced bronchospasm. It is unique amongst anti-asthma agents in that it has no broncho-dilating or anti-inflammatory properties.

Theophylline is a potent bronchodilator which has lately been found to be safe and effective in controlling chronic asthma when given at regular intervals to maintain peak serum concentration of approximately $10-20$ μg/ml.

Intal is the primary drug for management of chronic asthma in childhood at Hammersmith Hospital, London, whereas theophylline is the primary drug for management of chronic asthma in childhood at two centres in Denver, U.S.A. Hambleton et al. (1977) have studied children in London and Denver to assess the relative efficacies of these two agents. Twenty-eight patients (13 from London and 15 from Denver), each with chronic asthma, were randomly treated for three periods of four weeks with Intal alone, theophylline alone, and then with both drugs in combination. The study was double blind and appropriate placebos were given in each single drug test period. These studied children received Intal in doses of 20 mg, q.i.d., and/or theophylline given four times daily in doses to achieve peak serum levels of $10-20$ μg/ml. (Mean dose 6 mg/kg/dose q.i.d.) Four children from Denver had to be withdrawn from the study for various reasons, 2 of them due to incidental illnesses.

They found that theophylline was associated with significantly more symptom-free days when given alone or in combination with Intal than was Intal alone (71 per cent symptom-free days versus 51 per cent respectively). In addition the increase in peak flow was statistically significant when theophylline was added to Intal. Thus theophylline when administered in individually adjusted doses at regular intervals prevented asthmatic symptoms at least as well as cromoglycate and appeared on average rather more effective though with considerable inter-patient variability.

Cromoglycate was rather more expensive, but unlike theophylline carried no risk of acute toxicity. The use of theophylline requires the obtaining of serum levels to establish an adequate dose and so requires more patient/doctor contact. Tolerance of theophylline was increased when the initial doses did not exceed the lesser of 4 mg/kg/dose q.i.d. or 100 mg/dose q.i.d. followed by incremental increases at not less than 3-day intervals up to the lesser of 7 mg/kg/dose q.i.d. or 250 mg/dose q.i.d.

They conclude that both drugs have a very useful effect and that 'there appears to be no indication for the *routine* use of both drugs simultaneously'. They noted that the patient who is inadequately controlled with cromoglycate may obtain some additional benefit when theophylline is added or substituted, but the reverse was not necessarily the case.

An Editorial Comment (1977) comments that there are many opportunities for establishing collaborative clinical studies between countries with differing therapeutic practices and that studies such as this will serve in the end to identify some of the reasons for these differing practices and ultimately lead to better treatment for all patients.

REFERENCES

Editorial (1977) *Pediatric Alert* **2**, 20.
Hambleton G., Weinberger M., Taylor J., Cavanaugh M., Ginchansky E., Godfrey S., Tooley M., Bell T. and Greenberg S. (1977) Comparison of cromoglycate (Cromolyn) and theophylline in controlling symptoms of chronic asthma. *Lancet* **1**, 381.

INFANTILE GASTROENTERITIS: SOME RECENTLY DISCOVERED CAUSES

Infantile gastroenteritis remains a major problem of child health. It accounts for about 250 deaths each year in infants under 1 year of age in England and Wales (Registrar General 1975), and about 25 000 infants and toddlers are admitted to hospital annually (Tripp et al., 1977). Despite careful searches for pathogens, in over half the cases no cause can be found and 'virus' is usually blamed. Where a pathogen is detected this is usually a bacterium, e.g. salmonella, shigella, or certain strains of *E. coli*. These strains are distinguished from the ordinary *E. coli* found in the stools by their possession of specific somatic antigens ('O' antigens)—to which numbers have been given, e.g. '055', '0114'—and these strains appear to cause gastroenteritis largely by the production of endotoxin.

Rotavirus

Whilst it was believed that most outbreaks and sporadic cases of gastro-enteritis were due to viruses, evidence has until recently been lacking. From time to time several viruses had been found in some cases of infantile diarrhoea, mainly enteroviruses and adenoviruses, but there was little evidence that they actually caused the illness. However, in 1973 things changed. Workers in Melbourne (Bishop et al., 1973) examined duodenal biopsies from 9 children aged 4 – 31 months who had gastroenteritis, using electron microscopy. They discovered virus particles in duodenal epithelial cells in 6 of the 9 patients, and the virus was not seen in duodenal biopsies after clinical recovery. Later the same virus particles were found by electron microscopy in the stools of cases of infantile gastroenteritis, not only in Melbourne but in many other centres throughout the world (Editorial, 1977).

This new virus, when seen under the electron microscope, has an outline like the rim of a wheel, and it has therefore been called the 'rotavirus'. It appears to be very closely related to two other viruses causing diarrhoea in young animals, namely the EDIM virus of mice (epizootic diarrhoea of infant mice) and a virus causing diarrhoea in young calves (Flewett, 1976, 1977).

Rotavirus can be found in more than half the cases of infantile gastro-enteritis. A recent report found the virus in one-third of a series of infants with intussusception (Konno et al., 1977). After the age of 7 years most people have antibodies to rotaviruses, and the virus does not appear to cause serious disease in adults. Second infections can apparently occur. Children aged 6 months to 3 years are especially susceptible to rotavirus infection, and the incidence of the disease is highest in the winter. It appears that infants in the first few days of life often have subclinical disease with asymptomatic infection despite the finding that human milk in the early puerperium contains rotavirus antibodies (these fall to undetectable levels by five days after birth) (Thouless et al., 1977). The newborn's protection from serious disease may be due to maternal antibody transmitted across the placenta, but it is worth noting that ordinary undiluted cow's milk also unactivates human rotavirus (Thouless et al., 1977).

Complete proof that the rotavirus is really causative of disease is lacking, but the case is generally regarded as being convincing. It has been nicely pointed out that the small intestine is a likely site for virus infection; 'If a maker of virus vaccines wished to devise an apparatus for propagating viruses in quantity he could hardly do better than invent the small bowel. Here is a flexible tube several feet long, lined throughout with susceptible cells, their available surface area vastly increased by a complex system of villous infolding; the cells being constantly renewed to maintain them in optimum condition, nourished by nutrients diffusing from the wall of the vessel; and with an in-built mechanism for moving any contents slowly from one end to the other. All he would have to do is to put the virus inoculum in at one end and collect the rich harvest at the other.' (Flewett, 1976.) Certainly direct electron microscopy of faeces has been a most promising new technique, which may allow a result to be telephoned through the same day.

Campylobacter

Looking for bacterial pathogens in adults or children with diarrhoea has always been important but not always terribly rewarding. There is no reason to think that a recent series from Manchester (Dale, 1977) is not representative. One hundred and eighty-two stools from cases of 'sporadic diarrhoea' were examined. There were 2 cases of shigella, one of salmonella, and 1 of an enteropathogenic *E. coli*— not a great yield. There were 5 cases of giardia, underlining the importance of looking for this organism, which can lead to chronic diarrhoea and which is easily amenable to specific treatment (for example, metronidazole). Giardia is an all too easily forgotten pathogen, and not by any means confined to the tropics as is sometimes wrongly imagined. Nine out of 182 specimens were positive for conventional pathogens, but by using a new technique a 'new' organism, campylobacter, was found in 14 cases (8 per cent).

The species *Campylobacter fetus (Fibrio fetus)* has been known to vets for many years as a cause of infectious abortion of cattle and ewes, and it has also been found in chickens, turkeys, sparrows, starlings and pigeons (Simmons and Gibbs, 1977).

Skirrow (1977), from the Worcester Public Health Laboratory, reported on a technique for the culture of campylobacters introduced by some Belgian microbiologists (Butler et al., 1973). The results were little short of dramatic. Out of 803 unselected patients with diarrhoea 57 (7 per cent) grew campylobacter in their stools. One hundred and ninety-four normal people's stools were studied—none grew campylobacter, but when 113 contacts of patients with campylobacter enteritis were studied 19 had positive stools. Infected people were of all ages, and half the patients with campylobacter were aged 15 – 44 years, though the incidence was highest in the very young.

A similar incidence has been found in other parts of England, and the use of this new technique for the culture of campylobacters has become routine for stool cultures in many laboratories. The principal clinical manifestations are diarrhoea (which may be severe for two or three days), general malaise and fever, a sore throat, and abdominal pain which is often prominent. It has been shown that the organism is sensitive to erythromycin stearate, but antibiotics, because of all their disadvantages in gastroenteritis, are likely to be reserved for very severe cases or where there is reason to suspect a septicaemia. Within a few months of campylobacter's re-discovery it has been confirmed as the commonest identifiable bacterial cause of infectious diarrhoea in England. It has been suggested that the reservoir of the organism is the wild bird population, with organisms being transmitted to humans by poultry and meat contaminated or infected with bird droppings (Simons and Gibbs, 1977), but this is unproven. Spread within households certainly occurs, and some cases have been acquired while travelling abroad (Skirrow, 1977). However, the full epidemiology of the disease is largely uncertain at present. (*See also* p.23.)

REFERENCES

Bishop R. F., Davidson G. P., Holmes I. H. et al. (1973) Virus particles in epithelial cells of duodenal mucosa from children with acute non-bacterial gastroenteritis. *Lancet* **2**, 1281.

Butler J. P., Dekeyser P., Detrain M. et al. (1973) Related vibrio in stools. *J. Pediatr.* **82**, 493.

Dale B. (1977) Campylobacter enteritis. *Br. Med. J.* **2**, 318.

Editorial (1977) Rotavirus gastroenteritis. *Br. Med. J.* **2**, 784.

Flewett T. H. (1976) In: *Ciba Foundation Symposium 42,* Amsterdam, Elsevier, p. 237.
Flewett T. H. (1977) *Recent Advances in Clinical Virology.* Edinburgh, Churchill Livingstone, p. 151.
Konno T., Suzuki H., Kutsuzawa T. et al. (1977) Human rotavirus and intussusception. *N. Engl. J. Med.* **297,** 945.
Registrar General (1975) *Statistical Review of England and Wales for the Year 1973.* London, H.M.S.O.
Simmons N. A. and Gibbs F. J. (1977) Campylobacter enteritis. *Br. Med. J.* **2,** 264.
Skirrow M. B. (1977) Campylobacter enteritis: a 'new' disease. *Br. Med. J.* **2,** 9.
Thouless M. E., Bryden A. S. and Flewett T. H. (1977) Rotavirus neutralisation by human milk. *Br. Med. J.* **2,** 1390.
Tripp J. H., Wilmers M. J. and Wharton B. A. (1977) Gastroenteritis: A continuing problem of child health in Britain. *Lancet* **2,** 233.

Surgical

A. W. WILKINSON ChMEdin, PRCSE, FRCS, FAAP(Hon) FRACS(Hon)

EXOMPHALOS AND GASTROSCHISIS

In the 10 years between 1964 and 1974 96 babies with exomphalos or gastroschisis were treated in the Children's Hospital, Sheffield. In 36 the lesion was a minor one, in 30 it was large, in 27 there was what was described as a ruptured exomphalos and 3 had gastroschisis. The overall mortality rate was 46·9 per cent which is far greater than has been recently claimed in some series but which is probably much nearer the true mortality rate for this group of conditions. Venugopal et al. (1976) found that survival was closely and inversely related to the birth weight, and was higher when the liver was within the sac and when there were also associated severe congenital anomalies in other systems. In exomphalos where there is a defect at the site of the umbilical cord, mortality rate was closely related to the size of this defect, and was only 20 per cent when it was less than 5 cm but over 50 per cent with larger defects.

This series illustrates again the difficulty in deciding whether a lesion should be called a ruptured exomphalos or a gastroschisis. In only 1 patient in this series did the sac rupture after birth, in all the other patients in whom the defect was classified as a ruptured exomphalos the rupture occurred in utero, and it is extremely difficult to distinguish accurately between an exomphalos which ruptures in utero and a gastroschisis. In exomphalos there is a defect of the whole opening at the umbilicus, whereas in gastroschisis by definition the defect is in the anterior abdominal wall separately from a normal intact umbilical cord, usually to the right and rarely to the left; in this series there were only 3 examples of exomphalos as narrowly defined in this way, and all these patients died. There were, however, 28 patients who were defined as having an intrauterine rupture of the exomphalos and 18 of them died.

It is to be expected that there should be some abnormality of fixation of the midgut when there is a major anomaly of the umbilicus in utero, and malrotation of the midgut is common in both exomphalos and gastroschisis. But other associated anomalies are also common in addition, and many of these are so severe that the patient dies with or without treatment of the umbilical lesion. Conservative treatment of exomphalos with 0·5 per cent mercurochrome and 65 per cent alcohol was associated with a mortality rate of 33·3 per cent, and since treatment in hospital is required for an average of 10 weeks, it is a very expensive method of doubtful value. The mortality rate of primary repair (39·6 per cent) was not much greater; but this method is usually feasible only when the whole abdominal wall can be closed, and when the skin alone could be closed over the extruding bowel the mortality rate was even higher (80 per cent). The mortality rate for the use of silastic sheeting as a primary repair of the lesion was over 60 per cent, most of the deaths being due to infection and septicaemia.

Other series have been reported in which the mortality rate is considerably lower than in this series from Sheffield, and it seems likely that the authors with the much lower mortality rates have been remarkably fortunate in their experiences and that the Sheffield results much more accurately represent the average experience of paediatric surgeons working in neonatal units.

REFERENCE
Venugopal S., Zachary R. B. and Spitz L. (1976) *Br. J. Surg.* **63**, 523.

OESOPHAGEAL ATRESIA

In about 10 per cent of patients born with oesophageal atresia the gap between the two portions of the oesophagus is too wide for a primary anastomosis to be made safely. A variety of solutions have been proposed for this surgical dilemma and the most commonly used has been the combination of gastrostomy and cervical oesophagostomy initially, combined at a later stage, usually when the child is about a year old, with the bridging of the gap by an isolated segment of transverse and left colon. More recently a gastric tube of the Heimlich type has also been used.

Howard and Myers (1965) suggested that the upper pouch should be lengthened by being stretched by the repeated passage of a stiff large gum elastic bougie, and that this should be followed by a delayed primary anastomosis. This has been used with some success by others, but it is not always effective. Hendren and Hale (1976) suggested that metal bougies should be put into the two ends of the oesophagus and then these bougies should be pulled together by intermittent pulses from an electromagnetic field. In this way both ends of the oesophagus could be elongated enough to allow a delayed primary anastomosis to be made without tension. They have employed this method successfully in 4 patients, in 3 of whom there was an oesophageal atresia without a tracheo-oesophageal fistula and in the remaining patient there was an associated oesophago-bronchus to the lower lobe of the right lung. Treatment with the electromagnetic bougies was carried out for 58 days in 1 patient but for shorter periods in the others. Hendren and Hale feel confident that with their method it is possible to avoid the use of colon to join the two ends of the oesophagus together when there is a wide gap. They recommend that a lateral pharyngostomy should be made to the upper pouch, because the prolonged period of stretching is more risky with nasal suction tube than with a pharyngostomy. Another advantage of their method is that the oesophageal segments are not only lengthened but are made considerably thicker because of hypertrophy by the time of the secondary operation. Their method involves the use of an alternating magnetic force which is on for 60 seconds and off for 60 seconds, 30 times an hour, 720 times a day, and about 20 000 times in a month.

The machine is expensive and will be worth while buying only in those institutions who deal with enough babies with oesophageal atresias to make its use economical, since it would be applicable in only about 15 – 20 per cent of babies with this anomaly. Since the treatment is started in the first few weeks of life and may continue for two months or more it is obviously expensive in the duration of hospital care. A stay of three months or more could cost £6000 in a London teaching hospital and very much more in North America. It also involves a lot of time of highly skilled nursing staff, and it remains to be established whether the overall risk of this method in a large number of patients is less than for oesophagostomy and gastrostomy combined with oesophageal replacement by a segment of colon or a gastric tube.

REFERENCES

Hendren W. H. and Hale J. R. (1976) *J. Pediatr. Surg.* **11**, 713.
Howard R. and Myers N. A. (1965) *Surgery* **58**, 725.

TORSION OF THE TESTIS

The diagnosis of torsion of the testis is one of the most worrying problems presented to the paediatric surgeon. The fate of the testis depends on the right decision as to whether an enlarged, tender, and discoloured scrotum is the site of a twisted testis or an epididymo-orchitis. Many surgeons believe that it is better to look and see than to wait and miss the chance of saving a testis which might otherwise have survived. This is a rare emergency, and Wright (1977) found that in the 25 years between 1950 and 1975 56 patients were admitted with proved testicular torsion to the Royal Newcastle Hospital, New South Wales. This hospital serves a population of about 300 000 at the present time. During the 25 years covered by this review there were 400 000 admissions, so that testicular torsion represented about 1 per 7 000 admissions. (During the same time 73 children were admitted with intussusception, about 1 in every 5 600 admissions.)

Wright found that the testis was removed in 15 patients, but that only 26 of the remaining 41 were followed up, 19 by personal examination, 5 from subsequent hospital records, and 2 from replies to a questionnaire. Wright makes the point that torsion occurs in children and young adults, and the peak incidence is between the ages of 10 and 15 years. Only 4 were over the age of 30 years and none over the age of 40, and Wright states (1966) that a man with a swollen and tender testis aged more than 40 years almost certainly has an epididymo-orchitis, which is most common in the fourth, fifth, seventh and eighth decades. During the same 25-year period 25 patients with torsion of an appendix of the testis or of the epididymis were operated on, and all of these were aged less than 15 years.

It is of interest that in 7 of the patients the twisted testis was undescended and in 5 of these the testis was excised. In one mentally retarded patient with bilaterally undescended testis, both twisted with an interval of 10 years between the episodes. This incidence of torsion in undescended testis (12 per cent) is far higher than Scorer (1964) gave for the male population as a whole (0·8 per cent).

Of the 56 patients 27 were admitted within 12 hours of the onset of pain, in none of whom was the testis removed; and of the 17 of these patients who were assessed at follow-up the testis was considered to be normal in 15, and 2 were thought to be atrophic; one of these was half of the normal size, and the other was said to be smaller than the normal opposite testis. Of the 7 patients who presented within 13 – 24 hours of the onset of pain, the testis was removed in 2, 1 testis which was thought to be viable at operation subsequently sloughed and was removed after severe wound infection, and the other 4 had normal sized testes at follow-up. Of the 4 patients who presented between 24 and 48 hours after the onset of pain, the testis was removed in 1, 1 testis atrophied, and 2 were lost to follow-up. Of the 18 patients who presented after more than 48 hours from the onset of pain, the testis was removed in 12, 4 other testes atrophied, I had an already hypoplastic descended testis, and another was lost at follow-up.

There is abundant evidence in this and in previous reports that the degree and duration of interference of the blood supply determines whether a twisted testicle will survive or not. The duration of pain is at best a crude assessment of the duration of the disturbance of the blood supply but is the best clinical indication that there is. Even at operation it is often difficult to decide whether the testis is alive or dead, and many surgeons recommend that a testis which is not obviously finally infarcted should be untwisted and put back. This theory confirms the conclusion of the earlier one by Skoglund et al. (1970) that the sooner the testis is untwisted the better is the chance of survival. From Wright's series it appears that the prognosis is hopeful when the patient presents within 12 hours of the onset of symptoms, less so if the duration is more than 12 hours, and if presentation is later than 24 hours the testis is almost certainly irreparably infarcted and orchidectomy is probably the best form of treatment. When an infarcted testis is not excised subsequent infection may occur, but this happened in only 2 patients of this series.

Hitch et al. (1976) have described a modification of the scanning procedure used in adults by Nadel et al. (1973) in the differential diagnosis of testicular torsion. Hitch et al. employed this method on 18 patients admitted to the Hospital for Sick Children, Toronto, during 10 months from August 1974. They used 99^m pertechnetate in 21 scrotal scans in 18 patients whose ages ranged from 1 to 16 years, most of whom were more than 10 years old. There were abnormal scans in 11 patients, of whom 7 had torsion of the testis and 4 had epididymo-orchitis, but in the others the scans were normal. They successfully diagnosed torsion in 7 of the 11 patients who had abnormal scans, and epididymo-orchitis in the remaining 4 who were not explored. In another patient who had a normal scan the testis was explored because, although the clinical diagnosis was torsion of the testis, this testis had untwisted spontaneously and had a good blood supply. In another patient the scan was normal, but the clinical evidence suggested epididymitis. These were the only two false negatives in the whole series. Of the remaining 5 patients, all of whom improved rapidly, there was an allergic inflammation of the scrotum in 1, torsion of an appendix in 3, and the last had no demonstrable disease. Hitch et al. have not used their technique in any patients with hydroceles, incarcerated hernias, or testicular tumours, although increased activity has been reported in a seminoma of the testis. They believe that the gamma camera is preferable to a rectolinear scanner because the perfusion of the scrotum may be followed from the moment of injection, duration of scan is minimal, multiple views may be quickly obtained, and resolution is good. They have since scanned a further 24 patients, and 11 accurate diagnoses have been made out of 13 of these. In the other 2 patients spontaneous reduction of the torsion had occurred in 1 and in the other there was partial rotation of the testis without vascular interference. It is obvious that in those institutions where scanning is available it will be of considerable value in resolving the clinical difficulties in making a diagnosis and it should be employed on all suspected testicular torsions.

REFERENCES
Hitch D. C., Gilgay D. L., Shandling B. and Savage F. P. (1976) *J. Pediatr. Surg.* **11**, 537.
Nadel N. S., Gitter N. H., Hahn L. C. and Vernon A. R. (1973) *Urology* **1**, 478.
Scorer C. G. (1964) The descent of the testis. *Arch. Dis. Child.* **39**, 605.
Skoglund R. W., McRoberts J. W. and Ragder H. (1970) *J. Urol.* **104**, 604.
Wright J. E. (1977) *Br. J. Surg.* **64**, 264.

BILATERAL RETRACTILE TESTES

A retractile testes is defined as one that may reside in the superficial inguinal pouch but can be pushed into the scrotum, though not always to the bottom of it, and which then slowly retracts up into the superficial inguinal pouch. A retractile testes does not jump back into the superficial inguinal pouch as soon as it is released, as does the inguinal ectopic testis, which can be pushed a short distance down, perhaps only to the pubic tubercle.

Puri and Nixon (1977) reviewed 164 boys with bilateral retractile testes seen in the Hospital for Sick Children, Great Ormond Street, between 1953 and 1960. In 145 of these patients treatment was not undertaken; the remaining 19 patients received one or two courses of hormone therapy. They sent questionnaires to 131 patients who were over the age of 25 years at the time of the review, and they were able to contact 43 of these patients, of whom 5 had had hormone treatment. The 19 patients who lived reasonably near were interviewed, of whom 2 had had hormone treatment, and an estimate of tubular function was obtained by using the testicular volume test with Prader's orchidometer (Prader, 1966). Twenty-three (74 per cent) of the 31 boys who had married had had children. Of the remaining 8 patients the wives of 2 had been taking the contraceptive pill since marriage, one couple did not wish to have any children and the other 5 boys had been married 1, 2, 3 and 4 years respectively and had not had any children. Of the 5 patients who had had subsequent hormone treatment 4 were married and 3 had children. Of the 19 patients who were interviewed the testes were palpable in the scrotum at the time of the examination in all, and only one complained that one of his testis occasionally ascended into the groin. The testicular volume of these 19 patients ranged from 17·5 to 25 ml which is within the normal adult range.

In 1968 of men under the age of 45 who had been married 5 years 78·9 per cent had had fertile marriages (Registrar General, 1973). This suggests that the fertility of boys who in childhood had bilateral retractile testes was not significantly different to that of the general population. The administration of 500 International Units of chorionic gonadotrophin weekly for 6 weeks obviously had not caused any ill-effects on testicular development. This study clearly indicates that there is no indication for operation on retractile testes and furthermore that they are likely to develop normally if left alone.

REFERENCES
Prader A. (1966) *Triangle* **7**, 240.

Puri P. and Nixon H. H. (1977) *J. Pediatr. Surg.* **12**, 563.
Registrar General (1973) *Statistical Review of England and Wales 1971,* Part II, Tables, Volume Table QQ. London, H.M.S.O.

LESIONS OF THE BREAST IN CHILDREN AND ADOLESCENTS

In childhood lumps in the breast cause anxiety out of all proportion to their nature. Mothers think that the lump in their daughter's breast is a cancer. Boys with gynaecomastia are greatly distressed and often demand excision because of the embarrassment which is caused when they have to change for games or physical exercise at school. Yet malignant disease in the breast of a child is extremely uncommon. Bower et al. (1976) reviewed 207 children with lumps in the breast who were treated in the St Louis Children's Hospital between January 1964 and December 1974. These patients ranged in age from 1 week to 16 years, and 161 (78 per cent) were girls. Of the 134 (64 per cent) who were treated by operation 84 had fibro-adenomas, 76 per cent of all lesions in the breast in their group of girls. Sixty-five (74 per cent) of these girls were black, an indication that fibro-adenoma is commoner in the Negro than in the rest of the population in St Louis. Twelve girls (15 per cent) had multiple fibro-adenomas, some of which were of considerable size.

A 10-year-old white girl had a simple mastectomy in 1967 for an invasive carcinoma of the breast and was well and alive 9 years later; a 15-year-old girl also had a simple mastectomy for an infiltrating duct carcinoma in 1968 and was alive and well at the time of review 8 years later; and one other child had a metastasis of rhabdomyosarcoma in the breast; but these were the only children with malignant disease out of the whole series. Bower et al. make the point that enlargements of the breast in the first 4 years of life are probably due to premature thelarche, whereas between 6 and 11 years they are considerably less common and due to precocious puberty, and from 10 years on they become increasingly common and are then due to fibro-adenoma, which is by far the commonest neoplasm in the adolescent female breast but has rarely been described before the menarche.

Cystosarcoma phylloides is uncommon but is the second most frequent cause of massive breast enlargement in adolescent females. It usually presents as a firm, smooth, but perhaps irregular or lobulated, well-circumscribed mass. The overlying skin may be stretched and shining, and there may be distended veins and great distortion of the nipple and areola. Benign cystosarcoma phylloides in adolescents does not usually recur after complete excision and metastases are most uncommon.

Juvenile hypertrophy of the breast may affect one or both breasts, which undergo rapid enlargement out of proportion to the general growth of the body, and this is probably due to pubertal hormonal stimulation. The breast is symmetrically enlarged and pendulous but diffusely firm without nodules and without much lobulation, and this condition is rare.

Gynaecomastia is most common in boys at the time of puberty. It is believed that this enlargement is due to hormone secretion, and the lesion usually regresses in 6 months to 2 years from the onset. Hormone-induced enlargement of the male breast is also found soon after birth and is probably due to maternal hormone. This also occurs in girls. Gynaecomastia may very rarely be associated with hermaphroditism and Beckwith's syndrome, testicular turmours, or hepatoblastoma.

Enlargement of the breasts of a girl during the first 4 years of life after the neonatal period is thought by Bower et al. to be due to a premature thelarche, with early development of the corpus mammae alone without any other manifestations of sexual precocity such as hair growth and genital enlargement, and is commonest about the third year of life. The enlargement may not progress and may disappear or persist until puberty. In true precocious puberty enlargement of the breasts is usually associated with premature genital development and the production of pubic and axillary hair, a growth spurt, and sometimes menstruation. Although in most patients there is no obvious cause for precocious puberty, in some it may be due to disturbance of hypothalamic function in association with an intracranial tumour, head injury, meningitis, or encephalitis, and a few are associated with McCune – Albright's syndrome. Sometimes the breast enlargement and the development of secondary sexual characteristics are due to an ovarian tumour, or an oestrogen-producing adrenocortical tumour, or exogenous hormone administration.

The surgeon's attitude to lumps in the breast of young girls and boys should be conservative, since most are caused by either neonatal enlargement in response to maternal hormone, premature thelarche, or precocious puberty, and biopsy in such children is not indicated. The bone age should be estimated from a radiograph of the wrist, and, if normal, and if no cause can be found for the enlargement of the breast, it should be treated conservatively. Unilateral lesions of the breast at the time of puberty should also be treated conservatively because usually other signs of puberty soon appear and the opposite breast also enlarges. Discrete lumps in the adolescent girl should be biopsied in order to exclude malignant disease, which possibly occurs in not more than 1 per cent of a large series of patients, to improve the appearance of the breast, and to calm the child and her family. Mastectomy is not indicated. In boys, neonatal breast enlargement is usually self-limiting, and reassurance and observation are what are needed; but in the older boy a discrete mass should be excised. Gynaecomastia before puberty ought to be treated with suspicion because rather more boys than girls with this abnormality have an underlying endocrine or other abnormality. A buccal smear should be examined for sex chromatin in all patients, and while reassurance about the temporary nature of the enlargement should be enough in most patients, subcutaneous mastectomy will be necessary in some.

REFERENCES
Bower R., Bell M. J. and Ternberg J. L. (1976) *J. Pediatr. Surg.* **11**, 337.

NEURAL TUBE DEFECTS

The incidence of open spina bifida ranges from about 1·5 per 1000 live births in the South East of England to 4·5 per 1000 in Northern Ireland. Those who survive this condition are usually severely handicapped physically and a quarter of them mentally as well. The results of a collaborative study in 19 centres has recently been published (Report, 1977), and it is of great interest that out of almost 19 000 pregnancies examined defects of the neural tube were found in 301 cases, that anencephaly was a little more common than open spina bifida, and encephalocele was comparatively rare. All babies born with anencephaly died, but this anomaly is so common that it must be included in a consideration of neural tube defects as a whole. Since only about 10 per cent of all babies born with neural tube defects are produced by women who have had a previous child with one of these defects, 90 per cent of them are unexpected. Once a woman has produced a child with a neural tube defect the risk of subsequent sibs being afflicted in the same way is considerable, about 1 in 40 for a child with open spina bifida and about 1 in 20 for any kind of defect of the central nervous system.

When Brock and Sutcliffe (1972) described an abnormally high concentration of alphafeto protein in the amniotic fluid in a pregnancy where the fetus had a spina bifida it seemed that there might be some hope of making the diagnosis early enough in pregnancy for termination to be a clinical possibility. The recent collaborative study has established that the determination of the serum alphafeto protein concentration may be of considerable value in identifying abnormal fetuses between the sixteenth and eighteenth week of pregnancy; but this may also be associated with a normal fetus, and there is considerable overlap between normal values and those found in association with fetuses with neural tube defects. When the concentration of alphafeto protein in the serum is high the concentration in the amniotic fluid should at once be measured. In association with open spina bifida or anencephaly the amniotic fluid alphafeto protein is usually at least 10 standard deviations above the normal mean. The results of the collaborative study indicate that there is considerable variation between different laboratories in the results of estimation of alphafeto protein in amniotic fluid, and that a value of $2\cdot5$ times the median value for normal pregnancies in any particular laboratory should be chosen as the critical level rather than a single figure nationally for all laboratories. When such a level is employed the study indicates that almost 80 per cent of fetuses with open spina bifida and 90 per cent with anencephaly can be detected by the original estimation of alphafeto protein in the serum. It is clear that these encouraging results are merely a beginning and that much remains to be done before these severe neural tube defects can be detected in the majority of the women who are carrying them in their pregnancy.

REFERENCES
Brock D. J. H. and Sutcliffe R. C. (1972) *Lancet* **2**, 197.
Report of U.K. Collaborative Study on alphafetoprotein in relation to neural-tube defects (1977) *Lancet* **1**, 1323.

COMMUNITY MEDICINE AND EPIDEMIOLOGY

RALPH E. MIDWINTER BSc, MD, MFCM, DPH, DCH

MORTALITY AND THE PILL

Two major prospective studies are under way in the United Kingdom to try to assess the magnitude of possible risks associated with the use of oral contraceptives. Both have issued interim reports which tend to confirm the findings of previous retrospective studies, that risks of death from cardio-vascular diseases are increased. The Royal College of General Practitioners' oral contraceptive study is following-up 46 000 women of childbearing age. Observations began in 1968 and 1400 practitioners are co-operating by recording all new episodes of illness in the study population. Beral and Kay (1977) have now reported on the findings up to June 1976. Among ever-users of oral contraceptives there was a 40 per cent increase in the age-standardized mortality rate compared with non-users. Standardized mortality rates for circulatory diseases were 4·7 times those of the control group. Rates for non-rheumatic heart disease and hypertension were 4·0 times greater and for cerebrovascular disease 4·7 times greater than those experienced by non-users. These categories account for nearly all the excess deaths. Mortality for all circulatory diseases combined was 4·9 times that of the controls. Among ex-takers of oral contraceptives the circulatory disease mortality rate was 4·3 times that of the non-takers. Death rates among smokers taking oral contraceptives were higher than among non-smokers, although within each category the relative risk was about the same. Excess mortality rose sharply with increasing age and with increasing length of time of oral contraceptive use. As yet, few young women have been at risk for long enough periods for the effects of these two factors to be separated. Women who use oral contraceptives have other characteristics which are different from those who do not. This may help to explain the excess deaths from accidents and violence that was found in the user group. The excess mortality from all causes amounts to 1 death per 5000 ever-users per year. This is more than twice the mortality rate for accidents in the study population and is about 11 times greater than that associated with the larger number of pregnancies that occurred in the control population. The excess mortality ranges by age from 1 in 20 000 ever-users aged 15 – 34 to 1 in 700 aged 45 – 49. Excess mortality by length of use ranges from 1 in 8000 among women users of less than 4 years' duratio to 1 in 2000 for users of more than 5 years, and by smoking habit from 1 in 10 000 non-smoking ever-users to 1 in 3000 ever-users who smoke.

Vessey et al. (1977) have published the findings to date on the follow-up of 17 032 participants in the Oxford Family Planning Association contraceptive, study. This study also started in 1968 and is taking place in 17 Family Planning Clinics throughout England and Scotland: 56 per cent of the entrants were using oral contraceptives, 25 per cent a diaphragm and 19 per cent an intra-uterine device. The women in each group tend to have similar characteristics apart from the fact that there is a higher percentage of heavier cigarette smokers among the pill-takers. So far, 43 deaths are known to have occurred in the study population. There have been 9 deaths attributed to cardiovascular diseases: all 9 occurred in the oral contraceptive group.

Both sets of findings support those of earlier case-control studies but widen the range of vascular diseases associated with oral contraceptive use. It also seems that the risks persist after the pill is discontinued. Because the follow-up period is still relatively short, it is not possible to say whether any induced vascular changes are permanent or are reversible in the long term. In both studies, while risk of death from cardiovascular disease is increased, overall death rates are lower than for the general population. This apparent anomaly arises because both study populations tend to consist of active, motivated women initially selected as being healthy and who smoke as a group less than the average number of cigarettes. There is a need to minimise the excess cardiovascular risk associated with oral contraceptive use by careful selection, especially by age and smoking habit, and by regular supervision which should include blood pressure monitoring.

REFERENCES

Beral V. and Kay C. R. (1977) Mortality among oral contraceptive users. *Lancet,* **2,** 727 – 31.
Vessey M. P., McPherson K. and Johnson B. (1977) Mortality among women participating in the Oxford/Family Planning Association contraceptive study. *Lancet* **2,** 731 – 33.

DIET AND HEART DISEASE

Some interesting associations have come to light from Professor J. N. Morris's detailed research into coronary artery disease among London busmen during 1956 – 66 (Morris et al., 1977). The Medical Research Council's Social Medicine Research Unit were looking at means of assessing diet in the hope that a prospective study of diet and coronary disease might be possible. Some detailed diet recording was undertaken but it proved impossible to develop a simple enough technique for large scale use. However, the pilot study had involved 337 healthy busmen and bank staff aged 30 – 67, and each had taken part in a 7-day individual-weighed dietary survey. The morbidity experience of these men has been recorded at regular intervals since then and details of any deaths have been notified through a 'tagging' procedure. By the end of 1976, 45 had developed clinical coronary heart disease before the age of 70 and 26 of these had died.

There was a significant but unexpected association between energy intake and the likelihood of developing coronary disease. High energy intake was found to be associated with a lower risk of disease and vice versa. This association persisted after allowance was made for age difference and it was also present within each occupational group. It has been shown previously that short men are more prone to developing coronary disease than tall men: short men eat less than tall men but the two effects appear to act independently. There were more cigarette smokers among men with a low energy intake but once again these two factors appear to exert separate effects. Men whose diets were low in fibre were more likely to develop coronary disease. The association is with ceral fibre and not with fibre from other fruit or vegetable sources. Dietary sugar intake ranged from 10 to 260 g daily. No relationship was apparent between sugar intake and heart disease, neither was any relationship apparent with dietary cholesterol. The ratio of polyunsaturated to saturated fatty acids in the diet was significant: men whose diets contained more polyunsaturated acids were less at risk. Those who took more physical activity in their leisure time were similarly less at risk.

There are many pitfalls involved in detailed dietary studies and in the application of the necessary multivariate analysis techniques to identify relationships. Nevertheless, the authors seem to have revealed a possible pattern for healthy living. A high energy intake and output, a high consumption of cereal fibre and avoidance of cigarette smoking are associated with a reduced likelihood of developing coronary heart disease. Low energy intake, little physical activity, low dietary cereal fibre and cigarette smoking seem to predispose to increased risk.

REFERENCE
Morris J. N., Marr J. W. and Clayton D. G. (1977) Diet and heart: a postscript. *Br. Med. J.* **2**, 1307 – 1314.

MEASLES AND VACCINATION

Roden and Heath (1977) have reviewed the effects of the measles vaccination programme on the immunity state of the child population in England and Wales. Measles vaccination was first introduced nationally in 1968, as part of the schedule of routine immunization in the second year of life. The national acceptance rate for children under 3 years of age is now about 50 per cent. As a result of the vaccination campaign, the regular biennial cycle of notified measles cases, while still apparent, shows much smaller oscillations (*Fig.* 1).

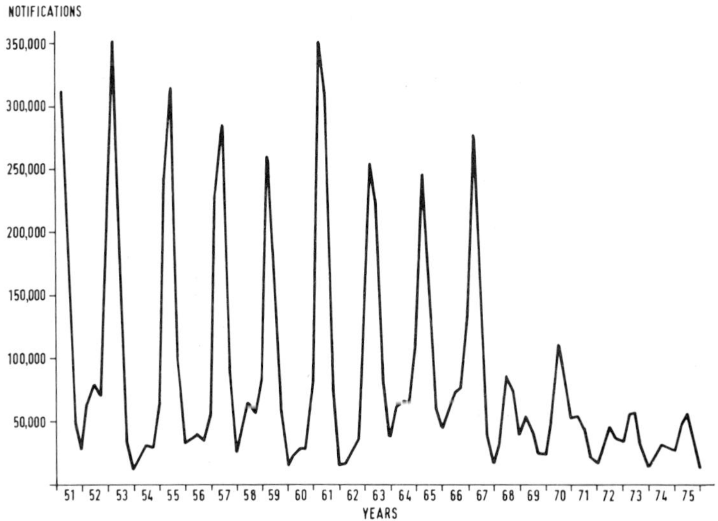

Fig. 1. Quarterly corrected notifications of measles for England and Wales, 1951 – 75. (By kind permission of *Health Trends.)* (Reproduced with the permission of the Controller of Her Majesty's Stationery Office.)

The reduction in measles incidence has been greater in Southern England than elsewhere and is greater among 1 – 4-year-olds than in children aged 5 or more. The effect of vaccination on the immunity state of the child population has been examined. The accuracy of the estimates is difficult to determine, as a number of assumptions have to be made with little supporting evidence to justify them. One such assumption is that notification is 66·6 per cent complete. It seems that vaccination has raised the level of immunity in the fourth year of life from 1 in 3 of those children born in 1965 or before to about 2 in 3 of those born in 1969 or after. In the eighth year of life immunity states have remained about the same. However, in the twelfth year of life there is a slow decline in the level of immunity. This is a consequence of the decline in the numbers of children immunized by the natural disease. If vaccination acceptance rates remain at their present level of about 50 per cent, the number of persons in the community susceptible to measles will tend to rise. There is already evidence that measles is becoming a disease of later rather than earlier childhood. Other evidence suggests that 80 – 90 per cent acceptance rates are necessary to prevent the disease from spreading when introduced into a community from which it has previously been eliminated. If measles is not to become a disease of adult life and if, ideally, it is to be eliminated, then the vaccination campaign must be intensified.

REFERENCE
Roden A. T. and Heath W. C. C. (1977). Effects of vaccination against measles on the incidence of the disease and on the immunity of the child population in England and Wales. Health Trends 9, 4, 69 – 72.

SMOKING IN PREGNANCY

Simpson (1957) showed that babies born to mothers who smoked during pregnancy tended to be of lower birthweight than those born to non-smokers. Many subsequent studies have confirmed this finding and the difference in mean birthweight is of the order of 200 g. The reason for this difference is the subject of considerable debate. Two possible explanations have their ardent supporters. One is that smoking in pregnancy is the cause of lowered birthweight. The other is that mothers who smoke are also in some other way, perhaps genetically, different from those who do not and that it is this secondary association and not the smoking that is responsible. Goldstein (1977) has reviewed the findings of relevant studies to attempt to determine which of the two hypotheses is the more likely. The birthweight distribution of babies in each group is similar except for the shift in the mean value (*Fig.* 2).

It should be noted that the mean birthweight of low-birthweight babies (i.e. under 2500 g) is lower in the non-smoking group than in the smoking group, as the latter is weighted by more babies being pushed over the borderline by the 200 g average lowering. The calculation of mean birthweights for parts of samples below arbitrary cut-off points on normal distributions is open to question. However, the fact that there are relatively more babies in the smoking group who fall into the low birthweight category does help to explain some of the inconsistencies in perinatal mortality measures among babies in the two groups. The weight difference is not accounted for by factors such as differences in maternal age, parity or social class. Standardizing for each of these factors still leaves the basic smoking/non-smoking difference unchanged. Many attempts have been made to falsify the causal hypothesis. So far, all have failed and each failure makes the hypothesis therefore more acceptable. There is an undisputed relationship between birthweight and perinatal mortality (*Fig.* 3).

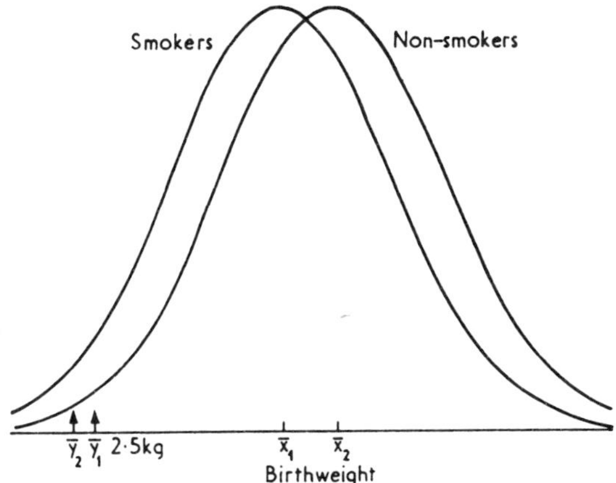

Fig. 2. Birthweight distribution for babies of mothers who smoke and of mothers who do not. (Not to scale.)
x_1 = mean birthweight for babies of smokers.
x = mean birthweight for babies of non-smokers.
y_1 = mean birthweight for smokers for births <2·5 kg.
y_2 = mean birthweight for non-smokers for births <2·5 kg.

(*Figs.* 2 and 3 by kind permission of the *British Journal of Preventive and Social Medicine.)*

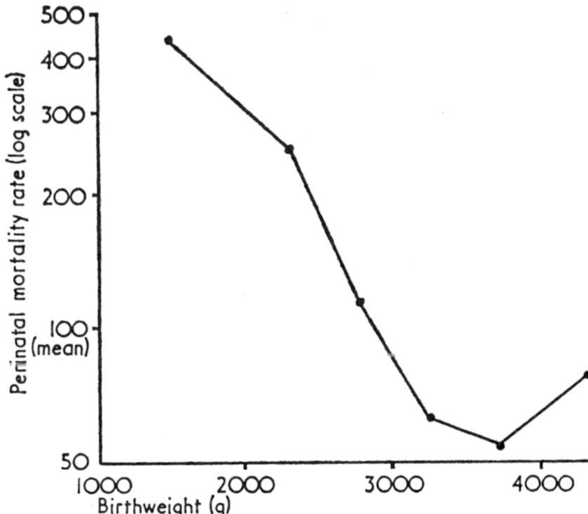

Fig. 3. Perinatal mortality rate by birthweight. (1958 British Perinatal Mortality Survey, mean = 100.)

Reduction of birthweight from 3500 to 3300 g increases perinatal mortality risk by less than 10 per cent. Reduction from 2500 to 2300 g results in a 30 per cent increase in risk. Hence the greatest risk from maternal smoking is to the baby whose mother is already at risk of producing a low-birthweight baby by reason of other factors such as high parity, small stature or low social class. It is estimated that in Britain about 1500 babies in this category die each year because their mothers smoke.

Donovan (1977) has carried out a randomized controlled trial of intensive anti-smoking advice in pregnancy. Because most women do not present themselves for antenatal care very early on in pregnancy, the campaign was of necessity directed towards altering smoking habits later rather than earlier in pregnancy. There was evidence to show that anti-smoking counselling reduced smoking to some extent but little to show that this resulted in increased birthweight. The study does illustrate the difficulties inherent in trying to measure smoking by history-taking and the degree of inconsistency of replies when patients were re-questioned after delivery. It was not possible to determine whether the anti-smoking advice was largely unheeded, was irrelevant or was given too late in pregnancy to be effective.

REFERENCES

Donovan J. W. (1977) Randomised controlled trial of anti-smoking advice in pregnancy. *Br. J. Prev. Soc. Med.* **31,** 6 – 12.

Goldstein H. (1977) Smoking in pregnancy: some notes on the statistical controversy. *Br. J. Prev. Soc. Med.* **31,** 13 – 17.

Simpson W. J. (1957) A preliminary report of cigarette smoking and the incidence of prematurity. *Am. J. Obstet. Gynec.* **73,** 808 – 815.

EAR, NOSE AND THROAT DISEASES
JOHN GROVES FRCS

MENIÈRE'S DISORDER
Fluctuant sensorineural deafness and tinnitus are complaints so common and of such varied aetiology that in isolation neither can be taken as specific for diagnosis of Menière's disease (labyrinthine hydrops). Nevertheless, either symptom may occur and even progress, in isolation, without, for a long time, the appearance of vertigo, in what later may be recognized as 'Menière's disease'. Clinical experience suggests that in a practical sense it is not wise to diagnose 'hydrops', unless the classic attacks of paroxysmal (rotatory) *vertigo* recur within a pattern compatible with the classic condition.

These criteria must be observed in any critical study of current literature, and in the clinical application of modern therapies. It is not unfair to point out that, in the prevailing state of ignorance of the causation of Menière's disorder, biochemical, endocrine, allergic, auto-immune, pyschogenic, and vasomotor factors all retain some plausible relevance. Heredity, otosclerosis, and even Eustachian tube dysfunction are implicated in various ways by different authors.

House (1975) discusses some of the observed abnormalities of the labyrinth and suggests how these may explain the protean variety of symptoms in this troublesome disease.

He suggests that the earlier stages of the disease with classic fluctuant low-tone sensorineural deafness, variable tinnitus and episodic vertigo may correlate with intermittent crises of labyrinthine disorder, with no more than moderate, reversible endolymphatic distension. A spontaneous rupture of the membranous labyrinth may produce relief and prolonged remission. On the other hand, permanent distension, with obliteration of the scala vestibuli (by Reisner's membrane), prolapse of the helicotrema, and saccular apposition to the stapes footplate, result in persistent disequilibrium, with severe and unchanging deafness, a pattern which can be quite unlike classic Menière's syndrome. He does not discuss the possibility that these two distinct states might even be separate 'diseases'—just one more conceivable theory in this almost infinitely complex area for speculation.

Many therapies are advised. The following is a representative but by no means complete list:

1. *Medical*
    Dietary—Low sodium/restricted fluid intake. Diuretics
    Vasodilator drugs—Nicotinic acid, betahistine hydrochloride, naftidro-
            furyl
    Sedation—e.g. Barbiturates
    Vestibular sedatives—e.g. cinnarizine
    Histamine desensitization injections

2. *Conservative surgical*
    Stellate ganglion block
    Stellate ganglionectomy
    Insertion of grommet
    Saccus operations (decompression, drainage)

3. *Destructive surgical*
    Ultrasonic selective labyrinth destruction
    Labyrinthectomy
    Vestibular nerve section

Most of the surgical therapies carry undesirable hazards which must be called unacceptable, unless good prospect of benefit is on offer. The fact that good results have been reported for so great a diversity of techniques must in itself cause concern. The apparent success of a wide variety of conservative medical measures based on opposing theories may even give rise to cynicism. Some authors have commented upon the frequently observed improvement or even remission seen in Menière's disorder which follows upon sympathetic consultation, investigation and reassurance only.

Diagnosis

Compounding these difficulties are the basic problems of differential diagnosis. Menière's disorder may be mimicked by otosclerosis, destructive middle-ear disease, syphilitic labyrinthitis, acoustic neuroma, posterior fossa tumour, brain-stem vascular disorder, disseminated sclerosis, and epilepsy. The fact that sensorineural deafness from any cause is so common, and can be coincidental and irrelevant to both tinnitus and vertigo, completes the diagnostician's nightmare. Again and again devoted otological and neurological skills in combination fail to achieve confident diagnosis.

Newer aids to diagnosis

Recently electrocochleography, polytomography, and the glycerol dehydration test have slipped unobtrusively ahead of better-known, established investigative measures such as caloric testing and audiometric tests for recruitment. This is not to say that the latter have become obsolete. Their fallibility has never been under-estimated but they remain useful as relatively inexpensive screening procedures.

Electrocochleography provides a fairly reliable diagnosis for an end-organ disorder (of hearing) when the cochlear microphonic responses are abnormal. It also provides good evidence of a retrocochlear lesion when the 8th nerve action potential is impaired. Expertly performed and interpreted it gives helpful differentiation between peripheral (sensory) hearing loss and retrocochlear (neural) deafness (e.g. from acoustic neuroma). Since this distinction is one that troubles clinical otologists very frequently, and is not dependably resolved by tests for recruitment (including S.I.S.I., Bekesy and tone decay tests) it is reasonable that electrocochleography should receive wider recognition, assessment and application. Already it is evident that the necessary transtympanic insertion of a needle-electrode to contact the promontory is essentially harmless. Whenever the test might be helpful it may ethically be used, even if, (uncommonly), general anaesthesia is necessary.

Polytomography. Quite apart from the necessary use of accurate radiological methods in differential diagnosis (e.g. tomography of internal auditory meatuses to help exclude acoustic neuroma), precision radiography of the canal for the ductus endolymphaticus has lately acquired some relevance to menière's disease. Valvassori, and also others, pursuing theories of ductus lesions in Menière's disorder, have described narrowing or obliteration of the bony canal shown by polytome X-rays. This point demands elucidation and as a 'non-invasive' investigation the technique will, it is hoped, be further explored.

Glycerol dehydration test. The effects of dehydration upon the hearing in Menière's disorder were studied and first exploited by Klockhoff and Lindblom (1976). Significant change in plasma osmolarity may be achieved by oral administration of glycerol $1\cdot2$ g per kg body-weight (in equal dilution with normal saline and flavoured with lemon juice). A salt-loading regime (sodium chloride g 1 q.d.s. for 5 days) precedes the test. Pure-tone and speech audiometry performed before and after this 'provocation' may show transient hearing improvement. It is supposed that any such improvement would occur only if the patient has cochlear deafness due to Menière's disorder (endolabyrinthine hydrops). Regarded in this light, the test may be thought of as a diagnostic procedure. Considering the frequent difficulties in diagnosis (and therefore prognosis) we may be glad to have this additional approach to our problem.

Management

Reversibility of deafness, confirmed by the glycerol test, with amelioration of tinnitus and vertigo, represents the challenge for conservative managers of Menière's disorder. Whereas there is no usefulness in conservative treatment of an irreversible condition (and it may be better in such cases to look for relief of symptoms by labyrinthectomy, or vestibular neurectomy), reversibility of symptoms is a strong inducement to persevere with conservative measures, whether medical or surgical.

The surgical alternatives present a difficult choice. For 50 years the saccus operation of Portman has been in and out of fashion, with one or other technical variation. We are still a long way from knowing why it appears to work, or fail, in different hands, and in different cases. The dehydration tests give a new dimension, a reasonably objective criterion, of reversibility and are now being correlated with results of saccus surgery (Gibson, 1977). Indeed, it is already widely assumed that results of saccus surgery are predictably better in patients who have shown improved hearing with dehydration. A great deal more experimentation on patients than has so far been reported will be necessary to achieve a true understanding because there are so many variables in the equation. Doubtless this will occur with the appropriate ethical safeguards.

At the present time no easy escape from these problems can be envisaged. The impossibility of treating vertigo of unknown aetiology, deafness of unknown aetiology, and tinnitus of unknown aetiology, is self-evident. Each patient involved has his own priorities, which are not necessarily the same as the clinician's proper and conscientious objectives. The latter would deserve more respect if they were dictated by a more dependable, scientific knowledge of the long-term prognosis (not to mention pathology and diagnosis). Current research is directed towards correlations between electrocochleography findings, dehydration effects, and operations on the saccus endolymphaticus. This is necessary but disheartening because the 'variables' appear to be increasing, not diminishing. The crucial 'break-through' observations, whether still to come, or already made, are still out of reach, or unrecognized.

REFERENCES

Gibson W. P. R. (1977) Personal communication.

House W. F. (1975) Menière's disease: management and theory. In: Fluctuant Hearing Loss. *Otolaryngol. Clin. North Am.* **8**, 515.

Klockhoff I. and Lindblom U. (1976) Glycerol test in Menière's disease. *Acta Otolaryngol. (Stokh.)* Suppl. 224, 449 – 451.

ENDOCRINE GLANDS

IVAN D. A. JOHNSTON MCH, FRCS

Recent developments in endocrinology include the identification for the first time of high levels of hormones in the plasma linking some endocrine tumours with symptoms which have so far been unexplained.

Tourniaire et al. (1977) have reported the first proved case of a prolactin secreting adenoma of the pituitary in association with the multiple endocrine adenoma syndrome. Galactorrhoea and secondary amenorrhoea were the symptoms associated with the pituitary tumour. The evidence that the pituitary tumour contained prolactin cells was obtained from electron microscopy and innumofluorescent studies. Koracs and his associates in Toronto (Horvath et al., 1977; Koracs et al., 1977) have added a further 2 cases. The frequency with which prolactin-secreting tumours are present in multiple endocrine adenopathy has yet to be determined. Raised blood prolactin levels have been noted in between 25 and 70 per cent of patients with pituitary tumours, indicating that many pituitary tumours will be producing prolactin as well as other hormones.

Some non-insulin secreting tumours of the pancreas are associated with refractory watery diarrhoea, hypokalaemia and hypochlorhydria. Secretin, glucagon and gastrin have been among the hormones suggested as the cause of these symptoms. It is now clear that the vasoactive intestinal polypeptide (VIP), which is found in many tissues and for which no physiological role has been identified, is the cause of the W.D.H.A. syndrome (Modlin et al., 1977). VIP stimulates small intestinal secretion and inhibits gastric acid production. The infusion of VIP into pigs produces profuse gastrointestinal fluid losses. Thirty-nine patients with watery diarrhoea and high levels of VIP in the plasma were found to have pancreatic tumours by Bloom and his group.

The early detection of a raised plasma VIP is of great clinical importance. The syndrome develops slowly and half the tumours have metastasized when the diagnosis is eventually made. A case is described (Modlin et al., 1978) which illustrates the importance of finding raised plasma VIP levels in a patient with unexplained watery diarrhoea. A tumour was localized in the pancreas by selective arteriography and removed successfully, after which all the symptoms disappeared. The polypeptide VIP is thus a specific marker for the presence of a vipoma.

The first case of a tumour producing the growth hormone release inhibiting hormone somatostatin has been reported (Larsson et al., 1977). The clinical abnormality was steatorrhoea, a diabetic type glucose tolerance and hypochlorhydria. A pancreatic tumour was found composed of cells similar to islet D cells.

REFERENCES

Gagel R., Costanza M. and De Leslis R. (1976) Streptozotocin treated Verner Morrison syndrome. *Arch. Intern. Med.* **136**, 1429 – 1436.

Horvath E., Koracs K., Rayan N., Sarger W. and Ezrin C. (1977) Incidence of prolactin-producing adenomas. *IRCS Medical Science* **5**, 447.

Koracs K., Horvath E. and Kereny N. A. (1977) Prolactin cell adenomas associated with multiple endocrine tumours. *IRCS Medical Science* **5**, 446.
Larsson L. I., Holst J. J., Kubl C., Lindquist G., Hirsch M. A., Ingemansson S., Jensen S., Rehfeld J. F. and Schwartz T. W. (1977) Pancreatic somatostatinoma: clinical features. *Lancet* **1**, 666.
Modlin I. M., Bloom S. R., Barnes A. and Welbourn R. B. (1978) Care of intractable watery diarrhoea by excision of a vipoma. *Br. J. Surg.* **65**, 234–236.
Modlin I. M., Bloom S. R. and Mitchell S. J. (1977) The role of VIP in diarrhoea. *Gut* **18**, 418.
Tourniaire J., Tronillas J., Mallet P., David L., Pallo D., Mink V. T. and Bressol C. (1977) Prolactin cell adenomas in multiple endocrine adenopathy. *Ann. Endocrinol. (Paris)* **38**, 141.

ADRENAL MEDULLA

Phaeochromocytoma is a dramatic cause of hypertension and can be extremely dangerous if unsuspected during the management of acute illness or injury and phaeochromocytomas are still uncovered for the first time at autopsy.

The incidence of phaeochromocytoma has been estimated to range from 0·4 to 2 per cent of all patients with hypertension. The tumour is usually single and suprarenal in position, but the Mayo Clinic group (1974) found that 10 per cent were extra-adrenal and 10 per cent were multiple. The incidence of malignant change ranged from 11 to 13 per cent in the experience of Scott and his colleagues (1976) and ReMine et al. (1974) at the Mayo Clinic, but this figure is probably rather high.

Seventy-two patients with phaeochromocytoma were encountered in Hammersmith Hospital, London, Belfast and in Newcastle between 1955 and 1975 (Modlin et al., 1978). Twelve were found incidentally at post mortem emphasizing the danger of unrecognized tumours.

Tumours were localized radiologically in over 80 per cent of patients. The operative mortality before pharmacological blockade was 10 per cent and this has been reduced to 2 per cent by the introduction of α blockade in the preoperative preparation.

After operation 40 per cent became normotensive and required no drugs, while additional drug therapy produced normal blood pressure in a further 40 per cent.

REFERENCES
Modlin I. M., Farndon J., Welbourn R. B., Johnston I. D. A., Shepherd D., Kennedy T. L. and Montgomery D. A. D. (1978) Phaeochromocytomas in 72 patients—diagnosis, management and long term results. *Br. J. Surg.* In the press.
ReMine W. H., Chong G. C. and Van Heerden J. A. (1974) Current management of phaeochromocytoma. *Ann. Surg.* **179**, 740.
Scott H. W., Oates J. A., Nies A. S., Burke H., Page D. L. and phamy R. K. (1976) Phaeochromocytoma—present diagnosis and management. *Ann. Surg.* **183**, 585–592.

THYROID

Cancer of the thyroid is uncommon and it is very difficult on clinical grounds to distinguish it from the much more common benign conditions. Papillary carcinoma accounts for half the adult thyroid cancers. It is multifocal in about 20 per cent of patients, with a peak incidence between 20 and 40 years of age. Papillary cancer is usually a relatively benign tumour, but occasionally it can be rapidly fatal.

There is still considerable debate about the extent of the surgery required and the need for supplementary radio-iodine and thyroid hormone therapy after surgery.

Massaperri and his group (1977) have been able to examine the effect of different forms of treatment in 576 patients treated by the United States Airforce Medical Service, and a review of such a large number of patients is valuable.

Poor prognosis was associated with tumours which were greater than 2·5 cm in diameter which had extended beyond the capsule, particularly in patients in the older age groups. Recurrence was twice as common after subtotal as after total thyroidectomy. They conclude that local lymph node excision was entirely appropriate and radical surgery of nodes did not influence the outcome. Support was also forthcoming for thyroid hormone therapy and radio-iodine ablation of residual functioning tissue.

Surgery continues to be indicated strongly for the solitary cold nodule of the thyroid. Katz and Zager (1976) have found, in over 900 patients, that the incidence of malignancy was greatest in patients over 70 years of age, and in a selected group of patients considered to be at risk over 20 per cent were found to have malignant disease.

A study (Clark and Demburg, 1976) of cold nodules in patients over 60 years of age indicates that evidence of increased risks of cancer, such as a growing lesion in a man with some lymph node involvement, should lead to thyroidectomy irrespective of age. There were no operative deaths in a group of 100 patients over 60 years of age and only one significant complication.

The decision when to explore a non-functioning thyroid nodule is sometimes difficult, particularly as many apparent solitary nodules are in fact part of a multi-nodular goitre, and of course the majority of true solitary nodules are benign. Continued efforts are being made to refine the selection process for patients who need operation. The addition of ultrasonography to radioactive scintiscanning has permitted the safe conservative management of cystic lesions of the thyroid (Miskin et al., 1975). Scandinavian workers have advocated for some time needle aspiration biopsy, using a fine needle as a useful diagnostic method to assist in patient management (Ljungberg, 1972). There has, however, been resistance by both pathologists and clinicians due to difficulties of interpretation for the wider use of needle biopsy in the thyroid.

The results of a prospective study of combined aspiration biopsy and ultrasonography in the assessment of the cold thyroid nodule by Toronto workers (Walfish et al., 1977) could, however, change the minds of many. Adequate material for cytology was obtained in 94 per cent of patients and the correlation with subsequent histology was 82 per cent. There were no false positive results and no complications. Emphasis is placed on not accepting normal or negative cytology as the sole basis for not exploring all cold nodules. Ultrasonography should precede aspiration cytology. Wang and his colleagues (1977), at the Massachusetts General Hospital, report their experience of 1200 needle biopsies of the thyroid. The diagnosis made on needle biopsy specimens was confirmed at surgery in 90 per cent of cases. The diagnosis was inconclusive in 5 per cent and wrong in 5 per cent. There was no evidence of any dissemination of malignant cells or compromising of the prognosis by needle biopsy. Haematoma occurred on only 4 occasions. There is no doubt that there will be a cautious increase of needle or aspiration biopsy in the assessment of thyroid lesions prior to surgery.

There have been further reports on the value of angiography in the assessment of thyroid nodules (Mojab and Ghosh, 1976). Solitary adenomas and nodular colloid goitres were distinguished easily on the angiogram. Some cardinomas were associated with an increased and abnormal vascularity, but it is hardly likely that angiography will replace other methods of assessment.

It is recognized that the presence of a medullary carcinoma of the thyroid is associated with a high level of calcitonin in the plasma. Elevated plasma calcitonin levels have led to exploration of the thyroid on a number of occasions when no lesion could be detected. A group of Boston workers (Leape et al., 1976) now describe total thyroidectomy in 19 children with familial and clinically undetectable medullary carcinoma on the basis of raised calcitonin levels. Eight of the children had C cell hyperplasia of the thyroid. The value of raised basal or stimulated calcitonin as a basis for surgical exploration of the thyroid is now clearly established.

The greater precision which has developed in the selection of patients with possible malignancy for exploration and the adaptation of operations to the histological type and extent of disease have improved considerably the results of treatment, and the prognosis for operable differentiated thyroid cancer can now be described as good (Block, 1977).

REFERENCES

Block M. A. (1977) Management of thyroid cancer. *Ann. Surg.* **185**, 133.
Clark O. H. and Demburg R. (1976) Management of thyroid nodules in the elderly. *Am. J. Surg.* **132**, 615.
Katz A. D. and Zager W. J. (1976) The malignant cold nodule of the thyroid. *Am. J. Surg.* **132**, 459.
Leape L. L., Miller H. H., Graze K., Fieldman Z. J., Gagel R. F., Wolfe H. J., Delellis R. A., Tashjian A. H. and Relchlin S. (1976) Total thyroidectomy for occult familial medullary carcinoma of the thyroid in children. *J. Pediatr. Surg.* **11**, 831.
Ljungberg O. (1972) Cytological diagnosis of medullary carcinoma of the thyroid. *Acta Cytol.* **16**, 253.
Massaperri E. L., Young R. B., Oertel J. E., Kemmerer W. T. and Page C. P. (1977) Thyroid cancer in the U.S. Armed Forces. *Medicine (Baltimore)* **56**, 177.
Miskin M., Rosen I. B. and Walfish P. G. (1975) Ultrasonography of the thyroid gland. *Radiol. Clin. North Am.* **13**, 479.
Mojab K. and Ghosh B. S. (1976) Thyroid angiography. *Am. J. Surg.* **132**, 620.
Walfish F. G., Hazani E., Strawbridge H. T. G., Miskin M. and Rosin I. B. (1977) A prospective study of combined ultrasonography and needle aspiration biopsy in the assessment of the hypofunctioning cold thyroid nodule. *Surgery* **82**, 474–482.
Wang C., Vickery A. L. and Maloof F. (1977) Needle biopsy of the thyroid. *Surg. Gynecol. Obstet* **143**, 365.

PARATHYROID GLANDS

Radiation has been linked with neoplasia of the thyroid for 50 years, but evidence for parathyroid involvement has so far been scanty. Prinz and his colleagues (1977), however, have found that 30 per cent of 89 patients with primary hyperparathyroidism had had neck irradiation in the past. Half of the involved patients had hyperplasia and half had single adenomas. Ten patients also had benign or malignant disease of the thyroid. Parathyroid disease appears to be increasing, but the role of irradiation in this increase remains uncertain. However, those patients who have had previous neck irradiation should be included among those groups in whom serum calcium should be measured.

The debate on the conservative versus liberal approach to parathyroid neck exploration continues with a significant contribution from the Mayo Clinic (Edis et al., 1977). The radical approach is justified by reports of an increasing incidence of primary chief cell hyperplasia as the cause of the disease. A high rate of recurrent hyperparathyroidism following the removal of a single adenoma and no serious management problems after the removal of three and a half glands would also support a radical approach (Haff and Armstrong, 1974).

One surgeon at the Mayo Clinic adopted the liberal or radical approach removing up to three and a half glands, while another used a conservative approach removing only grossly enlarged glands. Symptomatic hypocalcaemia was a problem in 24 per cent of patients after liberal exploration compared with 4 per cent in the conservatively treated group.

The liberal approach did not produce a higher cure rate, which was 99 per cent in the whole series.

In the usual case of primary hyperparathyroidism a single adenoma will be found. if one other parathyroid gland of normal size is found the surgeon can be reasonably sure that he is not dealing with hyperplasia. He must, however, make sure that a second adenoma is not present by attempting to identify four glands.

Similar patterns of presentation of findings and results of conservative operative treatment are reported from a recent series involving 200 patients by Coffey and his colleagues (1977) from Georgetown University, Washington D.C. They had an incidence of hyperplasia of 6 per cent with no recurrence in any patient at the time of reporting. The finding of unsuspected hyper-calcaemia accounts for an increasing number of diagnoses in the majority of recently published reports.

The successful management of persistent hypoparathyroidism after radical neck surgery has taken a significant step forward by the first report of the successful transplantation of frozen parathyroid tissue into the forearm in man (Wells et al., 1977) from Duke University. Successful animal experiments have demonstrated that parathyroid isografts will function after preservation at $-200\,°C$ for nine months. A patient with severe, poorly controlled renal osteodystrophy had 5 large parathyroid glands removed and some tissue was cryopreserved in liquid nitrogen at $-200\,°C$. The serum calcium fell sharply and six weeks later an autograft was placed in a forearm muscle. The graft was soon producing parathyroid hormone and the patient subsequently underwent a successful renal transplantation. He remains normo-calcaemic more than 2 years after receiving his parathyroid autograft. The long term survival of this graft will be watched with interest.

It is thus not too fanciful to suggest that all patients in whom 3 or more parathyroid glands are being removed should have some tissue placed in cryopreservation, for replacement should persistent postoperative hypo-calcaemia occur.

It is unusual to have details of the outcome of re-exploration of the parathyroids for persistent or recurrent disease. Wang (1977), in Boston, reports on the results of second and subsequent operations on 112 patients. A total of 110 abnormal parathyroid glands was found, 19 per cent of these as a result of mediastinal exploration. A fifth gland was found on four occasions.

Ultimate success in the treatment of primary hyperparathyroidism rests with the surgeon who must be able to explore thoroughly all the possible sites for parathyroid tissue.

REFERENCES

Coffey R. J., Lee T. C. and Canary J. J. (1977) The surgical treatment of primary hyperparathyroidism. *Ann. Surg.* **185,** 518.

Edis A. J., Becks U. J., Heerden J. A. and Akloari O.E . (1977) Conservative versus liberal approach to parathyroid neck exploration. *Surgery* **82,** 466 – 472.

Haff R. C. and Armstrong R. G. (1974) Trends in the current management of primary hyperparathyroidism. *Surgery* **75,** 715.

Prinz R. A., Paloyen E., Lawrence A. M. et al. (1977) Radiation-induced hyperparathyroidism. *Surgery* **82,** 296 – 302.

Wang C. A. (1977) Parathyroid re-exploration: a clinical and pathological study. *Ann. Surg.* **186,** 140.

Wells S. A., Gunnells J. C., Gutman R. A., Shelbourne J. D., Schneider A. B. and Sherwood L. H. (1977) The successful transplantation of frozen parathyroid tissue in man. *Surgery* **81,** 86.

EYE DISEASES

J. I. McGILL MA, DPhil, FRCS

CHOROIDAL MALIGNANT MELANOMA

In the ophthalmological world a great deal of interest has been shown in the diagnosis and managment of choroidal malignant melanoma. Over the last two years many papers and a recent symposium have highlighted both the difficulty in the differential diagnosis between benign and malignant choroidal melanoma, and the management of malignant melanoma, particularly the small posteriorly placed lesion.

In the past many authors have correlated mortality with pathological changes on the basis of the Callender classification (Callender, 1931), but many experienced ocular pathologists have great difficulty in agreeing amongst themselves as to the classification of cells in a choroidal melanoma (MacRae, 1953). Furthermore, Gass (1977) has pointed out that such classifications are based on only a few sections of a tumour, whereas if other cell types were present elsewhere in the tumour, the mortality figures would be biased and many tumours thought to contain only spindle A cells could have other cell types present in other parts of the tumour. Therefore, the previous studies (e.g. Paul et al., 1962) which have shown a definite but low mortality in spindle A and spindle B tumours (81 and 73 per cent surviving in each group after 15 years) may reflect the difficulty in pathological classification in such tumours rather than any definite mortality associated with spindle A cell types. Also, the eventual mortality rates of many series are often based on figures relying more on clinical impressions for the cause of death than on biopsy or autopsy confirmation. The fundamental flaw using a cytological classification is that firstly there is no absolute pathological criterion for malignancy, secondly in many cases clinicians probably do not observe the tumours for long, so that there is an incomplete clinical observation, and thirdly that the pathologist's report is based on the clinical observation of biological activity. None of Callender's 35 patients with spindle A or spindle B tumours died of the tumour, leading Gass (1977) to believe that the Callender classification is not a classification of malignant melanoma but rather a cytological classification of melanocytic tumours, 'some of which are benign'. In Hagler's series of 92 patients (Hagler et al., 1977) there were 6 with spindle A tumours, none of whom died from the tumour.

Therefore, the diagnosis, management and prognosis of choroidal melanoma will be reviewed in the light of recently published papers.

Clinical diagnosis of choroidal melanoma

The choroidal melanoma has to be particularly differentiated from a choroidal secondary or a choroidal haemorrhage. The clinical differentiation between a benign and a malignant melanoma of the choroid is based on the appearance of the tumour, its rate or absence of growth on continued observation, and the use of specialist investigations such as fluorescein angiography, ultrasonography or radioactive phosphorus (^{32}P) uptake.

Gass (1977) has pointed out that clinical features favouring a benign lesion include normal vision, a small flat lesion with white drusen on the surface (colloid bodies), absence of feeder vessels or a serious retinal detachment, and the absence of orange (lipofusin) pigment on the surface of the lesion. Furthermore, such benign lesions can be associated with hypopigmentation of the retina, with cystoid retinal changes on the surface or even a neovascular membrane between the retina and the choroid due to a break in Bruchs membrane and growth of the choroidal vessels through it to lie beneath the retina. Such pigmented lesions do not grow under observation or grow only slowly. *Malignant lesions,* on the other hand, tend to affect vision, are larger, elevated more than 2 mm, deeply and unevenly pigmented with irregular clumps of orange (lipofusin) pigment on their surface, with pigment breaking through the retina and associated with a serous retinal detachment. On continued observation such lesions usually show growth (Gass, 1977).

On fluorescein angiography the presence of a malignant melanoma is suspected if there are spots of hyperfluorescein which increase in intensity during the course of the angiogram. This has been thought to be due to changes in the pigment epithelium, and to abnormal highly permeable and irregular vessels (Singh Hayreth, 1970; Gass, 1977). However, McMahon, Tso and MacLean (1977) histologically localized fluorescein injected intravenously some 2 – 20 minutes before enucleation of an eye with a melanoma. Immediately after enucleation the eye was freeze-dried and the fluorescein was identified in sections of the tumour. The intensity of the fluorescein staining was greatest in the extracellular spaces. In spindle tumours there was a great deal of cohesion between the cells with minimal extracellular spaces, so that these lesions tended to fluoresce very little. There was a dense fluorescence in those tumours that had necrosis, macrophages present, or extracellular spaces in which there was extravisication of plasma. In addition, there was marked hyperfluorescence in tumours filled with epithelioid cells, due to the lack of cohesion between individual cells and the wide extracellular spaces resulting. So it would appear that hyperfluorescence of malignant tumours is due to pooling of the fluorescein.

The radioactive phosphorus test has been used to try to differentiate between benign and malignant melanomas. It has had a recent revival after a period of disfavour due to a high number of erroneous results, and inability to place the probe accurately over posteriorly placed lesions. The uptake is compared between the suspected tumour area and a non-involved area, and the percentage uptake depends on:

$$100 \times \frac{\text{average counts over the tumour: average counts over the non-involved quadrant of the globe}}{\text{average count over the non-involved quadrant of the globe}}$$

Shields et al. (1975) considered that a value of more than 50 per cent was positive and diagnostic of a tumour, whereas Char et al. (1976) considered 60 per cent diagnostic. Shields et al. (1975) reviewed the results of the test on 100 consecutive cases of histologically proved malignant melanomas, on which the ^{32}P test was performed prior to enucleation. The test was positive in all 100 cases, and there was a significant difference between these uptakes and those from 30 benign lesions; with no false positives encountered. Char et al. (1976) correlated the results of radioactive phosphorus uptake with histopathological observations in 29 patients who had had an enucleation for ocular malignant melanoma. There was enough scatter in the results to make individual analysis unreliable, though the higher uptakes were found in the more malignant lesions. Lower ^{32}P tests were found in spindle cell melanomas than in those with mixed cell melanomas. There was no correlation between the ^{32}P tests and the tumour volume, age and sex of each patient, duration of symptoms before enucleation, fluorescein angiograph findings or involvement of the overlying retina. In their series of 92 consecutive patients, seen between June, 1965, and June, 1971, Hagler et al. (1977) found no statistically significant correlation between the ^{32}P test results and cell types, nor between ^{32}P uptake and size of the tumour. They were unable to predict either the degree of malignancy or the 5-year prognosis for the patient using the test.

However, the ^{32}P test carries the criticism that the patient is exposed to radioactivity and the investigative dose is close to the therapeutic one. The therapeutic use of ^{32}P has a definite morbidity. In addition, especially for posteriorly placed choroidal lesions, a surgical procedure is necessary as the probe of the counter has to be placed over the lesion and such manipulation can lead to vitreous haemorrhage or central retinal artery occlusion, as Burton (1976) has shown in a series of 13 cases. Robertson (1976) also observed bleeding into and under melanomas in such circumstances. As both Robertson (1976) and Char and Hogan (1977) have pointed out, such manipulation could influence tumour dissemination. Char and Hogan (1977) found a 10 per cent incidence of ocular complications after the ^{32}P test.

False negative results can be recorded over lesions later found to be malignant melanomas. Robertson (1976) reported on 2 such cases, one of which was thought to be negative due to an increased distance between the counting probe and tumour due to a haemorrhagic detachment. In an extensive series Shields (1977) reported on 500 cases of melanoma investigated with the ^{32}P test. After i.v. injection of the ^{32}P the uptake was measured after 48 hours, with greater than 50 per cent regarded as positive. One hundred and seventy-two patients were measured using the transconjunctival route, but the accuracy was much less than if the probe was placed directly on the sclera. In 328 such patients 98·8 per cent of malignant tumours and 96·9 per cent of benign tumours were correctly diagnosed.

Some benign lesions may have a positive ^{32}P test, and some malignant lesions a negative result. Because of this unreliability, and because of the theoretical and established complications of this test, Char and Hogan (1977) do not recommend the ^{32}P unless an enucleation is planned anyhow in the event of a positive result.

For these reasons the advent of *ultrasonography* has been of great use in the diagnosis of solid choroidal tumours. In a recent series Shields et al. (1977) reported on 358 eyes enucleated for malignant melanoma, of which 31 had opaque media. Between 1962 and 1971 before the advent of radioactive phosphorus and ultrasonography, one-third of the enucleated eyes with opaque media had unsuspected melanoma, and there was a 36-month average delay in diagnosis of such tumours. They pointed out that the diagnosis of such tumours in eyes with cataracts or a hazy vitreous was much faster with the use of these diagnostic tools, and of the 13 patients seen between 1971 and 1975 there was only a 4-month delay, and the combined use of these diagnostic tools was positively successful in all cases. Of the 19 patients with melanoma patterns shown on either A or B scan ultrasound, 12 had a positive radioactive phosphorus uptake and all were proved histologically to have malignant melanoma. The 7 that had a negative radioactive phosphorus uptake, however, were all documented later on follow-up to have had benign lesions such as a subretinal haemorrhage. The authors concluded that ultrasonography and radioactive phosphorus were useful diagnostic aids in eyes with opaque media. They advocated the use of the B scan to detect possible intra-ocular tumours and, if this was positive, then to use the A scan to pinpoint the exact location and to obtain more information of the tissue diagnosis. Hodes and Choromokos (1977) in 19 cases found that the A scan gave an accurate picture of tissue texture and enabled them to diagnose correctly malignant melanoma in 18 of the 19 cases, the false positive being due to an atypical retinoblastoma.

Pathological prognostic factors

Recent studies of enucleated eyes have tried to predict which cytological changes are significant in assessing mortality rates. McLean, Foster and Zimmerman (1977), in a series of 217 patients with small melanoma, found that there was an overall mortality of 25 per cent in 6 years, rising to 36 per cent in 10 years. They found that if the tumours were small mortality occurred later than if the tumours were large. In all they found seven risk factors which were significant. The *first,* and most important, was *the cell type.* If the tumour was less than 10 mm in diameter, there was a 6·5 per cent mortality if spindle cells were present, but this rose to 47 per cent if the cell types were either mixed or epithelioid. Similarly, if the tumour was larger there was an 18 per cent mortality for spindle cells, rising to 64 per cent if mixed cell type or epithelioid were present. The *pigmentation* of the tumour was important, for if it was light the prognosis was better than if it was heavy (9·5 − 63 per cent mortality respectively over ten years). Overall, if the tumour was *less than 8 mm in size* there was only a 15 per cent mortality, but *greater than 14 mm* carried an 86 per cent mortality. Other important factors included *scleral extension of the tumour,* for if there was none there was a 27 per cent mortality, if half the sclera was invaded there was a 54 per cent mortality, but if the episclera had been reached then the mortality climbed to 68 per cent. The degree of *mitotic activity* was important as well if the optic nerve had been invaded. If there was no *optic nerve invasion* there was only 31 per cent mortality, but 60 per cent if the posterior lamina had been invaded. The *position of the tumour* was also found to be important, for if it involved the ciliary body there was a 58 per cent mortality, whereas if it were posterior to the equator there was only a 23 per cent mortality. Shammas and Blodi (1977) also correlated mortality with cytological changes in enucleated specimens in a series of 293 cases with a minimum 5-year follow-up. They found that *the age* of the patient was important, for if the patient was under 60 there was a 27 per cent mortality, which rose to 47 per cent if the patient was more than 60. They too found that the *type of cell* present was vital in determining the prognosis, with a 6 per cent mortality for spindle A tumours rising to 64 per cent with epithelioid tumours. Other factors that they found important were in agreement with McLean et al. (1977), such as the *position of the tumour,* its *size* and the *degree of pigrentation.* They also pointed out that the greater the *height of the tumour* the higher the mortality, and that if *Bruch's membrane* was invaded, and the tumour was less than 2 mm in height, there was only a 7 per cent mortality, which rose steeply if Bruch's membrane had been ruptured. Overall, they found that if Bruch's membrane was intact and the tumour was lightly pigmented, small and relatively flat, there was a much better prognosis than if the tumour was heavily pigmented, large and breaking Bruch's membrane.

Overall, the data would suggest that the cell type is the significant feature and that the presence or absence of epithelioid cells is one of the most important progostic factors. Small tumours containing epithelioid cells have mortality rates similar to that of larger tumours with similar cells.

Management of small melanocytic tumours of the choroid

In the past many have advocated enucleation of small malignant melanomas, but there is no good clinical evidence that enucleation in these cases increases the survival rate. Recently, several authors, e.g. Gass (1977), Zimmerman and McLean (1975), and Char and Hogan (1977), have taken a more conservative approach, on the grounds that such small tumours are difficult to differentiate from benign ones, and that the various investigations, such as ^{32}P and fluorescein, are unreliable in these cases. Furthermore, Zimmerman and McLean (1975) have shown in a series of 105 small choroidal lesions that most were spindle cell tumours, and the mortality from such tumours were very low. Davidorf and Lang (1974), in their series of 43 small melanomas, found that 20·9 per cent were of mixed and epithelioid cell types, but overall there was only a 7·1 per cent mortality over 5 years, but others have found that the mortality from small tumours with the same cell type, being 50 per cent (Zimmerman and McLean, 1975), suggesting that metastasis, if it is going to occur in these tumours, occurs early (McLean et al., 1977), and that early enucleation is ineffective. Furthermore, enucleation can increase the intra-vascular spread of a malignant melanoma. Fraunfelder et al. (1977) studied the longevity of hamsters with experimental ocular melanoma. One group had their eyes atraumatically enucleated with special care not to manipulate the tumour, or cause a rise in intra-ocular pressure, and the tumour was isolated before surgery began by means of freezing it. Another group had their eyes conventionally enucleated. They found that compared to controls (untreated) the atraumatically enucleated group fared better than the traumatically enucleated group, suggesting that the intravascular spread of malignant cells at the time of surgery is an important factor in the prognosis of the condition.

It is for these reasons that some clinicians now merely observe patients with small asymptomatic malignant melanomas, particularly if there is no evidence of growth. Gass (1977) studied 38 patients with small (less than 15 mm) tumours of uncertain aetiology, for periods ranging from 1 to 10 years. Two patients showed tumour growth, and had an enucleation, and both had spindle B tumours. All 38 are alive and well. Another 20 had small melanocytic tumours diagnosed as malignant melanoma, which were observed for periods ranging from 4 months to 11 years. Thirteen tumours grew, 12 were enucleated, but no patient has yet developed evidence of metastatic melanoma. Char and Hogan (1977) studied 20 patients with small elevated pigmented choroidal lesions for from 2 to 20 years. Diagnostic tests such as ^{32}P test and ultrasonography were often misleading, and enucleation was only carried out in 9 of their patients whose tumour was found on serial observation to have increased in size. None of the 20 patients has developed detectable metastatic disease. They also found that close serial examination without therapeutic intervention is safe in such patients with small melanomas. Hogeweg et al. (1976) followed 2 patients with small pigmented choroidal lesions, and only enucleated when definite growth was observed.

As Gass (1977) has pointed out, 'Observed growth is the only reliable clinical indication of possible malignancy.' However, others disagree with this conservative approach. Hagler et al. (1977) carried out early enucleation in 84 out of 92 patients having malignant melanoma of the choroid, diagnosed on clinical grounds and using the ^{32}P test. Enucleation was performed as soon as the diagnosis was made, without waiting for evidence of tumour growth. With all types of tumour (large and small) they had a 14 per cent 5-year mortality, which compares with the 50 – 80 per cent rates reported from other series (*see* e.g. Yanoff and Fine, 1975), and is in agreement with the experimental evidence of Fraunfelder et al. (1977) that early enucleation is beneficial.

Treatment

If a malignant melanoma is diagnosed and treatment decided upon, enucleation has been the classic treatment. However, in some patients this is not advised, either because the tumour may not have affected the vision or because it is an only eye or because the patient may refuse enucleation. Alternative treatments that have been tried have included diathermy, radium discs, cobalt gamma ray applications, cryotherapy and light coagulation and local excision.

Recent work has assessed the use of the *cobalt plaque*. The complication rate of this form of treatment is high. McFaul (1977) has pointed out that the complications include loss of brow and lashes, changes in the lacrimal gland producing a dry eye even up to 16 months later, or telangiectasia and iris atrophy, which can be accompanied by scleral necrosis. More importantly, complications can result producing loss of vision due to retinal vascular occlusion and optic nerve ischaemia. These vascular changes can develop up to 2 years after treatment, and it is throught that when regression of a tumour takes place it is due to these ischaemic processes. However, many tumours treated with cobalt plaque therapy do not respond to treatment, and McFaul and Morgan (1977) have reported on 100 patients treated this way, of whom 23 had eyes enucleated after cobalt therapy. Enucleation took place on an average of 32 months after treatment because of failure of treatment with evidence of continued tumour growth or because of radiational complications leading to a painful blind eye. In 17 of the 23 eyes there was no evidence of tumour necrosis, though irradiation changes were apparent in the adjacent tissues. Necrosis was found in only 6 cases and was marked in 2 of these. Yet, despite this, the 5-year survival rate was 86 per cent, compared with 50 per cent when treatment was enucleation, which suggests that irradiation can enhance survival. McFaul (1977), reporting on those patients who did not require enucleation after the cobalt therapy, found that only 20 had vision of 6/18 or better, and 4 were blind.

Other disadvantages of cobalt therapy are that not only does it require a surgical procedure for the implantation of the disc, but also there is a considerable scatter to the surrounding normal tissue. Constable and Gragoudas (1977) have reported on the use of proton irradiation. They point out that the optimal requirements for external beam irradiation of eye tumours are minimal scatter, tissue sparing on the site of entry and finite penetration of the beam with minimal irradiation of tissue beyond the tumour target. These physical requirements can be met with high energy proton beams which can be colonated into very small beams that retain their shape when penetrating to the target, and have a well defined range in tissues with a density of ionization delivered to tissues, which is maximal as the particles stop. Such beams were directed at a simulated ocular tumour in the owl monkey eye when a silicone sponge was sutured to the sclera. As much as 20 000 rads in single doses were delivered to a localized area of choroid without producing clinical side-effects in follow-up periods of up to 3 years, neither in the cornea or sclera at the entrance point of the rays, nor in the lens if the mitotically active cells at the equator were not irradiated. The authors found that if 2 major branch veins were included in the lesion very close to their branching near the optic disc, then secondary retinal oedema and exudation may occur in unirradiated areas six months to three years later. They developed a technique of applying this irradiation method to a human. A special apparatus was required for precise head fixation and the ocular target was positioned by sterotactic radiography of tantalum markers on the scleral surface. Immobilization of the eye itself was achieved either by voluntary fixation on a target or by retrobulbar anaesthesia. A television camera monitored minor eye movements. The first patient was treated in 1975, and the tumour showed signs of regression after 4 months. So far 5 have been treated, with no definite tumour regression, but changes of colour have been observed (Gragoudas et al., 1977). A long follow-up of this form of treatment may be of extreme interest.

Local excision of a choroidal tumour has been advocated. Foulds (1977) has recently reported on the elaboration of this technique. Of 22 patients with choroidal lesions 4 were in the ciliary body or iris. The remainder had uveal lesions. Prior to surgery he treated around the tumours with photocoagulation to seal the retina down and to prevent cell emboli from invading the tumour. At a later date a local excision of the mass was carried out by means of turning down a scleral flap to expose the tumour and overlying retina. The retina itself was separated from the tumour in some cases, but in others had to be removed as well. Three eyes were enucleated due to technique difficulties, but of the remainder the lesions were successfully excised and all patients were alive and well up to 8 years later with 10 of the 15 having useful vision. This highly skilled technique could well be used in future for local excision of small malignant melanomas.

Future developments

Fraunfelder et al. (1977) have pointed out that during ^{32}P testing scleral depression of a globe during routine examination of the globe, or even vigorous rubbing of the eyes, can significantly increase intra-ocular pressure. In the hamster, when tumours were inoculated into the eye, ocular massage statistically reduced the longevity of the animals. As those animals atraumatically enucleated had a longer survival than those traumatically enucleated, these results are in agreement with the principle of the no-touch-isolation technique practised in the surgery of colonic cancer, and could well influence the ophthalmological use of such investigations requiring ocular manipulation, such as the ^{32}P test or ultrasound.

In the future, conservative management of small ocular choroidal melanomas may well be more widespread, and the ^{32}P test used less and less. Treatment methods such as photocoagulation, which causes a rise in intra-ocular pressure, and cobalt therapy, which requires surgical manipulation, could thus theoretically lead to intravascular spread of the tumour. Future methods of investigation and treatment will have to take this into account, and a controlled trial is required of the effect on survival rate of the ocular no-touch technique.

REFERENCES

Burton T. C. (1976) Iatrogenic breaks in Bruch's membrane in choroidal melanoma. *Trans. Am. Acad. Ophthalmol. Otolaryngol.* **81**, OP841.

Callender G. (1931) Malignant melanotic tumours of the eye: A study of histologic types in 111 cases. *Trans. Am. Acad. Ophthalmol. Otolaryngol.* **36**, 131.

Char D. H., Brooks Crawford J., Irvine A. R., Hogan M. J. and Howes E. L. (1976) Correlation between degree of malignancy and the radioactive phosphorus uptake test in ocular melanomas. *Am. J. Ophthalmol.* **81**, 71.

Char D. J. and Hogan M. J. (1977) Management of small elevated pigmented choroidal lesions. *Br. J. Ophthalmol.* **61**, 54.

Constable I. and Gragoudas E. (1977) Proton irradiation for small malignant melanomas of the choroid. In: Brockhurst R. J., Boruchoff S. A., Hutchinson B. T. and Lessell S. (ed.), *Controversy in Ophthalmology.* Philadelphia, Saunders.

Davidorf F. H. and Lang J. R. (1974) Small malignant melanomas of the choroid. *Am. J. Ophthalmol.* **78**, 788.

Foulds W. S. (1977) The results of choroidectomy in the treatment of malignant melanoma of the choroid. *Trans. Ophthalmol. Soc. U.K.* In the press.

Fraunfelder F. J., Boozman F. W., Wilson R. J. and Thomas A. H. (1977) No touch technique for intraocular malignant melanomas. *Arch. Ophthalmol.* **95**, 1616.

Gass J. D. (1977) Problems in the differential diagnosis of choroidal nevi and malignant melanomas. Jackson Lecture. *Am. J. Ophthalmol.* **83**, 299.

Gragoudas E. S., Koehler A. M., Verhey L., Tepper J., Suit H. D., Brockhurst R. and Constable I. J. (1977) Proton irradiation of small choroidal malignant melanomas. *Am. J. Ophthalmol.* **83**, 655.

Hagler W. S., Jarrett W. H. and Killian J. H. (1977) Use of ^{32}P test in the management of malignant melanoma of the choroid. *Trans. Am. Acad. Ophthalmol. Otolaryngol.* **83**, OP49.

Hodes B. L. and Choromokos E. (1977) Standardized A-scan echographic diagnosis of choroidal malignant melanomas. *Arch. Ophthalmol.* **95**, 593.

Hogeweg M., Bas P. J. M., Greve E. L. and DeHaar A. B. (1976) Malignant melanomas of the choroid that on fluorescein angiograph and perimetry gave the impression of naevi. *Doc. Ophthalmol.* **40**, 301.

McFaul P. A. (1977) The results of local radiotherapy in the treatment of malignant melanoma of the choroid. *Trans. Ophthalmol. Soc. U.K.* In the press.

McFaul P. A. and Morgan G. (1977) Histopathological changes in malignant melanomas of the choroid after cobalt plaque therapy. *Br. J. Ophthalmol.* **61**, 221.

McLean I. W., Foster W. D. and Zimmerman L. E. (1977) Prognostic factors in small malignant melanomas of choroid and ciliary body. *Arch. Ophthalmol.* **95**, 48.

McMahon R. T., Tso M. O. M. and McLean I. W. (1977) Histological localization of sodium fluorescein in choroidal melanomas. *Am. J. Ophthalmol.* **83**, 836.

MacRae A. (1953) Prognosis in malignant melanoma of the choroid and ciliary body. *Trans. Ophthalmol. Soc. U.K.* **73**, 8.

Paul E. V., Parnell B. L. and Fraker M. (1962) Prognosis of malignant melanomas of the choroid and ciliary body. *Int. Ophthalmol. Clin.* **2**, 387 – 406.

Robertson D. M. (1976) Radioactive phosphorus uptake testing of choroidal lesions. *Br. J. Ophthalmol.* **60**, 835.

Shammas H. F. and Blodi F. C. (1977) Prognostic factors in choroidal and ciliary body melanomas. *Arch. Ophthalmol.* **95**, 63.

Shields J. A. (1977) Diagnostic methods in intraocular malignant melanoma. *Trans. Ophthalmol. Soc. U.K.* In the press.

Shields J. A., Hagler W. S., Federman J. L., Jarrett W. H. and Carmichael P. L. (1975) The significance of the ^{32}P uptake test in the diagnosis of posterior uveal melanomas. *Trans. Am. Acad. Ophthalmol. Otolaryngol.* **79**, 297.

Shields J. A., McDonald P. R., Leonard B. C. and Canny C. L. B. (1977) The diagnosis of uveal malignant melanoma in eyes with opaque media. *Am. J. Ophthalmol.* **83**, 95.

Singh Hayreth S. (1970) Choroidal melanomata. Fluorescence angiographic and histopathological study. *Br. J. Ophthalmol.* **54**, 145.

Yanoff M. and Fine B. S. (1975) *Ocular Pathology.* New York, Harper & Rowe.

Zimmerman L. E. and McLean I. W. (1975) Changing concepts of the prognosis and management of small malignant melanomas of the choroid. *Trans. Ophthalmol. Soc. U.K.* **95**, 487.

GENERAL PRACTICE

J. D. E. KNOX MD, FRCP, FRCGP

INTRODUCTION

During the past few years, the volume of medical literature has markedly increased: general practice, which formerly contributed little, has gradually been adding to what has now become a flood of information. Several attempts are now made to systematize general practice bibliography; for example, *'New Reading for General Practitioners'* is a helpful list published quarterly by the Royal College of General Practitioners. The Department of Health and Social Security also publish a bibliography, *'Current Literature on General Medical Practice'*, which is up-dated monthly.

Despite these and other aids, any attempt to give a concise and comprehensive account of recent work in general practice is difficult enough; to make such an account coherent is almost impossible, if the 'general' nature of general practice is to be preserved. Bringing together various topics, at first sight unrelated to one another, may result in a disjointed contribution. Perhaps the kaleidoscopic effect may be minimized by viewing the collected papers against a broad background of *patient care*.

REFERENCES

Department of Health and Social Security. *Current Literature on General Medical Practice*. London, HMSO.

Royal College of General Practitioners. *New Reading for General Practitioners*. London, BMA.

FROM MEDICAL CURE TOWARDS HEALTH CARE

Can good medical care be provided at reasonable cost? The McKinsey Company (Maxwell, 1975) has reviewed the situation in Western Europe, the USA and the USSR, attempting to relate to various indices of health the available resources and how they are deployed. Included in the report is a most telling figure, showing the diminishing returns resulting from increases in expenditure.

A somewhat similar approach has been employed by the Health Departments in the UK, in *Prevention and Health: Everybody's Business* (DHSS, 1976). This document advocates action to promote the concept of the individual assuming responsibility for his own health and for that of his family, as well as placing emphasis on prevention.

Both the publications referred to in this section highlight the increasing relevance of the low-technology and relatively high cost-effective problem-orientated characteristics of UK general practice.

REFERENCES

Department of Health and Social Security (1976) *Prevention and Health: Everybody's Business. A consultative document prepared jointly by the Health Departments of Great Britain and Northern Ireland*. London, HMSO.

Maxwell R. (1975) *Health care: The Growing Dilemma. Needs v. Resources in Western Europe, the US and the USSR*, 2nd ed. New York, McKinsey.

SELF-CARE

What factors determine who visits the doctor and who does not? It might be thought that the presence of a symptom was the determinant. Yet studies show that the situation is much more complex: there exist in the community more people with symptoms who might consult than those who actually contact the doctor. What factors are responsible for seeking medical help?

To answer this question, Anderson et al. (1977) designed a study using 'matched pairs' with the following characteristics:

1. Both members of the pair had suffered a similar complaint in the past 2 weeks.
2. One member (termed 'the user') had consulted a doctor for the complaint.
3. The other member ('non-user') had not consulted a doctor for the complaint nor for any other reason in the past year.

Ten general practitioners collaborated, selecting in each practice 100 patients who had attended in a 2-week period. Each was matched with the first non-user of the same sex and 5-year age group in the case files. After much elimination at interviewing, 60 pairs were found, each member having a similar complaint, being registered with the same practice and so on. Differences between the matched pairs were the subject of special study, and among the results the following features emerged: Those who visited the doctor

1. Perceived themselves as less healthy.
2. Fewer had attempted self-treatment.
3. None reported serious personal problems.
4. Fewer reported obstacles to visiting the doctor.

As the authors point out, for self-care to be encouraged, it must be done through a doctor – patient relationship which fosters health education, if serious under-use of necessary medical care is to be avoided. Studies are needed on how over-users can be educated to different patterns of behaviour.

A worth-while narrative account by a patient of how he went about changing his 'unco-operative general practitioner' is given by Bowshill (1977). The reactions of the BMA, the Post Office, the public library, and the doctors he approached make salutary reading for the medical profession. The patient had to overcome hostility and make a considerable effort—and in the end found himself a general practitioner of the kind he felt he needed.

REFERENCES

Anderson J. A. D., Buch C., Danaher K. and Fry J. (1977) Users and non-users of doctors—implications for self-care. *J. R. Coll. Gen. Pract.* **27**, 155 – 159.
Bowshill D. (1977) Choosing a doctor. *J. R. Coll. Gen. Pract.* **27**, 125.

PROVIDING MEDICAL CARE: A PROFESSIONAL CRITIQUE

AUDIT

If the patient comes to the doctor, how may a high quality of service be ensured? The idea that clinicians (including general practitioners) should keep a critical eye on what they are doing is not new; yet for a number of reasons it has been developed less fully in general practice than in other disciplines, possibly because it may be seen as a threat by the more professionally isolated general practitioner. If it is *self-imposed* and aims at achieving a measurable improvement in the quality of care through education, activity analysis may become generally more acceptable. That this can be one way in which colleagues in community medicine can help the general practitioner is demonstrated by a paper from Gruer and her colleagues (1977). They started by examining all patients referred urgently for surgical problems to one hospital. Since abdominal pain accounted for 10 per cent of all new patients, they reviewed this problem in detail, studying diagnostic accuracy, proportions of patients not admitted, percentage of admissions operated upon, and so on. It became clear that there was room for improvement in diagnostic accuracy by all doctors, both in hospital and in general practice. They were able to influence the situation in hospital and measure the resulting improvement (mainly in terms of a decrease in proportions of patients admitted). The next and most significant stage of their work was to extend the audit to include one large group practice, with the full and willing cooperation of the general practitioners. It was at this stage that the community medicine specialist came into the picture and 'held the ring'. A descriptive analysis of the practice's use of the hospital for acute abdominal pain led to an analysis of abdominal pain presenting in primary care. Feedback of this information educated the hospital surgical staff in several respects, e.g., the reasons behind some of the apparently 'unnecessary' referrals (21 per cent referrals were not admitted).

The authors plan to extend their study in a number of ways, crossing the hospital – general practice interface, with the aim of producing a statistically significant increase in the proportion of cases where the general practitioner is certain about the diagnosis, the proportion of patients referred who are admitted, and the proportion where initial diagnosis agrees with final hospital diagnosis.

Much can be done by the general practitioner himself, however, and frequently he is the only one who is in a position to capture the data and relate the findings at different stages in the evolution of a clinical problem.

An important paper published from the Birmingham Research Unit of the Royal College of General Practitioners sets out the case for evaluation in some detail (Royal College of General Practitioners, 1977). This advocates a method of continuous clinical and administrative self-audit or self-evaluation in which the reference standard is not some arbitrary absolute, but is determined by the observations and discussions of others involved in the same situation (a peer group). Such a scheme needs information in a form which identifies and highlights differences, without value judgements about which is right or best. Examples are given of how, by making a start with an examination of the prescribing by members of a group practice, practice policy on repeat prescriptions came to be altered. Building on this work, the Unit has invited general practitioners to take advantage of its computing facilities and provide standardized information on various practice activities which can be analysed and fed back rapidly.

Such observations fed in from different practices can be of help not only to practitioners cooperating in the system, but also those concerned with teaching undergraduates, training postgraduates, and carrying out research.

Competence to practise

Concern to ensure the maintenance of standards of professional competence is expressed not only in the current preoccupation with medical audit but also by the publication of the Alment Committee's report (Alment, 1976). Set up 'to review the present methods of ensuring the maintenance of standards of continuing competence to practise and of the clinical care of patients and to make recommendations', the committee includes the following among its recommendations: 'In our view it is a necessary part of a doctor's professional responsibility to assess his work regularly in association with his colleagues.' The committee came down against any form of compulsory re-examination at present in the UK. The report also includes a thought-provoking report by a working part on records which, among other things, relates the business of recording what the doctor does to quality and standards of care.

REFERENCES

Alment E. A. J. (1976) *Competence to Practise. The Report of a Committee of Enquiry set up for the Medical Profession in the United Kingdom.* London, CECP.
Gruer R., Gunn A. A. and Ruxton A. M. (1977) Medical audit in practice. *Br. Med. J.* **1,** 957 – 958.
Royal College of General Practitioners (1977) Self-evaluation in general practice. *J. R. Coll. Gen. Pract.* **27,** 265 – 270.

RECORDS, RECORDING, AND MEDICAL CARE

Among the many reasons for keeping clinical records in general practice, two can be singled out as important: (1) for providing good care at the level of the individual patient, and (2) for advancing knowledge about general practice. These aspects are illustrated by two recent publications. The first by Froggatt (1977) is related to the growing use made by patients of free contraceptive advice, introduced into the National Health Service in 1975. His paper describes a contraceptive record-card and flow-sheet, with the aim of assisting general practitioners to produce better surveillance. By careful design, the card groups together information important for clinical decision-making and is intended for use over a 6 – 9 year period. One side of the card is devoted to on-going arrangements for care, while the reverse side is reserved for information which is relevant but may not be needed at each consultation. The author has still to show that the use of his eminently sensible card in fact increases the quality of care in general practice.

The second aspect of record-keeping is illustrated by a publication which is of international significance (Royal College of General Practitioners, 1976). It is the result of several years' intensive work by a group of general practitioners drawn from such different countries as the USA, Canada, the UK, Norway, and Australia, but united by a common goal of helping general practitioners and others to classify the various conditions met in everyday work in general practice. In the past, it has been possible only to record *diseases,* yet, increasingly, patient contacts with general practice are concerned with *health* care. Furthermore, the routine work of general practice is related to solving *problems;* diagnosis, in the sense of a disease label, is often impossible or even irrelevant at the first contact stage. The working group of general practitioners, convened by the World Organisation of National Colleges and Academies of General Practice (WONCA) has produced a document which will allow for the classification of all the commoner problems encountered in day-to-day general practice without forcing the recorder into a straight-jacket of viewing all patient problems solely in terms of diseases. This classification has proved workable in four different countries; it is also compatible with the World Health Organisation's International Classification of Disease. It should prove to be a useful tool in further international collaboration among general practitioners.

REFERENCES
Froggatt C. (1977) A contraceptive card for use in general practice. *J. R. Coll. Gen. Pract.* **27**, 107 – 109.
Royal College of General Practitioners (1977) *An International Classification of the Health Problems of Primary Care by WONCA.* Occasional Paper No. 1, London, BMA.

PROVIDING HEALTH CARE

DEPUTIZING SERVICES AND OUT-OF-HOURS CALLS

The use of deputizing services continues to grow: they raise controversial issues—is there firm evidence that the care they provide has serious short-comings? Further studies reported from Sheffield by Dixon and Williams (1977) examine the workings of some 18 deputizing services in England. Using a 1 in 5 sample of nearly 500 000 patient contacts, they showed that there were considerable differences in the ways calls were handled e.g. proportions of patients referred to hospital varied between 9 per cent and 16 per cent, and proportions of calls judged to require no visit by a deputy varied between 3 per cent and 19 per cent. The authors conclude that their survey presents a reassuring picture and call for the removal of limitations on the use of deputizing services.

Lockstone (1976) analysed 163 night calls made on a group practice over one year. True emergencies accounted for 48 per cent, while 45 per cent were classified as unnecessary but reasonable, and only 7 per cent were regarded as irresponsible. This paper provides an interesting background against which to view the findings of a hospital doctor employed by an emergency call service. Gabriel (1976) analysed 153 home visits; only 14 per cent were regarded as medically essential and he records that 21 per cent of patients had no symptoms when visited. Most out-of-hours calls involve patients already under care or those whose view of the seriousness of their condition may differ from a doctor's. It could be argued that the patient's own doctor (or member of a partnership or group practice) is better placed to understand and relieve the real cause of anxiety.

REFERENCES
Dixon R. A. and Williams B. T. (1977) Twelve months of deputising: 500 000 patient contacts with eighteen services. *Br. Med. J.* **1**, 560 – 563.
Gabriel R. (1976) Emergency call service. *J. R. Coll. Gen. Pract.* **26**, 74 – 75.
Lockstone D. R. (1976) Night calls in a group practice. *J. R. Coll. Gen. Pract.* **26**, 68 – 71.

CARE OF CHILDREN AND THE FAMILY DOCTOR

Among the many recommendations of the Report of the Committee on Child Health Services (Court, 1976), two are especially important from the point of view of general practice. First, the preventive aspects of child health formerly administered by local health authorities and their successors under re-organisation of the National Health Service, should be merged with general practice. How feasible is it for general practitioners to undertake such work? Morris and Hird (1977), in Tayside, carried out a small-scale study in which two practices in a small community undertook school-health work on a seasonal basis. Their results were compared with those obtained from similar schools within the district where routine examinations were carried out by community health doctors. No practical problems arose, and, while the family doctors recorded less total morbidity than the community doctors, the significant morbidity was much the same in the two groups. The authors make a plea for the freeing of school doctors in the near future from the chore of unproductive screening for defects and for greater emphasis to be placed on 'Educational Medicine'.

A second important recommendation of the Court Report is that some general practitioners, perhaps one in three or one in four, should have extra training in paediatrics and become designated general practitioner paediatricians (GPP's). This recommendation has not met with a favourable reception from the majority of general practitioners, and it could be argued that there is still a lack of information about the extent to which general practice already meets the needs of child health.

Curtis Jenkins (1976) sampled the views on child health services of 5 general practitioners, 20 hospital-based doctors and 2 community health doctors. Findings in relation to such questions as 'Who should be responsible for surveillance?' and 'What steps need to be taken before a nationwide programme can be realized?' differed widely. The author expressed concern lest the experience of paediatric specialists working in areas with particular difficulties should unduly influence future patterns of child care in the UK. He warns that screening at the expense of providing a comprehensive paediatric illness service must be avoided at all costs.

New towns with large populations of children present ideal opportunities to study and implement extended primary care services for children. Bain (1977) visited some 10 new towns in a survey of general practitioner-based child care. He confirmed the high workload in these new situations and gained the impression that practices were 'overwhelmed by the demands from patients at the expense of innovations'. There was a general scepticism among general practitioners about the value of developmental screening clinics. The doctors themselves were strongly divided in their views as to how they can act most effectively in child health; for example, on how much could and should be delegated to the nursing sister and health visitor, on what role the general practitioner might play in care of the handicapped child, and on how social-work services might be improved. Bain recognizes the limitation of age-band specialization and the abhorrence expressed by some at the idea of a GPP, yet he feels that the objections may be less applicable in the new-town setting. He also considers that there is a case for separate funding of support services in new towns to allow full advantage to be taken of the opportunities and challenges they pose.

REFERENCES

Bain D. J. G. (1977) Child care in the new towns in the UK. *J. R. Coll. Gen. Pract.* **27,** 556 – 557.
Court S. D. M. (1976) Report of the Committee on Child Health Services. *Fit for the Future.* London, HMSO.
Jenkins G. Curtis (1976) Developmental and paediatric care of the pre-school child. *J. R. Coll. Gen. Pract.* **26,** 795 – 802.
Morris J. B. and Hird M. D. (1977) Employment of local general practitioners in the school health service. *Health Bull.* **35,** 119 – 128.

WORKING TOGETHER IN HEALTH CARE

Nursing, as a developing discipline, has much in common with general practice. Both have been attempting to develop a clearer identity, and much remains to be done in terms of simple descriptive studies. Mrs McIntosh and Professor Richardson of Aberdeen have collaborated in a work study of District Nursing Staff (McIntosh and Richardson, 1976) in an attempt to provide a firmer base for knowledge of mutual roles and functions. A research worker observed and timed 1961 home visits by various district nursing personnel; in addition, observations were made of the work carried out by nurses at practice premises. The authors build up a picture of the work currently being done and show the false assumptions commonly made when considering nursing in primary care. Categories of visiting, for example, are not homogeneous—a house call for an injection in one set of circumstances is not the same as a house call for an injection in another, and home nursing care consists of much more than technical procedures and some social chat. The paper suggests ways in which efficiency in teamwork could be improved, and draws attention to the skills (especially in decision-making) that home nursing requires.

While this paper describes the routine work of traditional district nursing, another paper by Hally et al. (1977) from Newcastle upon Tyne describes a scheme recently introduced to provide specialized nursing care of sick children in their own homes.

Team care and the sick child

Special considerations like maternal deprivation, which the general practitioner has to take into account when faced with a decision to admit a sick child to hospital, led to the setting up in 1974 of a scheme to provide specialized nursing care for such children in their own homes in Gateshead. Selected district nursing sisters, who were specially trained in paediatric nursing, looked after 22 children as the alternative to hospital admission. Most of these children were under 3 years of age, suffering from self-limiting acute conditions. In addition, 39 children were looked after in a scheme of planned discharge from hospital. They were older and usually required long-term support and education for conditions such as stabilized diabetes. Although there were 4 deteriorations in each group necessitating admission (or re-admission) to hospital, the majority of the children made rapid recoveries or good progress. The authors, while being cautious about the interpretation of the results of their evaluation, indicate that, in general, this innovation was well received: mothers were satisfied with home nursing, and the scheme avoided special arrangements having to be made for other siblings and the disruption entailed in visiting hospital.

Team care and child abuse

Group therapy for established psychiatric conditions is not a new idea but the potential of this form of activity in prophylaxis of psychosocial problems is explored in a paper by Roberts et al. (1977), working in collaboration with a primary care team in Didcot Health Centre. Mothers identified as being at special risk of inflicting injury on their children were selected from a register which had been compiled in a group practice. They were invited to attend together on a regular basis in the company of therapists specially skilled in counselling. One of the general practitioners acted as a 'co-therapist'. In addition, opportunities were afforded for the children of these disturbed families to meet as a group, with appropriate therapists available to coordinate their activities. Senior pupils from the local comprehensive school also assisted in the project. This paper sets out the criteria used and gives an interesting account of the lessons learned in an interesting approach to problems of prevention. The results appear encouraging enough to warrant a trial of the method elsewhere. The work reported is part of a larger project by the research team mentioned above.

The patient as a team member

Discussions on the health care team usually include the professionals—doctors, nurses, health visitors, receptionists, etc.—but it is only within the last few years that the idea of *patient* participation seems to have been promoted. As Wilson (1977) points out, the Health Service is a national one: it does not belong to the doctors, it belongs to the people. Wilson describes his experiences at Aberdare, where the partnership, now based on a health centre, had a long tradition of involvement in the community. A Patients' Committee participates with the doctors in running the primary care service at the health centre, considers complaints and improvements, provides health education, and communicates patients' opinions to various bodies concerned with the health service. This interesting paper shows what can be achieved in the field of health education and in identifying patients' needs by creating a system in which doctors become accountable not only to their profession but to 'their' patients, whom they know.

REFERENCES

Hally M. R., Holohan A., Jackson R. H., Reedy B. L. E. C. and Walker J. H. (1977) Paediatric home nursing scheme in Gateshead. *Br. Med. J.* **1**, 762 – 764.
McIntosh J. B. and Richardson I. M. (1976) *Work Study of District Nursing Staff.* Scottish Health Service Studies No. 37. Edinburgh, SHHD.
Roberts J., Beswick K., Leverton B. and Lynch M. (1977) Prevention of child abuse: group therapy for mothers and children. *Practitioner* **219**, 111 – 115.
Wilson A. T. M. (1977) Patient participation in a primary care unit. *Br. Med. J.* **1**, 398.

HEALTH, HEALTH HAZARDS AND THE GENERAL PRACTITIONER CARE

LEAD IN THE ENVIRONMENT

There is a growing body of evidence that health may be harmed by long-continued exposure to lead in the environment at levels insufficient to produce classical symptoms of lead poisoning. General practitioners have collaborated in several studies, two of which are reported here. In the first, Goldberg and his colleagues (Campbell et al., 1977), in cooperation with 62 general practitioners throughout Scotland, sampled water from 970 houses thought to have lead pipes or storage tanks. Blood samples were then taken from 283 people living in houses identified as having lead levels of over 0·48 μmol/l. The authors found a highly significant correlation between lead concentrations in water and blood. More disturbingly, raised blood lead levels were associated with renal insufficiency as evidenced by various biochemical findings, although none of the affected people showed clinical disease.

Froom (1977) presents evidence from America that increased absorption of lead, as shown by raised blood levels in a sample of 333 children, is closely correlated with low socioeconomic status. None of the children showed clinical evidence of lead poisoning. Froom suggests that the findings strengthen the case for screening, and that any screening programme should be aimed selectively to cover those most at risk—the poor and those living in antiquated housing.

REFERENCES

Campbell B. C., Beattie A. D., Moore M. R., Goldberg A. and Reid A. G. (1977) Renal insufficiency associated with excessive lead exposure. *Br. Med. J.* **1**, 482–485.
Froom J. (1977) Lead screening by family physicians. *J. Family Pract.* **4**, 631–633.

HYPERTENSION

Evidence that 'treating' a moderately raised blood pressure lowers mortality and morbidity may be controversial; evidence that a persistently raised blood pressure in the absence of other subjective or objective changes is potentially lethal rests mainly on actuarial computations, but there is no dispute that untreated hypertension with disease of kidney, heart or blood vessel may be lethal. The general practitioner is frequently presented with opportunities to record blood pressures in the course of routine clinical practice. With what frequency is this done, and what are among the reasons for blood pressure recording in general practice? Beevers and his colleagues in Glasgow (Barlow et al., 1977) took advantage of a large-scale strategic screening project to examine these questions in 3001 subjects who were also patients of nine general practitioners in Renfrew. A recording, made before attendance at screening, was found in 37·9 per cent. The blood pressure levels recorded correlate well with those obtained by the screening unit, and the general practitioner results added further cases to the unit's yield—some having been missed by the survey. Common reasons for taking a blood pressure in general practice included chest pain, headaches, lightheadedness, and dizziness: surprisingly, these symptoms did not appear to be helpful in the diagnosis of hypertension. The authors conclude that hypertension, if it is to be found, must be actively sought in some form of screening—and this could well include the 'tactical' screening open to general practitioners whenever a patient presents at the consulting room.

Broadly similar findings are reported from London in a paper by Heller and Rose (1977). Examination of the notes of 697 patients in a random sample of seven general practices showed that 24 per cent had had a blood pressure recorded in a 5-year period. The authors express their concern that more definitive action had not been taken in the case of diagnosed hypertension: the commonest drug treatment appeared to be sedatives and tranquillizers, yet 'these drugs have never been shown to be effective in the management of hypertension' (authors' quotation).

REFERENCES

Barlow D. H., Beevers D. G., Hawthorn V. M., Watt H. D. and Young G. A. R. (1977) Blood pressure measurement at screening and in general practice. *Br. Heart J.* **39**, 7–12.
Heller R. F. and Rose G. (1977) Current management of hypertension in general practice. *Br. Med. J.* **1**, 1442–1444.

ANTIBIOTIC THERAPY AND PATIENT CARE

The changing spectrum of bacterial resistance to antibiotics and the development of new antibiotics pose challenges to the general practitioner wishing to do the best for his patient presenting with problems requiring rapid solutions.

Two recent studies from general practice attempt to examine the place of amoxycillin and co-trimoxazole in the managment of two symptom complexes common in general practice—presumed infection of respiratory and urinary tract.

Respiratory infections in children

A double-blind, randomized, controlled trial of amoxycillin, co-trimoxazole, and placebo in 197 children with presumed viral respiratory infections is reported by Taylor and his colleagues from New Zealand (Taylor et al., 1977). The children were patients of a five-doctor suburban group practice sampled over a 10-week period in late winter. Three disease categories studied (nasopharyngitis, pharyngotonsillitis, and bronchitis) showed a generally similar pattern of resolution irrespective of treatment. There was a higher withdrawal rate from the trial and a higher consultation rate among children receiving a placebo.

The authors conclude that benefits of antimicrobial treatment in presumed viral respiratory infections are marginal and that the antibiotics studied should not be routinely prescribed for conditions in which β-haemolytic streptoccal infection is excluded.

Urinary infections

The second study, reported from general practice in Surrey (Grob et al., 1977), was undertaken because of doubts recently expressed about the activity of both ampicillin and co-trimoxazole in urinary infections. Amoxycillin, an antibiotic resembling ampecillin, but thought to be more rapidly bactericidal against *Escherichia coli,* was compared with co-trimoxazole.

In this study, involving 138 patients with 188 courses of treatment of probably urinary tract infection, pretreatment culture of urine samples revealed the presence of a treatable bacteriuria in only 83 instances. There was no significant difference between amoxycillin and co-trimoxazole in the eradication of the organisms identified. While all the cases treated with co-trimoxazole remained free from infection 4 weeks after the end of treatment, 2 cases of infection treated with amoxycillin had an early re-infection, but with different organisms, within 3 weeks of the end of the treatment.

Side-effects serious enough to warrant discontinuing the antibiotic occurred with equal frequency in both groups.

REFERENCES

Grob P. R., Benyon G. P. J., Gibbs F. J. and Manners B. T. B. (1977) Comparative trial of amoxycillin and co-trimoxazole in the treatment of urinary tract infection. *Practitioner* **219,** 258 – 263.

Taylor B., Abbott G. D., Kerr M. M. and Fergusson D. M. (1977) Amoxycillin and co-trimoxazole in presumed viral respiratory infections of childhood: placebo-controlled trial. *Br. Med. J.* **2,** 552 – 554.

DRUGS—SAFETY AND PATIENT CARE

Most general practitioners issue a prescription at least at every other consultation, and the bulk of all prescribing by the medical profession occurs in general practice. Several studies have reported on the prescribing habits of general practitioners, yet much remains to be discovered. Sir Richard Doll and his colleagues (Skegg et al., 1977) report an analysis of the distribution of dispensed prescriptions among a population of 40 000 people, registered with 19 general practitioners. The information on drugs, provided by the Prescription Pricing Authority, was linked to data obtained in connection with the separate Oxford Community Health Project. During one year more than half of all males and two-thirds of all females had at least one drug dispensed, with psychotropics accounting for almost one-fifth of all prescriptions. The paper sets out in some detail the various therapeutic classes of drugs, and points out the special feature of the study, namely the making available of accurate information on the distribution of prescriptions to identifiable individuals in a defined population.

It could be argued that interesting though this information may be when presented in this way, what could benefit the prescribing general practitioner more would be the rapid feedback of appropriately analysed data on his individual prescribing habits for his own interpretation and action. The impact of such information might be heightened by linking the drug data to the reasons for prescribing—and by presenting this as an item in the context of similar information from other doctors contributing to a monitoring system. Such a system is being developed in association with hospital-based studies in Dundee (Dingwall, 1977).

The value of cooperation among general practitioners in studying drugs and morbidity is further illustrated by the announcement by the Presidents of the Royal College of General Practitioners and the Royal College of Obstetricians concerning the risks of the oral contraceptive pill, based on the Royal College of General Practitioners' oral contraceptive study, the death rate from diseases of the circulatory system in women who had used oral contraceptives was five times that of controls who had never used them; and the death rate in those who had taken the pill continuously for 5 years or more was 10 times that of the controls. The excess deaths in oral contraceptive users were due to a wide range of vascular conditions. The total mortality rate in women who had ever used the pill was increased by 40 per cent, and this was due to an increase in deaths from circulatory diseases of 1 per 5000 ever-users per year. The excess was substantially greater than the death rate from complications of pregnancy in the controls, and was double the death rate from accidents. The excess mortality rate increased with age, cigarette smoking, and duration of oral contraceptive use. (*See* also p.102.)

REFERENCES
Dingwall D. W. (1977) Paper to Conference on Drug Monitoring, Oxford, June 1977. Dundee, Scottish General Practitioner Research Support Unit.
Royal College of General Practitioners (1977) Mortality among oral contraceptive users. *Lancet* **2**, 727–731.
Skegg D. C. G., Doll R. and Perry J. (1977) Use of medicines in general practice. *Br. Med. J.* **1**, 1561–1563.

CONCLUSION

This contribution from general practice has deliberately focused attention on much that is properly the concern of health services research. Such an approach was chosen partly because the orientation of other chapters is more towards biomedical aspects of disease and partly because the opportunities for research in general practice are frequently to be found in the developing field of health service research. Further work remains to be done, and increasingly general practitioners need to cooperate with those in other disciplines, including many which are outside the strictly 'medical' field. Such cooperation can be of mutual benefit to, for example, nursing, the social sciences, and to general practice itself.

GERIATRICS

A. N. EXTON-SMITH MA, MD, FRCP

BARBITURATES AND FALLS AND FRACTURES

Macdonald and Macdonald (1977), of the City and Sherwood Hospitals, Nottingham, have demonstrated a significant correlation between the use of barbiturate hypnotics in the elderly and (1) the incidence of nocturnal fractures of the femoral neck, (2) confusional states, and (3) a history of falls and episodes of dizziness. Their study is based on an examination of 390 inpatients with femoral fractures whose ages ranged from 65 to 101 years, with a mean of 85·0 years. The patients were classified into three groups according to the time of occurrence of the fracture. The only striking difference between the groups when an analysis was made of the importance of a number of factors was found to be the use of barbiturates (*see Table* 1).

Table 1. PATIENTS WITH FEMORAL NECK FRACTURES

	Time of Fracture						*P* value
	10 p.m.-6 a.m.		6 a.m.-2 p.m.		2 p.m.-10 p.m.		
No. (%) on barbiturates	91	(93)	12	(6)	0		<0·001
No. (%) on any type of hypnotic	96	(98)	182	(84)	46	(61)	N.S.
No. (%) with history of frequent falls	39	(40)	54	(25)	17	(23)	<0.02
Total no. of patients	98	(100)	217	(100)	75	(100)	

Ninety-three per cent of the patients who suffered nocturnal fractures were taking barbiturate hypnotics compared with only 6 per cent of those with morning fractures and none of those with afternoon fractures (*P*<0·001). Wheras 46 (45 per cent) of the 103 patients taking barbiturates had a history of frequent falls (over 4 falls per week), only 64 (22 per cent) of the 287 patients not on barbiturates had had frequent falls (*P*<0·001). Time of fracture was not related to type of fracture, physical incapacity, concomitant disease, living alone or other kinds of medication.

On admission to hospital the fracture patients taking barbiturates were significantly more confused than patients not taking them, when assessed by a mental status questionnaire (MSQ). During their stay in hospital barbiturates were withdrawn from all but 6 patients; 85 patients were discharged on non-barbiturate hypnotics and 12 on no hypnotics. At discharge the MSQ scores of the patients who had originally been taking barbiturates had improved significantly, so that they were rather better than those of patients who had not previously taken barbiturates. For these latter patients the MSQ scores had not significantly changed during the course of their stay in hospital. Thus barbiturate withdrawal during admission reduced confusion and gave clinically important benefits.

In addition to the study of hypnotic use in patients with femoral neck fractures, the authors also investigated the use of barbiturates and other hypnotics in new outpatients referred to the geriatric department. While the use of non-barbiturate hypnotics declined from 50 per cent in 1973 to 41 per cent in 1976, the proportion of patients taking barbiturates increased significantly from 41 to 51 per cent during the same period. Falls or dizziness were the reasons for referral of 86 per cent of the patients seen in the out-patient clinic in 1973 if they were taking barbiturates, but in only 23 per cent of the new patients not taking barbiturates. The association between barbiturate medication and a history of falls or dizziness was highly significant ($P<0\cdot001$). The study of the fracture patients indicates that the greatest liability to falls occurs within about 8 hours of taking barbiturate hypnotics. Overstall and his colleagues (1977), of University College Hospital, London, investigated the effects of drugs likely to impair postural balance in elderly people by measuring body sway using a Wright ataxiameter. The amount of sway recorded 10 – 12 hours after taking night sedative drugs was no different from that recorded in elderly patients not receiving such drugs.

Brocklehurst and his colleagues (1977, 1978) have investigated the factors involved in fracture of the femoral neck in 384 patients admitted to three Manchester hospitals and two London hospitals. In 352 patients information was available on the time of the fall and whether or not they were taking hypnotics. Eighty per cent were not taking any hypnotic, 11 per cent were taking non-barbiturate hypnotics and 9 per cent were taking barbiturates. There was no association between those takining hypnotics (of either type) and nocturnal fractures. In this series only 14 per cent of fractures occurred at night (10 p.m. – 7 a.m.), compared with the 25 per cent in the Nottingham series occurring between 10 p.m. and 6 a.m. An age and sex matched control series of patients without femoral neck fractures showed that 90 per cent were taking no hypnotic, while 5 per cent were on barbiturates and 5 per cent on non-barbiturate hypnotics. The marked differences revealed by the two surveys of femoral neck fractures, both in prescribing habits and in the ill-effects which may follow the use of barbiturates, indicate the need for further studies of this kind in other centres.

REFERENCES

Brocklehurst J. C., Exton-Smith A. N., Lempert Barber S. M. and Palmer M. K. (1977) Barbiturates and fractures. *Br. Med. J.* **3**, 699.
Brocklehurst J. C., Exton-Smith A. N., Lempert Barber S. M., Hunt L. P. and Palmer M. K. (1978) Fracture of the femur in old age: a two-centre study of associated clinical factors and the cause of the fall. *Age Ageing* **7**, 7.
Macdonald J. B. and Macdonald E. T. (1977) Nocturnal femoral fracture and continuing widespread use of barbiturate hypnotics. *Br. Med. J.* **3**, 483.
Overstall P. W., Exton-Smith A. N., Imms F. J. and Johnson A. L. (1977) Falls in the elderly related to postural imbalance. *Br. Med. J.* **1**, 261.

A LONGITUDINAL STUDY OF ISCHAEMIC HEART DISEASE

Kitchin and Milne (1977), of the Western General Hospital and the Royal Victoria Hospital, Edinburgh, over a 5-year period, have investigated 215 men and 272 women whose ages ranged from 62 to 90 years. The object was to record mortality rates and the incidence of new manifestations of ischaemic heart disease in the 5-year period and to relate these to subject characteristics at the start of the study.

Mortality and cause of death

Of the original 487 subjects 138 died (28·3 per cent) during the 5-year period. Myocardial infarction or ischaemic heart disease was the cause in 37 and myocardial failure in 2; the remaining 99 were non-cardiac deaths with the exception of 2 from valvular heart disease. At the first examination (Kitchin et al., 1973), 10 per cent gave a positive response to Rose's questionnaire (Rose and Blackburn, 1968) in respect of angina or infarction. The 5-year mortality in those with a history of angina was 10/53 (19 per cent) and in those without such a history it was 122/427 (29 per cent). Death rate in those giving a history of infarction was 8/32 (25 per cent) compared with 125/449 (28 per cent) in those without this history. These rather surprising results are ascribed by the authors to the unreliability of the Rose questionnaire in elderly subjects as well as to the difficulty in relating chest pain to cardiac pathology in the individual case.

Taking levels of 160 and 100 mm Hg for upper values of normal blood pressure mortality was higher for both men and women with pressures above these levels. Ischaemic heart disease accounted for a large proportion of this increased mortality. For the overall mortality the effect of systolic hypertension was significant only in women during a 14-year study in the Framingham survey (Kannel et al., 1971), a raised systolic blood pressure was more strongly associated with the development of ischaemic heart disease than was raised diastolic pressure, and the importance of systolic pressure in this association was greater with increasing age.

All types of electrocardiographic abnormality present at the initial examination exerted an unfavourable effect on the death rate from ischaemic heart disease. Since both electrocardiographic abnormalities and mortality increase with age the analysis was carried out for separate age groups. This showed that the overall death rate and the death rate from ischaemic heart disease were significantly associated with ST depression ($P<0·02$), T inversion ($P<0·01$) and with atrial fibrillation ($P<0·02$), and these unfavourable effects were exerted independently of their association with age.

Changes in 5-year survivors

A re-examination was carried out of 252 (72 per cent) of the 349 subjects who survived 5 years. There was little overall change in the frequency of positive responses to the Rose questionnaire, but nearly half the subjects who gave a history of angina at the first interview did not do so at the second, while none of those who gave a positive response for infarction did so at the second. These findings indicate that episodes of pain associated with angina are likely to be forgotten by older subjects when questioned 5 years later.

Blood pressure fell from 151·6±2·4 mm Hg systolic and 79±1·3 mm Hg diastolic to 149·6±2·5 and 77·8±1·3 respectively for men, and from 163·3±2·2 systolic and 88·3±1·3 diastolic and 148·3±2·1 and 82·6±1·3 in women. The magnitude of the fall was related to height of the blood pressure at the initial readings.

There was an increased frequency of all electrocardiographic abnormalities at the second survey. The greatest increase occurred in T wave inversion, ST depression, left ventricular hypertrophy and left axis deviation. In each case the increase was at a rate of about 1·5 per cent per annum. There was found to be a close correspondence in the increase in prevalence rates derived from the longitudinal study and those revealed by an analysis on a cross-sectional basis of changes in different age groups at the start of the study.

REFERENCES

Kannel W. B., Gordon T. and Schwartz M. J. (1971) Systolic versus diastolic blood pressure and risk of coronary heart disease: the Framingham study. *Am. J. Cardiol.* **27**, 335.

Kitchin A. H., Lowther C. P. and Milne J. S. (1973) Prevalence of clinical and electrocardiographic evidence of ischaemic heart disease in the older population. *Br. Heart J.* **35**, 946.

Kitchin A. H. and Milne J. S. (1977) Longitudinal survey of ischaemic heart disease in randomly selected sample of older population. *Br. Heart J.* **39**, 889.

Rose G. A. and Blackburn H. (1968) *Cardiovascular Survey Methods.* Geneva, WHO.

POTASSIUM STATUS OF OLD PEOPLE

It is generally believed that primary dietary deficiency of potassium does not occur in man (Davidson and Passmore, 1969). This view has been challenged by Judge (1972), working in the Department of Geriatric Medicine, University of Glasgow. He found that 56 per cent of a random sample of elderly people in Rutherglen received less than 60 mmol of potassium in their diet each day. A controlled crossover trial in 19 of these subjects showed an improvement in muscular strength and in mental function when 60 mmol of supplementary potassium was administered daily. Judge concluded that many old people are potassium deficient and would benefit from potassium supplementation.

There have been three recent studies in which the potassium status of the elderly has been investigated. Burr and his colleagues (1975), of the MRC Epidemiology Unit, Cardiff and the Gwent Geriatric Service, Newport, found that 37 per cent of a sample of people over the age of 70 living in two adjacent villages in S. Wales had a daily potassium intake of 45 mmol or less. Forty-six of these old people with low intakes completed a controlled crossover trial of supplementary potassium 48 mmol per day for 2 weeks. The results are shown in *Table* 2. The most striking finding is the absence of any benefit of potassium supplementation over placebo in these old people.

Table 2. GRIP STRENGTHS, REACTION TIMES AND MEMORY SCORES (MEAN±S.E.) WHEN SUBJECTS RECEIVED POTASSIUM AND PLACEBO

	Grip strength arbitrary units	Reaction time, msec	Memory score
When subjects received potassium	53·78±2·72	342·6±14·2	19·39±1·45
When subjects received placebo	53·98±2·71	338·5±15·6	19·54±1·29
Differences within subjects (potassium-placebo)	−0·196±1·77	4·15±13·6	−0·152±1·47

Bahemuka and Hodkinson (1976), of the Geriatric Department, Northwick Park Hospital, London, investigated the potassium status of 103 healthy subjects over the age of 65 by measurement of red blood cell potassium. There was no correlation between red blood cell potassium and grip strength. By means of 'step down' multiple regression analysis it was shown that only age and sex were significant predictors of grip strength ($P<0\cdot001$ for each). The red cell potassium levels were found to be normally distributed and there was no suggestion of the existence of a hypokalaemic subgroup such as might be expected if potassium deficiency were common in elderly subjects.

In the third study conducted by MacLennan and his colleagues (1977), of the University of Southampton, the University of Manchester and the Institute of Naval Medicine, Alverstoke, potassium status was assessed by measurement of ^{40}K on a whole-body counter in 13 healthy elderly subjects whose weight, skinfold thickness and grip strength were also recorded. These measurements were repeated after a 3-month course of potassium supplements given in a dose of 36 mmol per day. There were no significant changes in the total body potassium content nor in the ratio of total body potassium to lean body mass. An increase in right hand grip strength occurred after three months' potassium supplementation, but this was thought to be a placebo effect since no similar increase in grip strength occurred in the non-dominant side. The mean value of the ratio of total body potassium to lean body mass was 57 mmol/kg, which is lower than the ratio of $62\cdot6$ mmol/kg for young and middle aged people reported in the literature. The authors conclude that old people on diets containing adequate potassium often have low total body potassium levels compared with younger people, but these cannot be corrected by potassium supplements.

Thus the results of these three studies on healthy old people are in substantial agreement; potassium status is best evaluated by measurement of red cell potassium levels or by the whole body counter, it is not related to grip strength and it is not influenced by potassium supplementation. Nevertheless, potassium depletion is of considerable clinical importance. In elderly inpatients it is caused by other factors, such as the use of diuretics, and it plays a major role in the high incidence of digitalis toxicity.

REFERENCES

Bahemuka M. and Hodkinson H. M. (1976) Red blood cell potassium and hand grip strength in healthy elderly people. *Age Ageing* **5**, 116.
Burr M. L., St Leger A. S., Westlake C. A. and Davies H. E. F. (1975) Dietary potassium deficiency in the elderly; a controlled trial. *Age Ageing* **4**, 148.
Davidson S. and Passmore R. (1969) *Human Nutrition and Dietetics* (4th ed.). Edinburgh, Livingstone, p. 137.
Judge T. G. (1972) Potassium metabolism in the elderly. In: Carlson L. A. (ed.), *Nutrition in Old Age*. Stockholm, Almquist & Wiksell.
MacLennan W. J., Lye M. D. W. and May T. (1977) The effect of potassium supplements on total body potassium levels in the elderly. *Age Ageing* **6**, 46.

EMEPRONIUM BROMIDE FOR THE TREATMENT OF URINARY INCONTINENCE

Cystometric studies show that the uninhibited neurogenic bladder is the most common abnormality giving rise to urinary incontinence in the elderly. Decreased cerebral inhibition produces a contracted bladder in which massive detrusor contractions occur at low filling pressures with small volumes of urine in the bladder. Urgency of micturition and resultant incontinence present a major problem in management. In the past 20–30 years numerous anticholinergic drugs have been used in an attempt to treat the condition and emepronium bromide is the drug which is now most often prescribed. The clinical results are usually disappointing and this may be due to poor absorption of the drug, lack of end-organ response or the inappropriate selection of patients.

Ritch and his colleagues (1977), of the Faculty of Medicine, University of Southampton, have investigated these possibilities by studying the effects of emepronium on cystometric patterns in a group of elderly patients with incontinence due to an uninhibited neurogenic bladder. Following cystometry, 7 patients were given an intramuscular injection of 50 mg emepronium bromide and the cystometry was repeated 1 hour later. All patients were then given emepronium bromide 200 mg orally three times a day and the cystometry was repeated in 6 after an interval of 7 – 10 days. Three were given a second intramuscular injection of 50 mg emepronium bromide and a further cystometry was performed 1 hour later. The results are shown in *Table* 3.

Table 3. RESULTS OF CYSTOMETRY (MEAN±1S.D.) BEFORE AND AFTER TREATMENT WITH EMEPRONIUM

	1	2	3	4
	Initial Cystometry	After 50 mg i.m.	After one week oral therapy	One week oral therapy + 2nd i.m. dose
No. of patients in group	9	7	6	3
Recorded bladder capacity (ml)	91±104	333±118 $P<0.01$	97±65	367±126
Volume at 1st sensation of desire to void (ml)	61±45	214±87 $P<0.01$	97±65	272±89
Volume at 1st bladder spasm (ml)	74±65	300±42* $P<0.01$	97±65	293±181
Pressure during bladder spasm (cm water)	69±22	38±11 $P<0.01$	74±27	15±6
Intravesical pressure at bladder capacity (cm water)	72±20	25±22 $P<0.01$	83±13	28±23

* Only 2 patients in group.
P values refer to comparison of 1 with 2.
i.m. = intramuscularly.

Intramuscular emepronium bromide increased significantly the mean bladder capacity and the mean volumes at the first sensation of desire to void urine and at the onset of bladder spasms ($P<0.01$). In 5 of the 7 patients bladder contractions were completely abolished and in a further patient their frequency was greatly diminished. The intravesical pressure was reduced both during contractions and when the bladder was full ($P<0.01$). Oral therapy had no significant effect on the measurements.

In this study a good end-organ response to the parenteral administration of emepronium bromide was demonstrated. The failure of oral therapy is most likely due to inadequate or irregular absorption from the gastointestinal tract which is known to occur when quaternary ammonium compounds are given by mouth. This hypothesis was confirmed when in the same study emepronium bromide was shown to reduce the peak levels of the plasma concentrations of simultaneously administered propranolol. Three patients received 40 mg propranolol orally before starting emepronium bromide and after 7 days therapy, and blood levels of propranolol were measured at timed intervals for 8 hours afterwards. In all 3 patients there was a delay and reduction in the peak plasma concentrations of propranolol and this effect was attributed to the oral emepronium bromide causing a delay in gastric emptying. The likely explanation of these results is that some emepronium bromide must have been absorbed to act on the cholinergic receptors in the gastric smooth muscle, thus reducing gastrointestinal motility, but the amount was insufficient to produce measurable effects on the cholinergic receptors in the bladder. It can be concluded from this study that anticholinergic drugs are of limited value in the management of urinary incontinence unless they can be given by a parenteral route, thus avoiding their effects on gastrointestinal motility.

REFERENCE
Ritch A. E. S., Castleden C. M., George C. F. and Hall M. R. P. (1977) A second look at emepronium bromide in urinary incontinence. *Lancet* **1**, 504.

GYNAECOLOGY AND OBSTETRICS

JOHN BONNAR MA, MD, FRCOG

DISORDERS OF MENSTRUATION

A problem which often presents to the family doctor is the young woman with infrequent or absent menses. In the last five years the disorders of menstruation have been the subject of intense research, which followed on the development of sensitive methods, using radioimmuno-assay to measure pituitary and ovarian hormones. Three gonadotrophin hormones are now identified: follicle stimulating hormone (FSH), luteinizing hormone (LH) and prolactin. The control and function of prolactin is yet uncertain, but abnormal prolactin production is now known to be an important cause of secondary amenorrhoea and infertility.

Hyperprolactinaemic amenorrhoea

Amenorrhoea, combined with abnormal breast-milk secretion (galactorrhoea), has been recognized for centuries and was mentioned in the Aphorisms of Hippocrates. Many cases of amenorrhoea, due to elevated prolactin, do not have obvious galactorrhoea and this appears to be due to the wide variation in the sensitivity of the glandular tissue of the breast to prolactin. Women with amenorrhoea and hyperprolactinaemia are typically oestrogen-deficient. This may be clinically manifest with atrophic changes in the lower genital tract and the absence of withdrawal bleeding following a progestogen challenge. Despite the low levels of circulating oestradiol 17 β which are seen in most cases with hyperprolactinaemia, the serum gonadotrophin concentrations are not usually elevated. The failure of gonadotrophin secretion to rise, despite the profound oestrogen deficiency, implies an abnormality of the feedback control of gonadotrophin secretion. Since these patients release normal amounts of gonadotrophin in response to an injection of gonadotrophin-releasing hormone, the disorder of feedback may represent a failure of the hypothalmic/pituitary unit to respond to oestrogen (Glass, 1975).

Dr. H. S. Jacobs of St Mary's Hospital Medical School, London, and Dr. S. Franks of the Middlesex Hospital, London, recently reported their experience of 60 women with amenorrhoea due to prolactinaemia (Jacobs and Franks, 1976). The incidence of pituitary tumours in association with hyperprolactinaemia has been difficult to establish and the findings of these authors is therefore of particular interest. Based upon the results of radiology (lateral skull X-ray, cone views and lateral tomography of the pituitary fossa in all cases) and in some patients on operative findings, the patients were placed into one of three groups, according to the presence, or absence of a pituitary tumour. The authors acknowledge that it is not possible to establish with certainty whether a very small tumour is present, that is not visible radiologically, but they postulate that the majority of hyperprolactinaemic patients with normal X-rays do indeed have micro tumours of the pituitary. Of the 60 patients, 36 had no radiological evidence of pituitary tumour (Group 1). Seventeen of the 60 patients had an enlarged pituitary fossa detected on X-ray (Group 2). Seven patients of the 60 had received pituitary ablative therapy before being referred to them (Group 3). None of the 60 was taking any drug to raise prolactin levels and hypothyroidism was excluded clinically and by measurements of serum thyroxin and free thyroxin index.

The serum prolactin concentrations in the patients confirmed the lack of correlation between milk production and prolactin secretion. Galactorrhoea had occurred in about one-third of the patients and if this symptom alone had been used as an index for requesting a prolactin measurement, the diagnosis would have been missed in two-thirds of cases. Jacobs and Franks consider that the probability of a tumour being present can be obtained from the prolactin measurement. In their experience radiologically visible tumours were unusual in patients with serum prolactin levels below 80 μg/l; conversely a level above 100 μg/l rarely occurs in a patient with a radiologically normal pituitary fossa. These conclusions have particular importance because of the great difficulty which can be encountered in interpreting X-rays of the pituitary region. The incidence of pituitary tumours in the series of Jacobs and Franks is acknowledged as being higher than would normally be encountered because of bias in referral. They point out, however, that pituitary tumours probably occur in about 5 – 7 per cent of all women with amenorrhoea.

In women with hyperprolactinaemia, a characteristic history of galactorrhoea, present or past, may be found and symptoms of oestrogen deficiency may usually be found also. Superficial dyspareunia, and particularly failure of the vagina to moisten during intercourse are especially common; flushing attacks may also occur. Examination of the breasts may reveal evidence of milk secretion. Speculum examination usually shows a thin vaginal epithelium with little or no mucus coming through the cervical os. The uterus is palpably small, and if an endometrial biopsy is taken scanty inactive endometrium is obtained. Confirmation of the oestrogen deficiency in these patients may be obtained from a progestogen challenge test. Medroxy-progesterone acetate, 5 mg per day for five days, will produce a withdrawal bleed from a well oestrogenized endometrium, and a failure to bleed indicates that oestrogen production has not been sufficient to maintain the endometrium. Jacobs and Franks had a negative response to the progestogen challenge test in 88 per cent of their patients.

The treatment of a patient with hyperprolactinaemia requires to be individualized. If a patient has a radiologically visible pituitary tumour and she desires to become pregnant, Jacobs and Franks recommend prior pituitary ablative therapy, either with external irradiation, followed by secondary treatment with bromocriptine, or with a transsphenoidal surgical removal of the tumour. The aim here is to avoid the sudden enlargement of a pituitary tumour which could occur during pregnancy. Primary treatment with bromocriptine is reserved for patients in whom careful radiological evaluation has produced no evidence of a pituitary tumour, and for those with tumours who have no wish to conceive, providing the encephalogram has excluded upward extension of the tumour. Repeat X-rays of the pituitary fossa should be obtained before the patient embarks upon pregnancy and during pregnancy careful supervision with assessment of the visual fields at regular intervals is advisable.

In patients with hyperprolactinaemia treatment with bromocriptine rapidly lowers prolactin level and normal menstruation recurs within 5/6 weeks. Previously these patients showed no response to clomiphene and required treatment with gonadotrophin to induce ovulation. Treatment with bromocriptine has replaced the use of gonadotrophin injections in two-thirds of women requesting induction of ovulation (Jacobs et al., 1975). The advantages of treatment with bromocriptine over gonadotrophin are considerable; in contrast to gonadotrophin therapy treatment with bromocriptine is simple and, since it is not associated with ovarian hyper-stimulation, it requires none of the expense of clinical and biochemical monitoring that is required with gonadotrophin therapy.

Side effects with bromocriptine are usually transient. They include nausea and vomiting and this can be avoided by taking the drug with food. Postural hypotension occurs in some women and this problem can be obviated by taking the drug immediately before retiring at night. The one disadvantage of treatment with bromocriptine is that the prolactin levels are controlled, only while the drug is taken. Serum prolactin concentrations return rapidly to pretreatment levels, as soon as the drug is discontinued. The requirement, therefore, of prolonged and expensive therapy could be considered to constitute a strong argument for definitive surgical removal of prolactin-producing pituitary tumours, especially as small micro tumours, which are not radiologically detectable, are likely to be present in many patients with hyperprolactinaemic amenorrhoea (Jacobs et al., 1976). The technique of transsphenoidal micro-surgical selective removal of pituitary adenomas has been described by Hardy (1973); as yet, however, this technique is not widely available. Whether long-term treatment with bromocriptine will prevent further enlargement of pituitary micro-tumours is at present unknown.

Weight loss amenorrhoea

Amenorrhoea developing in the context of severe imposed weight loss is now an extremely common condition in young women. This type of amenorrhoea which is associated with impaired gonadotrophin secretion and a concomitant oestrogen deficiency was recently reviewed by Jacobs (1976). A great deal of confusion still remains in this area, due to the problems of establishing strict diagnostic criteria relating to the presence of a psychiatric disorder, namely anorexia nervosa and its diverse forms. A spectrum of psychiatric and physical features exist and the particular one predominating will determine, to a large extent, the specialist to whom the patient is referred—psychiatrist, physician, endocrinologist or gynaecologist.

A triad of psychiatric disturbance, weight-loss and amenorrhoea constitutes the recognizable features of anorexia nervosa. The amenorrhoea is nearly always secondary as the disorder usually appears after puberty. Rarely self-imposed weight loss may cause primary amenorrhoea and delay the appearance of secondary sexual characteristics. The amenorrhoea can precede the weight loss, but more often accompanies it. In the British Isles, amenorrhoea appears to be almost the rule when weight falls below 45 kg. The existence of regular, ovulatory menstrual cycles seems to depend on maintaining body weight at a particular level and amenorrhoea will follow when the weight falls below a certain critical level.

During the phase of severe weight loss, gonadotrophin secretion is very low and may be undetectable. As a result of severe gonadotrophin deficiency, ovarian follicles fail to develop, as shown by low concentrations of oestradiol 17 β and atrophy of the breasts and the lower genital tract. Two other features have now been suggested which may contribute to the profound oestrogen deficiency that characterizes this disorder. First is that extra ovarian oestrogen production, i.e. by the conversion of androstenedione to oestrone in fat cells, is minimal because of impaired production of the precursor and also because of the loss of fat tissue. The second feature which may contribute to the oestrogen deficiency is the recently reported finding that the preferred catabolic pathway of oestradiol 17 β is weight-dependent: in thin people, as in patients with hyperthyroidism, the balance of catabolism favours a relatively greater production of 2-methoxy-oestrone and so less oestriol is produced (Fishman et al., 1975). Whereas oestriol has oestrogenic potency, 2-methoxy-oestrone has features of an anti-oestrogen, in that, although it will bind competitively to the uterine cytoplasmic oestrogen binding protein, it has no intrinsic biological activity.

The patient with anorexia nervosa and severe weight loss thus acquires gonadotrophin deficiency which causes failure of follicular maturation and consequent deficiency of oestrogen; the lack of fat tissue also denies the patient extra ovarian sources of oestrogen and what little oestrogen is made can be antagonized by the endogenous production of an anti-oestrogen.

As the patient gains weight gonadotrophin secretion recommences and a linear relationship between body weight and the FSH response to gonado-trophin releasing hormone has been shown (Warren et al., 1975). It appears that the hypothalamic pituitary production of gonadotrophin recovers first and later the ovary begins to respond to stimulation by the endogenous gonadotrophin. A period of apparent ovarian refractoriness is not uncommon and may result from the severe oestrogen deficiency that characterizes this disorder and the presence of anti-oestrogenic effects of 2-methoxy-oestrone.

The logical treatment of patients with weight-related amenorrhoea is for the woman to put on weight. If this can be achieved to the extent that the pre-morbid weight is regained, the majority of patients will ovulate and where anovulatory infertility has been the problem, pregnancy is usually readily achieved. The problems of such treatment are, however, considerable, and although the reproductive disturbance is closely related to weight, the overall disorder is primarily psychiatric. In a study of patients presenting with amenorrhoea, partially recovered anorexia nervosa was the commonest single cause of amenorrhoea and accounted for one-third of all the cases (Jacobs et al., 1975).

The appearance of the patient with partially recovered anorexia nervosa may be deceptive and the history of the previous severe weight-loss may be frequently suppressed. A return of the body weight to a level which is metabolically safe is usually inadequate to ensure the return of ovulatory cycles. Since these patients are usually oestrogen-deficient and even in a partially recovered form may rarely respond to clomiphene, ovulation induction with exogenous gonadotrophin is usually undertaken. Despite the extensive amounts of psychiatric and endocrine study to which these patients have been subjected, they remain a challenging group in terms of their resistance to therapy (Hull et al., 1976).

Primary ovarian failure

Menstruation normally ceases at or around the age of 50 years. The characteristic endocrine feature of the menopause is oestrogen deficiency and high gonadotrophin levels due to the natural depletion of the genetic endowment of oocytes. The events accompanying ovarian failure have recently been investigated by several workers.

In women with normal ovulatory cycles, oestrogen production is based upon oestradiol 17 β which is secreted by the developing ovarian follicle and reaches peak levels just prior to the LH surge which induces ovulation. During and after the menopause, when follicular maturation does not occur, the major oestrogen produced is oestrone. Although oestrone is secreted by the developing follicle during the reproductive years, it is produced almost exclusively in the postmenopausal woman by extraglandular aromatization of androstenedione, the sources of which are the postmenopausal ovarian stroma and the adrenal cortex. The major site of conversion to oestrogen is still uncertain, but present evidence suggests that fat tissue and hair folicles have the enzyme capacity to aromatize androstenedione (Nimrod and Ryan, 1975; Schweikert et al., 1975). Fat women are able to convert a greater proportion of the precursor androstenedione to oestrone than thin women. This probably explains how symptoms of oestrogen excess can occur in postmenopausal women despite cessation of ovarian function.

A gradual fall of the gonadotrophin levels is reported to occur with increasing age after the menopause and in some elderly women the levels may approach the pre-menopausal range (Chakravarti et al., 1976). This could be related to the increase of extraglandular oestrogen production which was shown to increase with age (Siiteri and MacDonald, 1973). Women who have had an early menopause often suffer more severely from symptoms of oestrogen deficiency than do women who have a late menopause, and this may be due to the greater overall deficit of oestrogen which develops in the younger woman (Jacobs, 1976).

In women with amenorrhoea due to primary ovarian failure, serum LH and FSH concentrations are high, but the LH level is also high at the time of the LH surge in the normal menstrual cycle. For diagnostic purposes, the level of FSH is more useful for distinguishing primary ovarian failure from the non-ovarian causes of amenorrhoea, as the levels are increased by four to five times that of normal (Jacobs, 1975). This provides a test, therefore, for the woman who has stopped menstruating and wishes to know if she has reached her menopause.

The diagnosis of primary ovarian failure or premature menopause in a young woman who wishes to become pregnant may be difficult to establish with certainty. Repeated assessment of both gonadotrophin and oestrogen production is required and laparoscopy is advisable to allow detailed inspection of the pelvic organs and ovarian biopsy. Chromosomal abnormalities, including mosaic forms causing primary ovarian failure, are well documented (Grumbach and van Wyk, 1974); full genetic investigation with karyotype analysis is required for a correct diagnosis.

Primary ovarian failure can also arise as a result of ovarian irradiation taking place inadvertently in women with disorders such as Hodgkin's disease. Thomas and colleagues (1976), in a recent analysis of 22 patients with Hodgkin's disease, found that doses of irradiation to the ovaries, about 500 rads, were commonly associated with ovarian failure. In 1 patient in the series, however, who developed a typical picture of primary ovarian failure—amenorrhoea, oestrogen deficiency and high serum gonadotrophin levels—after radiotherapy, pregnancy occurred some years later. It seems likely therefore that some oocytes may recover and subsequently respond to gonadotrophin stimulation. Damage to the ovaries may also arise from cytotoxic therapy. In rare situations, primary ovarian failure may arise in association with auto-immune disorders such as primary hypothyroidism and Addison's disease. Jacobs and Murray (1976) have emphasized the difficulty of diagnosing primary hypothyroidism in patients with a premature menopause, as thyroid function tests can be confusing.

When a diagnosis of primary ovarian failure (premature menopause) is established, the hormone deficiency should be treated by cyclical oestrogen administration, combined with a progestogen. Regular withdrawal bleeding provides protection from inducing hyperplasia of the endometrium and may offer protection against the long-term risk of endometrial neoplasia. Whether hormone therapy should be continued after the normal age of the menopause is questionable and must await more information on its advantages and disadvantages.

REFERENCES

Chakravarti S., Oram D., Forecast J. and Studd J. (1976) A study of gonadotrophins after the menopause. *Br. J. Obstet. Gynaecol.* **83**, 587 – 588.

Fishman J., Hoyar R. M. and Hellman L. (1975) Influence of body weight on estradiol metabolism in young women. *J. Clin. Endocrinol. Metab.* **41**, 989 – 991.

Glass M. R., Shaw R. W., Butt W. R. et al. (1975) An abnormality of oestrogen feedback in amenorrhoea-galactorrhoea. *Br. Med J.* **3**, 274 – 275.

Grumbach M. M. and van Wyk J. J. (1974) Disorders of sex differentiation. In: Williams R. H. (ed.), *Textbook of Endocrinology.* London, Saunders, pp. 423 – 501.

Hardy J. (1973) Transsphenoidal surgery of hypersecreting tumours. In: Kohler T. O. and Ross J. P. (ed.), *Diagnosis and Treatment of Pituitary Tumours,* pp. 179 – 185. (*Excerpta Med. Int. Congr. Ser.* 303.)

Hull M. G. R., Murray M. A. F., Franks S. and Jacobs H. S. (1976) Endocrinopathy of weight-recovered anorexia nervosa in women presenting with secondary amenorrhoea. *J. Endocrinol.* **66**, 43 – 44.

Jacobs H. S. (1975) Endocrine aspects of anovulation. *Postgrad. Med. J.* **51**, 209 – 214.

Jacobs H. S. (1976) Failure of components of the negative feedback system. In: Baird D. T. (ed.), *Clinics in Obstetrics and Gynaecology,* Vol. 3, No. 3. London, Saunders, pp. 522 – 524.

Jacobs H. S. and Franks S. (1976) Diagnosis and treatment of hyperprolactinaemic amenorrhoea. In: Bayliss R. I. S., Turner T. and MacLay W. P. (eds.), *Pharmacological and Clinical Aspects of Bromocriptine (Parlodel). Proceedings of a Symposium held at the Royal College of Physicians, London, May,* 1976. Tunbridge Wells, Kent, MCS Consultants.

Jacobs H. S., Franks S., Murray M. A. F., Hull M. G. R., Steele S. J. and Nabarro J. D. N. (1976) Clinical and endocrine features of hyperprolactinaemic amenorrhoea. *Clin. Endocrinol.* **5**, 439 – 454.

Jacobs H. S., Hull M. G. R., Murray M. A. F. and Franks S. (1975) Therapy orientated diagnosis of secondary amenorrhoea. *Horm. Res.* **6**, 268 – 287.

Jacobs H. S. and Murray M. A. F. (1976) The premature menopause. In: Campbell S. (ed.), *The Management of the Menopause and Post Menopausal Years.* Lancaster, England, MTP, pp. 359 – 368.

Nimrod A. and Ryan K. J (1975) Aromatization of androgens by human abdominal and breast fat tissue. *J. Clin. Endocrinol. Metab.* **40**, 367 – 372.

Schweikert H. U., Milewich L. and Wilson J. D. (1975) Aromatization of androstenedione by isolated human hairs. *J. Clin. Endocrinol. Metab.* **40**, 413 – 417.

Siiteri P. K. and MacDonald P. C. (1973) Role of extraglandular estrogen in human endocrinology. In: *Handbook of Physiology: Sect. 7, Endocrinology;* Vol. II, *Female Reproductive System,* Greep R. O., (ed. Part 1), pp. 615 – 630. Washington, D.C., American Physiological Society.

Thomas P. R. M., Winstanley D., Peckham M. J., Austin D. E., Murray M. A. F. and Jacobs H. S. (1976) Reproductive and endocrine function in patients with Hodgkin's disease: effects of oophoropexy and irradiation. *Br. J. Cancer* **33**, 226 – 231.

Warren M. P., Jewelewicz R., Dyrenfurth I., Ans H., Khalaf S. and van de Wiele R. L. (1975) The significance of weight loss in the evaluation of pituitary response to LH-RH in women with secondary amenorrhoea. *J. Clin. Endocrinol. Metab.* **40**, 601 – 611.

INFECTIOUS DISEASES

HILLAS SMITH MA, MD, FRCP

MORTALITY IN MENINGITIS

Bacterial meningitis is an eminently treatable disease, yet the overall mortality remains stubbornly high—an estimate of 20 per cent might not be too wide of the mark. It is possible within any group of patients with meningitis to recognize certain bad risk features—age of patient, type of infecting organism, presence of coma and presence of serious underlying disease, but even when all such factors are taken into account there remains an enigma as to why some patients with meningitis survive and others, apparently similar, do not. Does the standard of medical care, which differs from one institution to another, have any influence on the outcome? Some physicians have always felt that expert attention by specialists benefits patients and in the past the debate in regard to meningitis has been conducted at an unsatisfactory, even anecdotal, level which at best was inconclusive.

An attempt to alter this unsatisfactory situation has come from Goldacre (1976), an epidemiologist who reviewed 687 cases of acute bacterial meningitis identified in a defined population of children under 10 years of age. The study attempted to identify all cases of acute bacterial meningitis, meningococcal disease and acute meningitis of presumed bacterial aetiology occurring in the years 1969 – 73 in the North-West Metropolitan region of England (north-west London and adjacent counties, population 630 000 children). The results of treating these patients in three different groups of hospitals were assessed— infectious diseases hospitals, teaching hospitals and all other hospitals which were termed 'regional board' hospitals. Of the 687 patients 72 died, an overall case fatality rate of 10·5 per cent. There was no record of any diagnosed case of acute bacterial meningitis treated successfully without hospital care; 10 patients died outside hospital—the diagnosis being confirmed by autopsy. Surprisingly only 10 per cent of the surveyed patients were admitted to

Table 1. HOSPITAL OF ADMISSION BY ORGANISM

Organism	Type of hospital, number of cases (deaths) and proportion of cases						Total number	Case fatality rate %
	Teaching		Regional board		Infectious disease			
	Number	%	Number	%	Number	%		
Meningococcus	47 (1)	44·3	182 (24)	36·0	33 (1)	50·8	262 (26)	9·9
H. influenzae	27 (2)	25·5	147 (7)	29·0	17 (0)	26·2	191 (9)	4·7
Pneumococcus	8 (0)	7·6	53 (9)	10·5	5 (1)	7·7	66 (10)	15·2
Other named organisms	3 (0)	2·8	31 (9)	6·1	1 (0)	1·5	35 (9)	25·7
Organism unknown	21 (0)	19·8	93 (8)	18·4	9 (0)	13·8	123 (8)	6·5
Total	106 (3)	100·0	506 (57)	100·0	65 (2)	100·0	677 (62)	9·2

(10 patients died outside hospital)

(After Goldacre M. J., 1976)

infectious diseases hospitals, 16 per cent to teaching hospitals, but the regional board hospitals received 74 per cent. The mortality for the three groups of hospitals is also of interest—3 per cent, 3 per cent and 11 per cent respectively. Twenty-two per cent of all deaths (10 children died outside hospital and 6 were certified dead on admission) occurred before specialist care was reached. *Table* 1 taken from the paper gives details of hospital admissions and number of deaths.

Even when the different numbers of patients admitted to the different hospital groups is taken into account a mortality rate in the regional board hospitals almost four times that in the other two groups of hospitals is difficult to explain. The author suggests that the differences may reflect a higher proportion of gravely ill children admitted to the regional board hospitals or better medical care in infectious disease and teaching hospitals, or both. Other interpretations are possible.

REFERENCE
Goldacre M. J. (1976) Acute bacterial meningitis: where do children die? *Int. J. Epidemiol.* **5,** 343.

MENINGOCOCCAL MENINGITIS

There have been very considerable advances in recent years in the understanding of meningococcal infection, particularly in regard to epidemiology, the significance and control of the carrier state, and there have been a number of changes in therapy, particularly in view of widespread sulphonamide resistance resulting in a much wider use of penicillin as the major therapeutic agent, but the pathogenesis and appropriate management of major metabolic complications are as contentious as ever.

Table 2 shows the notifications at 10-year intervals together with the mortality rates for meningococcal infection from 1910 to 1970. The large fluctuation in incidence is reflected in notification (it is usually estimated that only 50 per cent of cases were notified (Goldacre and Miller, 1976) showing a high incidence during the war years. Before chemotherapy was introduced there was a very high mortality and in 1940 the mortality dropped to 20 per cent as a result of the introduction of sulphonamides; in subsequent decades the mortality has remained fairly constant at the 20 per cent mark. It is

Table 2. NOTIFICATIONS AND MORTALITY RATE FOR MENINGOCOCCAL MENINGITIS INFECTION AT 10-YEAR INTERVALS
(Extracted from Registrar General Reports, England and Wales)

Year	Notifications	Deaths	Mortality Rate %
1900	7 636	—	—
1910	5 006	—	—
1920	559	533	95
1930	661	631	95
1940	12 771	2 449	19
1950	1 150	283	24
1960	632	95	15
1970	525	143	25

important to realize that these figures relate to all notified cases of meningitis including those cases that died before admission to hospital. The mortality rate for cases of meningococcal infection treated in specialist units is much lower—probably under 5 per cent.

The 20 per cent mortality figure for acute meningococcal infection is therefore in large measure a reflection of the nature of meningococcal infection, emphasizing the untreatableness of acute fulminating cases by conventional current methods. As we do not know how to prevent invasion by the meningococcus, we can only try to prevent colonization; this in the past has been traditionally carried out by chemotherapy, sulphonamides being the most effective. Sulphonamide resistance has posed serious problems, for alternative drugs used to clear the carrier state, such as minocycline and rifampicin, have serious drawbacks. In outbreaks of meningococcal meningitis, particularly where the infection is due to serotypes A and C, vaccines have a role and this method has now been used successfully on a number of occasions.

REFERENCE
Goldacre M. J. and Miller D. L (1976) Completeness of statutory notification for acute bacterial meningitis. *Br. Med. J.* **2**, 501.

PNEUMOCOCCAL MENINGITIS

Pneumococcal meningitis differs from meningococcal meningitis in a number of important aspects—particularly in its higher mortality rate. This is now well documented in a large number of studies giving mortality rates usually in the 30 – 50 per cent range. In a number of studies from developed countries the presence of related diseases, a marked predilection and high mortality at extremes of age, have added up to a convincing clinical picture recognizable in many patients with pneumococcal meningitis. These predisposing factors have included—cirrhosis, pregnancy, nephrotic syndrome, hypogammaglobulin-aemia, cerebrospinal fluid rhinorrhoea, and particularly focal infection such as otitis, sinusitis or pneumonia. High mortality has been a feature of cases occurring at the extremes of life: nowhere does age seem to influence the outcome of an infection so much as in pneumococcal meningitis; the presence of coma on admission, bacteraemia and a low CSF white count are also poor prognostic features.

A recent detailed study of pneumococcal meningitis from Zaria by Tugwell and colleagues (1976) reports 42 patients from the Ahmadu Bello University Hospital. There was a mortality rate of 48 per cent despite treatment with large doses of penicillin. A fatal outcome was associated with impairment of consciousness on admission, a low CSF white cell count and a high CSF pneumococcal polysaccharide antigen titre.

All of these findings might be expected in any series of patients with pneumococcal meningitis, but the unusual features include an age incidence in which older children and young adults were particularly involved.

Few of the patients in the series showed any of the usual predisposing factors—one patient was pregnant, one had cirrhosis and another haemoglobin SC disease; all had immunoglobulin levels within the normal range. A high mortality rate of 48 per cent, despite adequate penicillin therapy, is disappointing and a little surprising (penicillin resistance almost certainly played no part in this feature). Bacteria persisted in the CSF for several days after starting treatment—a feature noted in other African series (Hutton et al., 1962) in marked contrast to usual findings in series reported from developed countries. The authors of this paper comment that these CSF findings suggest defective local phagocytosis, a defect that could be an important cause of failure of the infection to respond to treatment.

The disappointingly high mortality from pneumococcal meningitis in Africans is pursued further in another paper, also from Zaria, by Baird et al. (1976), who reviewed 207 patients. They quote recent reports showing mortality rates of 13 per cent in the United Kingdom, 22 per cent in Los Angeles, 29 per cent in Boston, but rates of 40 – 60 per cent for several African countries. Two studies from the United States in which there was a high proportion of Negro patients had mortality figures of 37 and 47 per cent. *Table* 3 taken from their paper gives details of the mortality rate.

Table 3. MORTALITY FROM PNEUMOCOCCAL MENINGITIS IN DIFFERENT COUNTRIES

Country	Mortality %
U.K.	13
Denmark	17
USA:	
Los Angeles	22
Boston	29
Philadelphia*	37
Harlem*	47
India	45
Egypt	33
Kenya	24
Malawi	43
Zambia	45
Uganda	51
Nigeria	51
Ghana	55
Upper Volta	60

*Series containing a high proportion of Negro patients.

(After Baird D. R. et al., 1976)

In assessing the clinical features and mortality these authors found, as have many others, that there was a strong correlation between the level of consciousness on admission and the outcome. This correlation is well demonstrated in *Table* 4, taken from their paper.

In trying to explain the high mortality rates in their patients the authors comment that it cannot be due to delay at presenting at hospital, as the highest mortality is found in patients with the shortest histories, and that poor medical and nursing care alone cannot be responsible since in their departments the mortality from meningococcal meningitis is about 5 per cent—comparable to European and American results. The fact that an American series of patients containing a high proportion of Negroes showed a much higher mortality than other American surveys supports the proposition that a genetic factor is possibly involved.

Table 4. OUTCOME OF PNEUMOCOCCAL MENINGITIS IN RELATION TO CONSCIOUS LEVEL ON ADMISSION

Conscious level grade	No. of patients	Deaths	Mortality (%)
0	19	6	32
1	70	28	40
2	69	37	54
3	18	17	94

(After Baird D. R. et al., 1976)

REFERENCES

Baird D. R., Whittle H. C. and Greenwood B. M. (1976) Mortality from pneumococcal meningitis. *Lancet 2,* 1344.

Hutton P. W., Shaper A. G. and Wilson A. M. M. (1962) Acute pneumococcal meningitis: the significance of mechanical factors in influencing mortality. *Trans. R. Soc. Trop. Med. Hyg.* **56,** 149.

Tugwell P., Greenwood B. M. and Warrell D. A. (1976) Pneumococcal meningitis: A clinical and laboratory study. *Q. J. Med.* **45,** 583.

'MENINGITIS BY THE SCORE'

Before leaving the subject of meningitis I would like to draw attention to a single case report by Macrae (1975) of a 38-year-old man who has had 21 different episodes of bacterial meningitis. The first attack occurred when he was 8 years of age and was of pneumococcal origin, and since that time there have been 14 other separate episodes caused by pneumococci of different types. The first episode due to *Haemophilus influenzae* took place at the age of 12 years; there were a total of six such attacks. Despite investigations and consultation with neurologists and neurosurgeons the attacks continue.

Treatment of individual attacks have been along conventional lines using penicillin with intrathecal injection for pneumococcal infections and chloramphenicol for the haemophilus. Long-acting penicillin (Penidural) did not prevent recurrence of pneumococcal infection.

From early in his most extraordinary life the patient learned to recognize a 'meningitis headache' and ignored all others; he recognized that he had a 'different headache' when he was first attacked by *H. influenzae* and thereafter calmly announced his newest episode as 'pneumococcal' or 'influenzal' and was never wrong in his self-diagnosis.

The author records this story including the details of investigations with a detached whimsicality. The individual episodes listed by him are given in *Table 5.*

Table 5.

	Dates in hospital		Infecting organism		Notes
	Admitted	Discharged	CSF	Blood	
1.	7 March, 1947	10 April, 1947	Pn	Pn	
2.	24 Nov., 1947	10 Jan., 1948	Pn	N.D.	Right mastoidectomy: 9th day after admission
3.	20 Oct., 1949	2 Dec., 1949	Pn	Pn	All sinuses explored: no pathogens. Child obese. Blood-sugar normal
4.	21 May, 1950	18 July, 1950	Pn	Nil	All sinuses explored: negative. Consultation: ENT surgeon, neurosurgeon and neurologist
5.	19 Feb., 1951	30 March, 1951	Pn	Nil	Consultation: neurosurgeon
6.	16 Oct., 1951	23 Nov., 1951	Pn	Nil	Consultation: neurosurgeon, ENT surgeon and neurologist. Pneumococcus untypable
7.	3 April, 1953	1 May, 1953	Pn	Pn	Pneumococcus untypable: CSF and blood different from episode 6
8.	2 Oct., 1953	28 Oct., 1953	Pn	Pn	Consultation: neurologist and eye surgeon. Visual fields normal. Same pneumococcus as episode 7. Right mastoid and sinuses explored: negative
9.	12 May, 1954	2 July, 1954	H	H	CSF and blood (formerly unknown): *H. influenzae* strain
10.	25 Oct., 1954	19 Nov., 1954	Pn	Pn	Type VI pneumococcus in CSF and blood. Normal immunoglobulin. Depot penicillin every 14 days
11.	6 April, 1955	20 May, 1955	Pn	Pn	Pneumococcus type XXI in CSF and blood. This episode 5 days after a depot dose of penicillin
12.	31 Dec., 1955	3 Feb., 1956	Pn	Pn	EEG normal

	Dates in hospital		Infecting organism		Notes
	Admitted	Discharged	CSF	Blood	
13.	11 March, 1956	18 April, 1956	Pn	Pn	Pneumococcus type XX in blood, CSF and nose
14.	2 Jan., 1958	7 Feb., 1958	H	Nil	Organism lost after identification
15.	10 Jan., 1959	8 Feb., 1959	Pn	Pn	Pneumococcus type XXIII
16.	17 March, 1959	21 April, 1959	H	H	Atypical organism, formerly unknown
17.	26 June, 1959	21 July, 1959	Pn	Nil	Pneumococcus type I
18.	10 Aug., 1961	5 Sept., 1961	H	N.D.	Pitman type 'B' organism
19.	25 Nov., 1961	19 Dec., 1961	Pn	Nil	Organism not types I, II or III. Depot Penidural (benzathine penicillin) weekly (intramuscularly)
20.	10 Jan., 1963	1 Feb., 1963	H	Nil	Pitman type 'B'. Mixed vaccine each autumn
21.	14 Feb., 1974	3 March, 1974	H	Nil	Minor amounts of penicillin in blood. Now on daily oral penicillin V (phenoxymethyl-penicillin). New strain of organism grown

Pn = Pneumococcus. H = *Haemophilus influenzae*. N.D. = Note done.
CSF = Cerebrospinal fluid. EEG = Electroencephalogram.

(After Macrae J., 1975)

REFERENCE
Macrae J. (1975) Meningitis by the score. *Practitioner* **215**, 641.

LEGIONNAIRES' DISEASE

First incident

In the summer of 1976 an American Legion Convention held in Philadelphia was marred by the outbreak of a serious respiratory illness affecting mainly those attending the convention. There were 180 cases and 29 deaths. Detailed investigation finally established that the illness was indeed an infection caused by a Gram-negative bacillus not previously recognized and with difficult growth characteristics.

Retrospective cases

Isolation of the organism led to the production of antisera which have been used to test sera from patients with pneumonia in a number of centres. These investigations suggest that Legionnaires' disease occurred in the District of Columbia in 1965, in Pontiac, Michigan 1968 and in Philadelphia in 1974.

In 1973 86 tourists, mainly from Scotland, who stayed at one hotel in Benidorm, Spain, developed respiratory symptoms: 3 died from penumonia. Fluorescent antibody titres to the Legionnaires' organism have been detected in four individuals including one of those who died. Another person who stayed in Benidorm in 1977 and who died on return to Scotland also showed a high titre.

Current situation

Since August, 1977, there have to date been 21 confirmed cases of Legionnaires' disease in Kingsport, Tennessee; there were 3 fatalities. In Vermont 27 cases have been confirmed since May; 15 patients died.

In late summer, 1977, physicians at the City Hospital Nottingham became concerned because of a severe pneumonia in a few patients which failed to respond to chemotherapy. Investigations at the Nottingham Public Health Laboratory failed to identify an aetiological agent, but sera from five of six tested at the Center for Disease Control, Atlanta, showed antibody titres suggesting Legionnaires' disease.

Information to date suggests that Legionnaires' disease is a serious pneumonia capable of causing severe outbreaks when large numbers of people appear to be infected from a common source. Case-to-case spread has not been established; isolated cases probably occur. So far no cases have been identified in children.

Clinical picture

The illness starts 2 – 10 days after exposure, malaise, muscle aches and headache are early symptoms. Within 24 hours there is high fever with chills and a non-productive cough is noted; abdominal pain and gastrointestinal symptoms have occurred in many patients. Physical examination at this stage shows an ill pyrexial patient, often with adventitious moist sounds in the lungs without evidence of consolidation. Chest X-ray shows patchy opacities which may progress to larger areas of consolidation. Pleural effusion may be noted but is not usually a marked feature.

As the illness progresses cough becomes productive but rarely purulent. In those who recover convalescence is prolonged.

The overall mortality is about 15 per cent—higher in those wth serious underlying disease. Patients die from shock or respiratory failure; upper gastrointestinal bleeding is not uncommon and renal failure has been noted.

Laboratory diagnosis

In the acute stage of the illness a polymorph leucocytosis is present and the erythrocyte sedimentation rate may be greater than 80 mm/hour. Proteinuria, mild azotaemia and a slight increase in serum transaminase are noted.

The causative organism has to date not been grown from sputum or blood, it has been cultured from post-mortem lung tissue using yolk sac inoculation of embryonated hens' eggs. In 2 patients the organism has been isolated from pleural fluid before the patients' deaths. Serological diagnosis with acute and convalescent sera is available in some centres and is the most likely method to confirm the diagnosis.

Chemotherapy

There are no formal trials of antibiotics in Legionnaires' disease on which to base rational therapy. Patients have been treated with many agents and on balance, at the moment, erythromycin appears to have been associated with low case fatality rates. This recommendation may alter as new information about this disease becomes available, but at the time of writing erythromycin is probably the agent most likely to be effective.

Many questions remain to be answered. Is this organism really 'new'? Why have we not encountered it before? Is there an animal reservoir of infection? Is it entirely a respiratory disease? Are children affected and what can chemotherapy offer? These are some of the questions to which we would like to have answers.

LEGAL DECISIONS AND LEGISLATION

NICHOLAS LYELL MA

The welcome reduction in general legislation resulting from the comparative stalemate caused by the Government's lack of overall majority during the past year has reflected itself in the medical field. There are, however, a number of interesting decisions at common law to report.

LEGISLATION

The National Health Service Act 1977 is the most extensive Act relating to medical practice to come into force in 1977. It is, however, merely a consolidating statute dealing with a number of provisions relating to the Health Service, including the controversial provisions relating to the withdrawal of paybeds and facilities for private patients as envisaged by the Health Services Act 1976, which are repeated.

The Medical Qualifications (EEC Registration) Order 1977 (No. 827) made under the European Communities Act 1972 provides for the registration as medical practitioners of nationals of Member States of the European Community who hold certain stipulated European qualifications. Applicants for registration do, however, have to satisfy the Registrar of the General Council that they have sufficient knowledge of English and if they fail to do so, either before or within six months of the date of their registration, the registration lapses. The Order also contains provision for temporary registration of visiting practitioners and the maintenance of a list of those registering in respect of specialist qualifications.

The Medicines Labelling Amendment Regulations 1977 (No. 996) amend the 1976 Regulations principally to require that the words 'keep out of reach of children' are displayed on containers for a number of relevant medicines.

The Medicines (Bal Jivan Chancho Prohibition) Order 1977 (No. 172) is of particular concern to witch doctors. This prohibits for a further period the sale or supply as a baby tonic of a dark brown aromatic solid substance to which were appended the following directions: 'Children diseases viz. varadh-capillor bronchitis, greenish diarrhoea, rikets, cough, convulsions etc. Rubbing the medicine with water or milk until it gets colour to be taken twice a day.'

CASES AT COMMON LAW

Income Tax

The case of *Mundy* v. *Furlong* [1977] 2 AER 953 establishes that a professional man, in that case a barrister, is entitled to tax relief on the cost of textbooks expected to last for some years, as 'plant' within the meaning of Section 41(1)(a) of the Finance Act 1971. The Court held that a professional man's 'plant' was not confined to things used physically, e.g. a dentist's chair, but extended to the 'intellectual storehouse' which a professional man uses in the course of carrying on his profession. There can be little doubt that this would apply as much to books needed by a doctor as a lawyer. Many practitioners may have been claiming this successfully in the past and will be glad to know that the practice has now been officially approved by the Courts.

Legal practice in personal injury cases

The right of a defendant to choose the medical specialist who examines the plaintiff on his behalf was considered in *Starr* v. *National Coal Board* [1977] 1 WLR 63. In that case the Plaintiff, a coal face worker, objected to being examined by the highly qualified neurologist appointed for the purpose by the National Coal Board. In balancing his civil liberties in objecting to such an examination against the defendants' right to obtain a report from the specialist of their choice the Court held that the defendants were entitled to nominate their own doctor unless in all the circumstances it would be unreasonable or unfair to choose a particular doctor; for example, if he were personally hostile to the plaintiff.

CRIMINAL LAW

The case of *R.* v. *Stone* [1977] 2 WLR 169, which came before the Court of Criminal Appeal, highlights in a tragic way the criminal responsibility which can be incurred by those who undertake the duty of caring for an infirm person and then recklessly disregard their needs. The tragic facts were that a 67-year-old widower, partially deaf, almost blind and with no appreciable sense of smell, lived together with his mistress and his mentally subnormal son. His younger sister came to lodge at the house. She was eccentric, suffered from anorexia nervosa and spent days at a time in her room becoming helplessly infirm. The defendants took her food and attempted to wash her but failed to take the advice of neighbours and a local publican to call in the Social Services or to take adequate steps to call a doctor. Their convictions were upheld on the grounds that whereas mere inadvertence was insufficient, criminal liability was established if indifference to obvious risks of injury to health were ignored.

Road traffic

Yet another 'breathaliser' case was considered in Attorney General's reference (No. 1 of 1976) 1977 1 WLR 646 in which it was held that the provision that a breath specimen cannot be demanded of a person who is in hospital as a patient, without notifying the doctor in immediate charge of the case, only applies at times before the treatment being given at the hospital is over. Once that treatment has been concluded and the patient is leaving the hospital he can be asked for a specimen without notifying the hospital or doctor. In a field rife with technicalities, common sense has once again prevailed. The same is true in the similar case of *R.* v. *Crowley* [1977] RTR 153 CA where a motorist had originally been asked to provide a breath specimen, following an accident, while he was sitting in the ambulance. In fact the ambulance drove him off to hospital before the kit could be provided but the enthusiastic police officer followed him to hospital and administered the breath test there while he was waiting at the casualty department before he was seen by any doctor. The prosecution submission that no doctor was in immediate charge of his case and therefore notification was unnecessary was rejected, the court taking the view that the doctor in 'immediate charge of his case' was the doctor directly responsible for him, who in such cases would usually be the duty casualty officer.

Assaults on mental patients

The case of *R.* v. *Runighian* [1977] Crim.L.R. 361 established an important distinction between the protection granted to staff in mental hospitals under Section 141 of the Mental Health Act 1959 in the case of patients formally admitted under the statute as compared to informal patients. It was held that the requirement that the leave of the High Court be obtained before proceedings either civil or criminal could be instituted did not apply to informal or voluntary patients and applied only to those admitted pursuant to an order or direction under the Act.

EMPLOYMENT

The proper use of medical reports by an employer when considering whether to dismiss an employee on medical grounds was considered in the case of *East Lindsey District Council* v. *Danbury, The Times* 26 April, 1977, which was heard by the Employment Appeal Tribunal. The respondent had been ill and absent from work for a considerable period and the Council's personnel director had asked his medical adviser to indicate whether he felt that the employee's health was such that he should be retired on grounds of ill health. The medical adviser asked another doctor to examine the employee and as a result of the report received advised the Council that the employee was unfit and should be retired. But the Council itself never saw any medical report and simply dismissed the employee on the basis of this advice. The employee was not notified that he might be dismissed at any time between receipt of the opinion from the Council's medical adviser and the notice of dismissal. The Employment Appeal Tribunal held that when considering a dismissal the duty of the employer, apart from ascertaining the true medical position, was at least to consult the employee and give him an opportunity to discuss and comment upon the proposed action. The absence of such consultation and the fact that the employee had no personal knowledge of the medical report indicated that the employers had not fulfilled their duty and the decision that the dismissal was unfair was upheld.

GENERAL MEDICINE
C. W. H. HAVARD MA, DM, FRCP

SEVERE AND RESISTANT HYPERTENSION

Last year the review of the year's work in general medicine was devoted to hypertension as this was a subject that had experienced a major reappraisal in our understanding of its physiology and its clinical importance and its management. Severe and resistant hypertension was not specifically discussed. The recent review of the subject in the *British Journal of Hospital Medicine* (Havard and Pearson, 1978) is therefore appropriate. The situations in which emergency reduction of high blood pressure is necessary are discussed. The major indications considered were:

1. Hypertensive encephalopathy
2. Hypertension causing left ventricular failure
3. Subarachnoid haemorrhage
4. Dissecting aneurysm
5. Eclampsia
6. Monoamine oxidase inhibitor interaction
7. Clonidine withdrawal
8. Phaeochromocytoma
9. Emergency surgery in a patient with uncontrolled hypertension
10. Prolonged epistaxis in a patient with uncontrolled hypertension
11. Myocardial infarction

The drugs available that were considered for the rapid reduction of raised blood pressure by the parenteral route are:

1. Diazoxide
2. Labetalol
3. Hydrallazine
4. Trimetaphan
5. Methyldopa
6. Clonidine intramuscularly
7. Nitroprusside
8. Reserpine
9. Guanethidine
10. Pentolinium

Diazoxide intravenously was considered to be the drug of choice at present. Labetalol is a promising new drug with alpha and beta receptor antagonist effects and may well prove to be an alternative to diazoxide. Methyldopa tends to cause drowsiness and this may create diagnostic confusion in disorders such as encephalopathy, and subarachnoid haemorrhage. Guanethidine should not be used in view of its propensity to induce hypertension initially. Pentolinium is only of historical interest and should not now be used as it may cause irreversible hypotension.

Resistant hypertension was then discussed and the reasons for resistance were divided into (1) apparent and (2) real. There are a number of apparent causes of resistance to treatment. Non-compliance with the regime is an obvious cause though often overlooked. Some hints for improving compliance are suggested. Drug interactions are also important. The concomitant administration of tricyclic antidepressants or chlorpromazine prevent the uptake of guanethidine and related antihypertensive drugs at the nerve ending and so antagonize their hypotensive effect. Other examples include the antagonistic effect of phenylbutazone on the antihypertensive effects of both diuretics and the sympathetic antagonists such as guanethidine; and also the antagonist effect of the sodium-retaining drugs, such as carbenoxolone, on the antihypertensive effects of diuretics and bethanidine. The coincident administration of drugs with hypertensive properties is also important. Examples of these include: (1) cold cures containing phenyl-epinephrine, (2) sympathomimetic drugs such as isoprenaline and amphetamines and proprietary remedies for dysmenorrhoea containing ephedrine, and (3) corticosteroids. The more important interactions are listed in *Table* 1.

Table 1. DRUG INTERACTIONS

1. Tricyclic antidepressants	with bethanidine
	clonidine
	debrisoquine
	guanethidine
Phenothiazines	with guanethidine
Antihistamines	with guanethidine
2. Phenylbutazone	with diuretics
Oxyphenbutazone	guanethidine
Indomethacin	
Salt	
Carbenoxalone	
3. Sympathomimetic drugs	with guanethidine
Amphetamine	bethanidine
Ephedrine	debrisoquine
Phenylephrine	
Phenylpropanolamine	
Phenteramine	

Genuine resistance to the effects of anti-hypertensive drugs is seen in severe primary hypertension especially when complicated by renal damage and in secondary hypertension associated with renal disease, pre-eclampsia and phaeochromocytoma. The means of countering genuine resistance are discussed under the headings of (1) increasing the dose of conventional drugs, (2) large doses of loop diuretics in cases in which the hypertension is volume-dependent, (3) large doses of beta-blockers in cases in which the hypertension is renin-dependent, and (4) the use of newer drugs.

The new drugs considered were (1) diazoxide, (2) minoxidil, (3) labetalol, (4) fusaric acid and (5) guanabenz. Their place in the management of resistant hypertension and their side-effects are discussed.

REFERENCE
Havard C. W. H. and Pearson R. M. (1978) *Br. J. Hosp. Med.* In the press.

AETIOLOGY OF MYASTHENIA GRAVIS

The last two years has seen great advances in our understanding of the aetiology of myasthenia gravis. This is the subject of a review in the *British Medical Journal* (Havard, 1978). There is now little doubt that this disorder is due to a reduced number of functioning acetylcholine receptors and that this comes about as a result of immunological damage to the acetylcholine receptor (ACh). The impetus to this exciting progress was the identification of bungarotoxin. Bungarotoxin is the protein contained in cobra venom and it interacts specifically with ACh receptors. It can thus be used to determine the number of ACh receptor sites, the number of bungarotoxin-binding sites being proportional and perhaps equal to the number of ACh receptor sites. Further progress was dependent on isolating the ACh antigen. This was done when Patrick and Lindstrom (1973) coupled cobra toxin to agarose beads and isolated the acetylcholine receptor from the rest of the homogenized muscle of an electric eel. The few milligrams of receptor isolated by Lindstrom were used to raise antibodies in the rabbit. A few weeks after immunization with AChR the rabbits became weak and died. They had developed antibodies to the electric eel AChR which cross-reacted with their own AChR. Furthermore, this muscle weakness could be transiently overcome by treatment with anticholinesterase drugs (Patrick and Lindstrom, 1973). This disorder is now called 'Experimental autoimmune myasthenia gravis' (EAMG). The disease has been induced in a number of different species, including the monkey, in which the clinical features of ptosis closely mimic human myasthenia gravis (Tarrab-Hazdai et al., 1975a). More recently the disease has been induced in rats by immunization with ACh receptor that is syngenetic and the ensuing myasthenia is associated with the formation of circulating antibodies to ACh receptors (Lindstrom et al., 1976). The proof that the circulating antibodies are the cause of the disease is provided by the fact that the serum of rats immunized with ACh receptor can cause the disease when injected into normal animals and the histological changes at the neuromuscular junction are similar (Lindstrom et al., 1976). Experimental autoimmune myasthenia gravis has, however, been most closely studied in the rat in which it develops in two phases. After about a week following immunization with AChR there is an initial stage of acute severe muscle weakness from which they recover and about three weeks later they develop a more insidious persistent weakness that is fatal within a few weeks. Electromicroscopic studies have shown that the first phase is associated with invasion of the neuromuscular junction by macrophages and a breakdown of the post-synaptic membrane at sites where AChR is most concentrated. In the later chronic phase there is a reduction in the number of acetylcholine receptors. The area of the post-synaptic membrane is decreased and its folded structure is simplified (Engel et al., 1976). It would seem that the circulating antibody to AChR damages the receptors and reduces their competence. Phagocytosis follows and the amount of ACh receptor is reduced. Thus both a reduction in the total amount of AChR and the formation of antibody AChR complexes contribute to the impairment of neuromuscular transmission. It appears that some regeneration of AChR can take place and the ability to synthesise new receptor will have an important effect on the prognosis (Lindstrom et al., 1976).

Nevertheless, despite the increasing evidence that a circulating antibody damages the post-synaptic acetylcholine receptor it is apparent that experimental myasthenia is T cell dependent for it will not develop in thymectomized animals and it can be passively transferred with cells (Tarrab-Hazdai et al., 1975b). Also the acute lesion at the myoneural junction in the experimental disease shows the lymphocyte infiltration characteristic of a cell-mediated immune response (Engel et al., 1976). Recently a high level of cell-mediated immunity to purified acetylcholine receptor has been demonstrated in human myasthenia gravis and an association noted between disease activity and the level of cell-mediated immunity to receptor. It does not seem likely that the cellular response is secondary to damage to the neuromuscular junction as these authors have shown it does not occur in amyotrophic lateral sclerosis in which breakdown of the neuromuscular junction regularly occurs (Richman et al., 1976). Clinical experience in man also implicates the 'T' cells in myasthenia. Both thymectomy and thoracic duct drainage deplete 'T' cells and improve the disease. The answer probably lies in the immunological situation whereby 'B' cell function is sustained by helper 'T' cells.

In 1974 it was shown that a circulating globulin in the serum of individuals with myasthenia blocked the binding of bungarotoxin to the ACh receptor extracted from denervated rat skeletal muscle (Almon et al., 1974). Recently the passive transfer of human serum fractions from individuals with myasthenia gravis has induced the disease in mice (Toyka et al., 1977). The active serum fraction was identified as IgG. Furthermore there was a rough correlation between the patient's clinical state and the potency of the serum factor in producing myasthenic features in the test animals, although disparities were seen in individual cases. Thoracic duct drainage has a beneficial effect in myasthenia gravis and re-infusion of the gammaglobulin fraction causes clinical deterioration (Lefvert and Bergstrom, 1976). There seems little doubt, however, that there is a myasthenia-producing IgG circulating in the blood of patients with myasthenia gravis. The action of this myasthenia-inducing IgG is influenced by the complement system for in the absence of C3 its effect is significantly lessened. Deficiency of C5 does not affect the results.

In human individuals with myasthenia gravis there are circulating antibodies to AChR. They can be demonstrated in 87 per cent of patients (Lindstrom et al., 1976). These antibodies have also been demonstrated in babies with neonatal myasthenia.

The antibody titres fall following thymectomy and indeed there is an inverse relationship between antibody titre and the interval following thymectomy (Scadding et al., 1977). A fall in antibody titre has also been reported following remissions induced by corticosteroids (Lindstrom et al., 1976). This suggests that clinical improvement is associated with a fall in antireceptor antibody titre which decreases over several years. It is, however, unlikely that thymectomy removes a major source of antibody as the titre should then fall more quickly. Thymectomy may therefore remove an antigenic stimulus or may cause a gradual decrease in 'T' lymphocytes necessary for antibody formation by 'B' lymphocytes. A fall in circulating 'T' lymphocytes has recently been demonstrated in myasthenic patients following thymectomy (Scadding et al., 1977), and this appears to be associated with an increase in the number of null cells, which are immature 'T' cells needing thymic hormone to complete their development.

There is no doubt that great advances have been made in the understanding of the pathogenesis of myasthenia gravis. The immunological basis of the disease is beyond question but the role of the thymus, though fundamental to the disease, has not precisely been defined. Its importance is twofold. It is the primary immunological source of 'T' cells and hence has a fundamental role in cell-mediated immunity. Secondly it is a source of myogenic cells with demonstrable acetylcholine receptors on their cell surface (Kao and Drachman, 1976). The recent work of Wekerle has shown the importance of this latter function. In long-term cultures of thymus reticulum cells from young adult rats and mice they detected skeletal muscle colonies in addition to the expected epithelial and mesenchymal reticular tissue types (Wekerle et al., 1975). These muscle cells were fully demonstrated by all morphological and functional criteria and possessed demonstrable amounts of acetylcholine receptors on their cell membranes (Ketelson and Wekerle, 1976). This finding is supported by the recent demonstration of bungarotoxin binding to epithelial cells of the thymus and an abundance of these cells in the thymuses of patients with myasthenia gravis (Engel et al., 1976). The fact that stem cells in the thymus can be induced to differentiate into striated muscle clones suggested the possibility that abnormal induction signals might occur in the human situation in response to pathological changes in the thymus, and Wekerle and Ketelsen (1977) have recently proposed a hypothesis for the pathogenesis of myasthenia gravis. They suggest that primitive intrathymic stem cells are induced by abnormal stimuli to differentiate into myogenic cells. Then immunologically competent 'T' cells start an immune reaction against these newly differentiated myogenic cells. Sensitized 'T' cells then leave the thymus and become killer 'T' cells infiltrating the neuromuscular junction and destroying it or cooperate with 'B' cells as helper cells to form antibodies to the acetylcholine receptor. The pathogenesis is under genetic control both at the differentiation of 'T' cells to myogenic cells and at the stage of immune responsiveness of the lymphocytes to these atypical muscle cells.

REFERENCES

Almon R. R., Andrew C. G. and Appel S. H. (1974) *Science* **186**, 55.
Engel A. G., Tsujihata M., Lindstrom J. M. and Lennon V. A. (1976) *Ann. N. Y. Sci.* **274**, 60.
Havard C. W. H. (1978) *Br. Med. J.* **2**, 1008.
Kao I. and Drachman D. B. (1977) *Science* **195**, 74.
Ketelsen J. P. and Wekerle H. (1976) *Differentiation* **5**, 185.
Lefvert A. K. and Bergstrom K. (1976) *Eur. J. Clin. Invest.* **6**, 334.
Lindstrom J. M., Einarson B. L., Lennon V. A. and Seybold M. E. (1976) *J. Exp. Med.* **144**, 726.
Patrick J. and Lindstrom J. M. (1973) *Science* **180**, 871.
Richman D. P., Patrick J. and Arnason B. G. W. (1976) *N. Engl. J. Med.* **294**, 694.
Scadding et al. (1977) In the press.
Tarrab-Hazdai R., Aharonov A., Abramsky O., Yaar I. and Fuchs S. (1975) *J. Exp. Med.* **142**, 785.
Tarrab-Hazdai R., Aharonov A., Silman I., Fuchs S. and Abramsky O. (1975b) *Nature (Lond.)* **256**, 128.
Toyka K. V., Drachman D. B., Griffin D. E., Pestronk A., Winkelstein J. A. and Kao I. (1977) *N. Engl. J. Med.* **296**, 125.
Wekerle H. and Ketelsen U. P. (1977) *Lancet* **1**, 678.
Wekerle H., Paterson B., Ketelsen U. P. and Feldman M. (1975) *Nature* **256**, 493.

GONADAL FUNCTION IN YOUNG ADULTS AFTER SURGICAL TREATMENT OF CRYPTORCHISM

The testes usually descend into the scrotum at about the 8th fetal month. Testes are undescended at birth in 3·4 per cent of full term male infants but in half these cases the testes are in the scrotum by the end of the first month and the incidence of undescended testes at the age of 12 months is 0·5 per cent. The textbooks tell us that maldescent may be due to mechanical abnormalities in the channel of descent of a normal testis or the cause may be an abnormality in the testis itself. Because the aetiology is uncertain the treatment is controversial. All men with bilateral undescended testes are infertile but the age at which the cryptorchid is damaged is uncertain. It is generally agreed that treatment must be started before puberty if irreversible damage to the testis is to be prevented.

The study of gonadal function in young adults with surgical treatment of cryptorchism is therefore of interest (Werder et al., 1976). These authors report a follow-up study of 48 young men who had been surgically treated for cryptorchism before puberty. Testicular function was assessed by examining the genitalia, testicular volume, secondary sex characteristics, semen, plasma LH and FSH after stimulation by the hypothalamic-releasing hormone LH.RH and the plasma testosterone concentration. Sixteen patients had been operated upon for bilateral and 32 for unilateral cryptorchism. In all surgery had been performed before the onset of pubert, the ages varying from 5 – 17 years with a mean of 11 years.

Secondary sex characteristics were normal. The mean testicular volume of both testes was in the low normal range in those who had had unilateral cryptorchism and below normal in those who had had bilateral cryptorchism. Of 14 patients who had had bilateral cryptorchism, whose sperm counts were recorded, 6 showed azoospermia, 4 severe oligospermia and 1 moderate azoospermia. Of 23 patients who had had unilateral cryptorchism none showed azoospermia, 1 had severe oligospermia and 9 had moderate oligo-spermia. In nearly all the patients who had had bilateral cryptorchism and in most of those with unilateral disease plasma gonadotrophin levels were increased. Four cases of possible partial LH deficiency were identified. Plasma testosterone levels were normal in all but 2 patients. In only 2 patients operated upon where the findings normal in all the investigations. The authors suggest that the common finding of raised gonadotrophin levels indicates that cryptorchism is generally a primary testicular disease. However, a minority may also be manifestations of deficient pituitary gonadotrophins, as suggested by the group of patients with LH deficiency. This possibility is supported by the fact that there is a high incidence of cryptorchism in patients with gonadotrophin deficiency (Santen and Paulsen, 1973).

REFERENCES
Santen R. J. and Paulsen C. A. (1973) *J. Clin. Endocrinol. Metab.* **36,** 47.
Werder E. A., Illig R., Torresani R., Zachmann M., Baumann P., Ott F. and Prader A. (1976) *Br. Med. J.* **2,** 1357.

EVIDENCE OF EXTRA PITUITARY ORIGIN FOR BETA-MELANOCYTE-STIMULATING HORMONE

Beta-MSH is found in the cerebrospinal fluid where unlike other pituitary hormones its concentration is greater than that in the plasma. Shuster has suggested that this hormone might, therefore, have a physiological role in the central nervous system in man (Smith and Shuster, 1976). Shuster and his colleagues have now studied 19 patients with hypopituitarism and found normal beta-MSH levels in both plasma and CSF (Shuster et al., 1977). They believe that the source of beta-MSH is unlikely to have been the pituitary as some patients had severe panhypopituitarism whilst others had had a surgical hypophysectomy. Residual pituitary tissue is in their view an unlikely explanation of the findings because there is no direct route for pituitary hormones into the CSF other than through the blood. They believe that beta-MSH is produced by and secreted from nervous tissue.

REFERENCES
Shuster S., Smith A., Plummer N., Thody A. and Clark F. (1977) *Br. Med. J.* **1**, 1318.
Smith A. G. and Shuster S. (1976) *Lancet* **2**, 1321.

METABOLIC DISEASES AND DIABETES MELLITUS
Pathogenesis of diabetic microangiopathy

Thickening of capillary basement membrane is one of the earliest pathological changes in diabetes mellitus. It can be detected in the renal glomeruli within a couple of years of the onset of juvenile diabetes mellitus (Osterby, 1975). As these micro-angiopathic changes advance capillary micro-aneurysms develop in the retina and provide the first physical sign of the complications of diabetes mellitus. Subsequently new blood vessels and connective tissue form and extend into the vitreous and in the form of retinitis proliferans provide one of the most distressing complications of diabetes mellitus. There seems little doubt that the micro-angiopathic changes are secondary to hyperglycaemia but the precise way in which they come about is uncertain. The proceedings of a conference on Diabetic Microangiopathy (McMillan and Ditzel, 1976) throw some light on the subject. Hyperglycaemia leads to increased incorporation of carohydrate into the basement membrane (Westberg, 1976). The capillaries become more permeable and the consequent exudation of protein varies with the length and the degree of hyperglycaemia. Poor control in previously well controlled diabetics is associated with a twofold increase in albuminuria (Parving, 1976). Hydrostatic pressure as well as capillary structure is important in determining the capillary leak so that systemic hypertension may well accelerate the progression of diabetic micro-angiopathy (Parving, 1976). The control of hypertension in patients with diabetes is therefore of great importance and may even delay the development of renal failure (Morgensen, 1976). Another factor that may affect hydrostatic pressure is blood viscosity and this has been found to be increased in diabetes mellitus. McMillan (1976) discusses the evidence that plasma protein changes in diabetics alter blood flow and play a role in the rate of progression of the micro-angiopathy. The role of growth hormone in the pathogenesis of diabetic micro-angiopathy is reviewed by Lundbaek (1976). The advocates of this hypothesis believe that growth hormone has a direct effect on the microvasculature.

Whether or not good diabetic control delays or prevents the complications of diabetes has been a vexed question for many years, but these studies do suggest that prevention of prolonged hyperglycaemia is important. Because randomized clinical trials in man would be lengthy, expensive and probably unethical, Fox, Lowy et al. (1977) have approached the problem in a different way. They induced diabetes in rats with streptozocin. They measured the glomerular basement membrane thickness in 23 rats with induced diabetes and in 12 age-matched controls. Diabetic rats were then randomly allocated to a normal or low carbohydrate diet. A highly significant positive correlation was found between the capillary basement membrane thickness and plasma glucose concentration for individual rats. They conclude that hyperglycaemia is the main determinant in the development of basement membrane thickening. In another study Fox, Darby et al. (1977) have found in the same group of animals that plasma glucose concentration correlates inversely with motor nerve conduction velocity so that hyperglycaemia is probably a major factor in the development of the neuropathy of diabetes mellitus. The message would seem to be clear.

REFERENCES

Fox C. J., Darby S. C., Ireland J. T. and Sönksen P. H. (1977) *Br. Med. J.* **2,** 605.
Fox C. J., Lowy C. and Sönksen P. H. (1977) *Clin. Sci. Molec. Med.* **52,** 24P.
Lunbaek K. (1976) *Diabetes* **25,** Suppl. 2, 845.
McMillan D. E. (1976) *Diabetes* **25,** Suppl. 2, 858.
McMillan D. E. and Ditzel J. (ed.) (1976) Proceedings of a Conference on Diabetic Micro-angiography. *Diabetes* **25,** Suppl. 2, 805.
Morgensen C. E. (1976) *Diabetes* **25,** Suppl. 2, 872.
Osterby R. (1975) *Acta Med. Scand.* Suppl. 574, 1.
Parving H. H. (1976) *Diabetes* **25,** Suppl. 2, 920.
Westberg M. H. (1976) *Diabetes* **25,** Suppl. 2, 805.

MENTAL DISEASE

J. S. PRICE DM, MRCP, MRC Psych,
DPM

PREMATURE EJACULATION

Delay in ejaculation or complete abolition of the reaction have frequently been reported as side effects of the phenothiazines, the tricyclic anti-depressants and the monoamine oxidase inhibitors. The exploitation of this side effect to treat premature ejaculation was suggested by Singh in 1963, but for some reason which is not entirely clear from the literature drugs have never come into favour and the treatment of premature ejaculation is now entirely psychological (Levine, 1976).

Possibly Singh's choice of thioridazine (Melleril) was unfortunate. Thioridazine appears to be more effective in delaying ejaculation than other phenothiazines, and had this effect in 49 per cent of a series of 57 patients studied at the University of California (Kotin et al., 1976); however, the patients on thioridazine had more difficulty in obtaining and maintaining erection than those on other tranquillizers, 19 of them reported an absence of ejaculate and 2 reported pain on ejaculation. The last two symptoms suggest retrograde ejaculation into the bladder, and it thus seems that thioridazine inhibits the strong contraction of the internal sphincter of the bladder which is a normal part of the ejaculatory response. Retrograde ejaculation is also reported with post-ganglionic sympathetic blocking agents, and it is a pity that the nervous control of ejaculation is still too obscure to permit this odd idiosyncracy of thioridazine to clarify the pharmacological profile of a phenothiazine which is already unusual in its excess of anticholinergic action, its low anti-emetic activity and its relative freedom from extrapyramidal side-effects.

More favourable results for the tricyclic antidepressants have been reported by Eaton (1973) who, in an uncontrolled trial, found low doses of clomipramine to be effective in almost 100 per cent of patients. However, this investigator was not on the look-out for retrograde ejaculation, and the promising findings do not appear to have been followed-up by a controlled trial. Delay in ejaculation is a known side effect of phenelzine (Nardil) and had an adverse effect on orgasm in both males and females in whom phenelzine was used to treat narcolepsy (Wyatt et al., 1971).

The currently accepted treatment of premature ejaculation requires the cooperation of both partners and is derived from the Masters and Johnson technique (Levine, 1976). The female is encouraged to stimulate the male manually and to respond to his signals that he is approaching orgasm by ceasing to stimulate and/or squeezing the penis firmly at the base of the glans. The sexual excitement of the male is allowed to die down for a while and then the procedure is repeated over and over again, and in this way he is helped to develop control over the onset of orgasm. Further lessons involve the use of a cream to simulate the lubricated state of the vagina, and then intercourse with the female in the superior position, adjusting her pelvic movements to the signals of the male.

A general physician presented with a patient whose partner will not cooperate and who for one reason or another does not wish to make a referral to a specialist in sexual disorders might be inclined to make a trial of one of the well-known tricyclic compounds such as imipramine, starting with a dosage of 10 mg t.d.s., and, bearing in mind the twentyfold individual variation in the rate of the 10-hydroxylation reaction which inactivates the drug, being prepared to increase the dosage at weekly or more infrequent intervals to 25 mg t.d.s. or even to 50 or 100 mg t.d.s. until there is therapeutic response or until side-effects, such as dry mouth, become uncomfortable.

REFERENCES

Eaton H. (1973) Clomipramine (Anafranil) in the treatment of premature ejaculation. *J. Int. Med. Res.* **1**, 432 – 434.
Kotin J., Wilbert D. E., Verburg D. et al. (1976) Thioridazine and sexual dysfunction. *Am. J. Psychiat.* **133**, 82 – 85.
Levine S. B. (1976) Marital sexual function: ejaculation disorders. *Ann. Intern. Med.* **84**, 575 – 579.
Singh H. (1963) Therapeutic use of thioridazine in premature ejaculation. *Am. J. Psychiat.* **119**, 891.
Wyatt R. J., Fram D. H., Buchbinder R. et al. (1971) Treatment of intractable narcolepsy with a monoamine oxidase inhibitor. *N. Engl. J. Med.* **285**, 987 – 991.

THE PINEAL GLAND

A recent review predicts that the pineal gland will shortly regain the pre-eminent place in psychiatry which it held for a century or more after Descartes identified it as the site of union of the body and the immortal soul (Mullen and Silman, 1977). English and Continental psychiatrists attributed insanity to calcification and other features of the pineal, and in 1676 the first postmortem to be carried out on a Bedlam patient concentrated almost exclusively on the state of the pineal.

One of the pineal hormones 5-methoxyindole acetic acid (melatonin) has been implicated in schizophrenia because of its chemical similarity to several psychotomimetic substances and also in depression as it has been observed to exacerbate depressive symptoms. Melatonin has a hypnotic action in a variety of species and it would not be surprising if an organ which is phylogenetically concerned with the light/dark cycle had some regulatory function in relation to sleep. Now that melatonin can be detected and measured in human plasma and CSF by gas chromatography mass spectrometry, the authors of this review may well be correct in their prediction. At the very least, it would be pleasant to have a more physiological alternative to Mogadon (nitrazepam).

REFERENCE

Mullen P. E. and Silman R. E. (1977) The pineal and psychiatry. *Psychol. Med.* **7**, 407 – 416.

EFFICACY OF ELECTROCONVULSIVE THERAPY

This year has seen the publication of the Royal College of Psychiatrists' Memorandum on the use of electroconvulsive therapy and a special section in the September issue of the *American Journal of Psychiatry* devoted to ECT. This interest is partly due to adverse comment about ECT in the lay and the medical press and on television. Writing in the *New Statesman* Mr Christopher Price MP (no relation to the present writer) claims that ECT should be as obsolete as clitoridectomy and hopes that 'fewer and fewer patients will give their consent to it'. An article in *On Call* states that '. . . with the rise of

Nazism and Fascism in the mid-thirties came the introduction of . . . electro-shock and psychosurgery' (Stern, 1977). Friedberg (1977) begins the conclusion of his neurological perspective of ECT as follows: 'From a neurological point of view ECT is a method of producing amnesia by selectively damaging the temporal lobes and the structures within them'. He describes this as a 'brain disease, with an estimated incidence of new cases in the range of 100 000 per year.' Attempts to reduce memory loss by giving unilateral ECT to the non-dominant hemisphere are dismissed by Friedman as exploitation of the anosognosia characteristic of lesions of the non-dominant hemisphere. In other words, the brain damage is so organized that the patient cannot compain about the results.

There can be little doubt that ECT is not only effective but more rapidly effective than antidepressive drugs in the severe endogenous/psychotic depressions of middle-aged and elderly patients. Strong clinical impressions have been supported by two large multicentre controlled trials, one in this country (MRC, 1965) and one in the United States (Greenblatt et al., 1974). Hopefully next year it will be possible to review three trials in which a course of ECT is compared with a course in which the application of electric current is omitted from some or all of the treatments; one of these has just given a preliminary report of a positive result (Editorial, 1977). However, there has been far too little good research into ECT, particularly in view of the attempts by pressure groups to have it abolished — as with the new stereotactic tractotomy operations (reviewed in last year's *Medical Annual*, p. 206) the clinician needs more than the usual scientific evidence of efficacy when he advises a treatment which is regarded by many as barbaric and degrading. We need more evidence of the efficacy of ECT in patients under the age of 40, and in patients whose depressions lie in the middle zone between the endogenous and neurotic categories. It would be useful to have more information on how long the benefit of ECT lasts, and on the use of maintenance ECT in those patients who tend to relapse. ECT is usually given two or three times a week but there is no comparative information on the efficacy and side effects of these two frequencies of treatment. Finally, it would be both interesting and helpful to know how ECT produces its antidepressant effect.

The mortality of ECT is in the order of 3 – 9 per 100 000 treatments (Royal College of Psychiatrists, 1977) which is low compared to the mortality from suicide in depressed patients inadequately treated by other methods. There is no evidence that ECT causes epilepsy. The only definite undesirable side-effect of ECT is memory loss, both subjective and objective. Squire (1977) has shown that the memory loss is greater with bilateral than with unilateral ECT, but could not be detected six to nine months after the completion of treatment; it affects particularly memory for the temporal sequence of popular television programmes in the years before the patients received ECT. There is no correlation between memory loss and therapeutic effect.

There is a need for more knowledge about the long-term effects of ECT on memory. The odd case report of long-lasting serious amnesia following ECT is probably due to the administration of ECT to patients with pre-existing dementing conditions, and it is known that depression is commoner than would be expected by chance in the early stages of dementia. Regarding milder degrees of memory loss there is more doubt, and some clinicians may hesitate before recommending ECT to those who live by their memories, such as academics and college porters.

REFERENCES

Editorial (1977) Treatment of depression. *Br. Med. J.* **4**, 1105.
Friedberg J. (1977) Shock treatment, brain damage, and memory loss: a neurological
   perspective. *Am. J. Psychiat.* **134**, 1010 – 1014.
Greenblatt M., Grosser G. H. and Wechsler H. (1964) Differential response of
   hospitalised depressed patients to somatic therapy. *Am. J. Psychiat.* **120**, 935 – 943.
MRC (1965) Report by Clinical Psychiatry Committee. Clinial trial of the treatment
   of depressive illness. *Br. Med. J.* **1**, 881 – 886.
Price C. (1977) Kicking the television set. *New Statesman,* 14 Oct., pp. 502 – 503.
Royal College of Psychiatrists (1977) Memorandum on the use of electroconvulsive
   therapy. *Br. J. Psychiat.* **131**, 261 – 272.
Squire L. R. (1977) ECT and memory loss. *Am. J. Psychiat.* **134**, 997 – 1001.
Stern M. (1977) ECT under attack. *On Call.* 10 Nov., p. 5.

ANOREXIA NERVOSA

Anorexia is a misnomer for this syndrome in which there is no real loss of
interest in food and eating—rather the reverse, the patients are morbidly
obsessed with food in a manner similar to subjects of experimental starvation
(Casper and Davis, 1977). The patients say that they do not eat normally
because they are fearful of becoming fat or of losing control over eating, or
that they experience unpleasant feelings of guilt after having eaten (Russell,
1967). They do not seek help and often deny there is anything wrong with
them in spite of gross emaciation, and their image of themselves tends to be
distorted and variable (Button et al., 1977). These phenomena suggest some
meaningful psychopathology. Crisp (1977) speculates that the anorectic girl is
deliberately thwarting her sexual development by reducing her body weight,
responding to fears about family and peer-group implications of puberty.
Casper and Davis (1977) see the syndrome as a desperate and unregulated
attempt by a depressed and insecure girl to make herself more attractive and
raise her self-esteem—she finds that dieting is the only thing she can succeed at
and she cannot stop. Similar psychopathology is suggested by the few males
who develop the syndrome (Hasan and Tibbetts, 1977). Others think that
some cases at least may be atypical affective disorders (Cantwell et al., 1977),
impressed by the amount of depression in the patients at follow-up and in their
relatives. Some cases remind one of the dysmorphophobias (Andreason,
1977). Dally (1977) points to the family pathology and to the high incidence of
depression in the mothers.

On the other hand, anorexia nervosa may be a primary disorder of the
hypothalamus (Lupton et al., 1976). Four recent cases of hypothalamic
tumour emphasize the fact that apparently 'psychogenic' behaviour may have
an organic basis, in that the patients had attitudes to their illness and to food
which were not at all dissimilar to those described in anorexia nervosa.

Lewin et al. (1972) describe a 25-year-old female who developed an aversion
to any form of carbohydrate following her father's death. Like a true anorexia
nervosa 'she was bright and cheerful despite her emaciated appearance (30·8
kg) and seemed unaware of the gravity of her illness'. Subsequently at post
mortem 'the brain contained a small circumscribed nodule measuring 0·5 cm
in diameter on the inferior surface of the hypothalamus posterior to the optic
chiasma and immediately posterior and to the right of the tuber cinereum'.

Heron and Johnston (1976) describe a 24-year-old male who had always
been a finicky eater but who received a diagnosis of anorexia nervosa after
losing weight for two years following his discharge from the army. His mother

devoted extraordinary attention to feeding him, cooked separate menus for husband and son, and had stocked a large pantry with excessive quantities of food. The patient's 'lack of concern about his illness was striking'. He sabotaged his treatment programme by 'sneaking candy while refusing a high calorie diet'. Even after direct instructions his mother refused to stop bringing home-baked snacks to him. 'The psychiatric staff concluded that this family could not tolerate interference with their shared psychopathology, in which conflicted feeding was a prominent feature.' He subsequently developed optic atrophy and pituitary deficiency, and biopsy of a mass in the hypothalamic area revealed an ectopic pinealoma.

One of Swann's (1977) patients was a 12-year-old boy who was active and uncomplaining in spite of losing 5·5 kg. He had started to diet on holiday because he thought he was becoming fat. He was noted to spit out his food at mealtimes and then rinse out his mouth with water. He admitted that food disgusted him and he was seen to vomit several times per day without discomfort. He ate normally after the removal of a large midline tumour (grade 2 astrocytoma) indenting the roof of the third ventricle.

Finally, a 15-year-old boy reported by White et al. (1977) illustrates some of the typical personal and family psychopathology of anorexia nervosa. He had always been a trouble maker and began to lose weight after entering junior high school at which time he was experimenting with drugs and alcohol. Following a fight with the patient, the father had a myocardial infarct which required cardiac surgery. 'Shortly thereafter, a woman neighbour who had been the patient's confidante for some time died suddenly from a malignancy. The patient immediately reduced his food intake dramatically and began to lose weight quickly.' In spite of weighing only 27·2 kg 'the patient persistently denied that there was anything wrong with his appearance or his eating behaviour and did not recognise the severity of his nutritional status. One of his overriding concerns throughout his psychotherapy was the rather oppressive control that was exerted in the family and his feeling that he had no control over himself or what happened to him. He also alluded to a fear of growing up and assuming adult responsibilities.' His appetite returned to normal after aspiration of a large cystic tumour (thought to be a low grade glioma) between the anterior cerebral arteries and above the optic chiasma.

Diagnostic difficulties exist in the reverse direction. Crisp (1977b) discusses various medical presentations of anorexia nervosa, many arising from the patients' abuse of purgatives and other potentially slimming agents such as carrots, amphetamines, diuretics and thyroxine. They may even have been able to purchase a sugar-coated cyst of *Taenia solium*.

REFERENCES

Andreason N. C. (1977) Dysmorphophobia: symptom or disease? *Am. J. Psychiatry* **134**, 673 – 675.

Button E. J., Fransella F. and Slade P. D. (1977) A reappraisal of body image disturbance in anorexia nervosa. *Psychol. Med.* **7**, 235 – 243.

Cantwell D. P., Sturzenberger S., Burroughs J., Salkin B. and Green J. K. (1977) Anorexia nervosa: an affective disorder? *Arch. Gen. Psychiatry* **34**, 1087 – 1093.

Casper R. C. and Davis J. M. (1977) On the course of anorexia nervosa. *Am. J. Psychiatry* **134**, 974 – 978.

Crisp A. (1977a) Diagnosis and outcome of anorexia nervosa: the St George's view. *Proc. R. Soc. Med.* **70**, 464 – 470.

Crisp A. (1977b) The differential diagnosis of anorexia nervosa. *Proc. R. Soc. Med.* **70**, 686 – 690.

Dally P. (1977) Anorexia nervosa: do we need a scapegoat? *Proc. R. Soc. Med.* **70,** 470 – 474.

Hasan M. K. and Tibbetts R. W. (1977) Primary anorexia nervosa (weight phobia) in males. *Postgrad. Med. J.* **53,** 146 – 151.

Heron G. B. and Johnston D. A. (1976) Hypothalamic tumour presenting as anorexia nervosa. *Am. J. Psychiatry* **133,** 580 – 582.

Lewin K., Mattingly D. and Millis R. R. (1972) Anorexia nervosa associated with hypothalamic tumour. *Br. Med. J.* **2,** 629 – 630.

Lopton M., Simon L., Barry V. et al. (1976) Biological aspects of anorexia nervosa. *Life Sciences* **18,** 1341 – 1348.

Russell R. (1977) The present status of anorexia nervosa. *Psychol. Med.* **7,** 363 – 367.

Swann I. (1977) Anorexia nervosa — a difficult diagnosis in boys. *Practitioner* **218,** 424 – 427.

White J. H., Kelly P. and Dorman K. (1977) Clinical picture of atypical anorexia nervosa associated with hypothalamic tumour. *Am. J. Psychiatry* **134,** 323 – 325.

ALCOHOLISM: INEFFECTIVENESS OF PROLONGED TREATMENT

Each of the last three centuries has seen a vast surge in the prevalence of drunkenness (Glatt, 1977), so that, for instance, in the 1830s Sydney Smith could write: 'Everybody is drunk. Those who are not singing are sprawling. The sovereign people are in a beastly state.' The nineteenth century surge did not in fact end until the First World War, and the amount of alcoholism then remained low during the depression and the Second World War. Now the rate is rising again. Convictions for drunkenness were 48 000 in 1950 and 104 452 in 1975, and other indices of alcoholism are rising *pari passu*. However, per capita consumption of beers, wines and spirits is still well below the level at the turn of the century, and convictions for drunkenness in 1900 numbered 200 000. However, even if things were worse in the past, there is no cause for complacency with an estimated 400 000 alcoholics in England and Wales, and an unusually high and rising incidence in young people and females.

If we are at the beginning of a twentieth century surge of alcoholism the remedy must be social rather than medical. As if to emphasize this point, Edwards and Orford (1977) have reported a trial of treatment in 100 married male alcoholics. The patients were divided at random into two treatment groups: one group had a single interview involving both husband and wife, and follow-up was carried out via the wife at monthly intervals with a joint follow-up at one year. The other group had the full package of current alcoholism treatment: the husband had an individual psychiatrist, the wife a social worker; where appropriate psychotropic drugs including Abstem were used, introduction was made to Alcoholics Anonymous and the patients who did not respond to outpatient care were admitted to a specialized alcoholism in-patient unit. At the end of a year there was no difference between the two groups, either in social adjustment or in drinking behaviour. The authors are careful to point out that this was a selected patient group and that the results should be generalized with caution. However, it does throw the onus of proof onto those who advocate lengthy and expensive regimes of treatment for alcoholism.

Over the past few years Goodwin and his colleagues in St Louis, Missouri have been carrying out a series of studies on the drinking behaviour of adopted children in Denmark, mainly comparing the alcoholism rates of the adopted children of alcoholic biological parents with the rates in the adopted children of control biological parents. The studies have now been completed (Goodwin et al., 1977). In line with expectation from twin studies, they found little evidence for genetic factors in social drinking, but there was a fairly strong genetic factor in alcoholism itself. The only other pathology manifested by the children of the alcoholics was a high divorce rate. The incidence of alcoholism among the daughters was, of course, much lower than among the sons, and it was unfortunate that the subjects were only in their mid-thirties; however, the drinking behaviour of the daughters appeared to be much more under the control of environmental factors than did that of the sons. Environmental factors include treatment, and therefore it would be of great interest to see a repetition of Edwards and Orford's excellent study, but on wives rather than husbands.

REFERENCES

Edwards G. and Orford J. (1977). A plain treatment for alcoholism. *Proc. R. Soc. Med.* **70**, 344 – 348.

Glatt M. M. (1977) The English drink problem through the ages. *Proc. R. Soc. Med.* **70**, 202 – 206.

Goodwin D. W., Schulsinger F., Knop J., Mednick S. and Guze S. B. (1977) Psychopathology in adopted and non-adopted daughters of alcoholics. *Arch. Gen. Psychiatry* **34**, 1005 – 1009.

NEUROLOGY

C. J. EARL MD, FRCP

HUW B. GRIFFITH MA, BM, BCh,
MRCP(Lond), FRCS(Eng)

Medical

C. J. EARL MD, FRCP

ISCHAEMIC STROKE

The eventual outcome of an ischaemic stroke will depend on the amount and situation of brain tissue irreversibly damaged by anoxia. The situation of the damage cannot of course be influenced directly by treatment but attempts have been made over a number of years to influence the amount of brain tissue destroyed. These attempts are justified by the fact that it is known that blood flow through collateral circulation may improve the chances of recovery of nervous tissue, which initially has not suffered irreversible damage. Matthews et al. (1976) reported the result of a blind control trial of the use of dextran. They used dextran because: 'The anticipated benefits from the use of this agent are based on its action in decreasing aggregation of platelets and erythrocytes, decreasing blood viscosity and preventing platelet thrombi, thus improving the micro-circulation in the areas of ischaemic brain.' They assessed patients suitable for the trial within a few hours of admission to hospital, recording the state of consciousness, the degree of neurological deficit and, as far as possible, the site of infarction as deduced from the physical signs. Cerebrospinal fluid was examined in all cases and any patient with more than 500 red cells per mm^3 was rejected. Other routine investigations included an electrocardiogram, skull and chest X-rays, blood count, ESR and WR, blood urea and LDH/GOT and examination of the urine. Carotid angiography was carried out only if there was doubt about the diagnosis of stroke or if the findings might influence subsequent treatment. Patients were randomly allocated to control and treatment groups. There were 52 in the dextran group and 48 in the control group. Those in the dextran group, received 500 ml of intravenous dextran 40 in 5 per cent dextrose over 1 hour and 500 ml every 12 hours for 72 hours thereafter. The controls were given similar volumes of 5 per cent dextrose without dextran. The survivors were assessed at between 3 and 4 weeks and at 6 months after the onset. The assessment was particularly directed at functional recovery with hand function, gait, visual field disturbance and bladder and bowel control being recorded. Neuro-psychological assessment was also carried out and at six months an estimate of the patients functional activities and daily living were recorded.

Analysis revealed that there were no significant differences in the severity or situation of strokes in the two groups, or in antecedent or concomitant features such as a previous history of stroke, myocardial infarction or the presence of hypertension. Analysis of the results of the trial revealed that when the groups were considered as a whole there was no significant difference in survival or subsequent disability of the survivors. However, where only the severe strokes were analysed it became apparent that the prospect of survival of a patient with severe stroke was significantly increased, though the ultimate degree of disablement was no less than that in the survivors who did not receive dextran. In commenting on their results, the authors review previous trials and point out that none reported so far has assessed patients over a long period. They feel that in one trial (Gilroy et al., 1969), where patients were admitted for trial only after 24 – 72 hours had elapsed, good results might not be expected because dextran, if helpful at all, might be expected to act within a few hours of the occlusion.

The importance of the assessment of 6 months is clear from the fact that in the present series assessment at 3 weeks would have pointed to clear evidence of improved rate of survival. They add: 'This reduction in acute mortality was, however, achieved at the cost of the survival of a number of severely disabled patients, very few of whom achieved independence and many of whom died of the effects of diffuse vascular disease during the next few months.'

Autopsies were performed on 13 of 14 patients who died. Two in the control group were found to have intracerebral haematoma. Those who died from hemisphere infarction within the first week were found to have swelling of one hemisphere sufficiently severe to produce secondary haemorrhages in the midbrain, which were the cause of death. The authors' view is that the increased survival in severe stroke must therefore have been due to a reduction in oedema. Shaw et al. (1959) published observations on the cause of death in cerebral infarction and drew attention to the importance of cerebral oedema in patients dying within a few days of the onset of the illness. In those dying later there was no oedema and no evidence of its effects on the brainstem. Attempts have been made to influence the development and severity of oedema since then. Thus Myer et al. (1971) used glycerol in an uncontrolled trial, and later (1972) they claimed a transient increase in cerebral blood flow with intravenous glycerol. Steroids have been used experimentally in the gerbil (whose cerebral vascular anatomy makes it easy to produce severe infarction by carotid ligation) (Harrison and Ross Russell, 1972). The mortality following carotid ligation was reduced and this was attributed to a reduction in cerebral oedema. In a clinical study, Patten et al. (1972) used dexamethasone 16 mg daily over 10 days in a controlled trial. In severe stroke the improvement with dexamethasone was striking and this would accord with the result of the trial of dextran by Matthews and his colleagues.

It is clear that the problem is far from a solution.

REFERENCES

Gilroy J., Barnhart M. I. and Meyer J. S. (1969) Treatment of acute stroke with dextran 40. *J. A. M. A.* **210**, 293 – 298.

Harrison M. J. G. and Russell R. W. R. (1972) Effect of dexamethasone on experimental cerebral infarction in the gerbil. *J. Neurol. Neurosurg. Psychiatry* **35**, 520 – 521.

Mathews W. B., Oxbury J. M., Granger K. M. R. and Greenhall R. D. C. (1976) A blind controlled trial of dextran 40 in the treatment of ischaemic stroke. *Brain* **99**, 193 – 206.

Meyer J. S., Chaney J. Z., Rivera W. M. and Mathew N. T. (1971) Treatment with glycerol of cerebral oedema due to acute cerebral infarction. *Lancet* **2**, 993 – 997.

Meyer J. S., Fukuuchi Y., Shimazu J., Ohuchi T. and Ericsson A. D. (1972) Effect of intravenous infusion of glycerol on cerebral blood flow and metabolism in patients with acute cerebral infarction. *Stroke* **3**, 168 – 180.
Patten B. M., Mendell J., Bruun B., Curtin W. and Carter S. (1972) Double blind· trial of the effects of dexamethasone on acute stroke. *Neurology* **22**, 377 – 383.
Shaw C. M., Alvord E. C. and Berry R. G. (1959) Swelling of the brain following ischaemic infarction with arterial occlusion. *Arch. Neurol.* **1**, 161 – 177.

DIABETIC FOOT ULCERS

Chronic foot ulcers in diabetes are a frequent and serious complication of the disease. The roles of vascular disease and sensory loss are both clear in the aetiology of such ulcers. A recent paper by Harrison and Faris (1976) elucidates the problem and points out the importance, not only of sensory loss but also of motor fibre involvement. Stokes et al. (1975) previously demonstrated that the distribution of weight in the diabetic foot was altered, more weight being thrown on to the forefoot, and a 'lateral shift' of the forefoot load. The load carried on the toes was decreased. Six patients who had diabetic foot ulcers were studied and it was found that the maximum load of the foot occurred at the ulcer site. The lateralization of relative load bearing in different parts of the foot were related in turn to foot deformity. Stokes et al. and Harrison and Faris both believe that the deformity is the result of weakness of intrinsic foot muscles and they demonstrated by electrophysiological examination that the muscles are certainly weak. For example, there was no recordable response from extensor digitorum brevis or the abductor hallucis brevis during stimulation of the medial and lateral popliteal nerves at the knee and the ankle.

Their clinical and electrophysiological findings demonstrated clearly that there is an association of sensory loss and intrinsic muscle weakness with diabetic foot ulcers. Although ischaemia may have a part to play in the aetiology it seems clear that the presence of a neuropathy, both sensory and motor, is the most important factor in the common type of ulcer.

REFERENCES
Harrison M. J. G. and Faris I. B. (1976) The neuropathic factor in the aetiology of diabetic foot ulcers. *J. Neurol. Sci.* **28**, 217 – 223.
Stokes I., Faris I. B. and Hutton W. C. (1975) The neuropathic ulcer and loads on the foot in diabetic patients. *Acta Orthop. Scand.* **46**, 839 – 847.

NEUROLOGICAL SYNDROMES IN RENAL FAILURE

A useful review of the neurological disorders seen in renal failure was published in the *New England Journal of Medicine* recently (Raskin and Fishman, 1976). They point out that as a result of haemodialysis and renal transplantation 'new syndromes have been defined as a consequence of both increased longevity and complications of therapy'.

Uraemic encephalopathy

Apathy, drowsiness, mental confusion and delirium with disorders of perception and hallucinations are constant features, although in a given case the symptoms vary in severity from one time to another. A disturbance of postural tone in the outstretched hands, identical with liver 'flap', is very common. Irregular tremor is often apparent and the well known 'classic' uraemic twitching, which, as the authors rightly point out, is myoclonic in nature, often occurs. They also point out that tetany is fairly common. Incoordination of the limbs, unsteadiness in walking and increased tone in the limbs is common, and even focal motor signs in the form of a hemiparesis may appear. Convulsions, either generalized or local often accompany uraemia but the authors make the point that the high incidence of convulsions in the older reports may well have been related to hypertensive encephalopathy, so common in the past with renal failure.

Phenobarbitone or phenytoin may be effective in the treatment of epileptic attacks and for status epilepticus, which they find is rare, they recommend intravenous diazepam 10 – 20 mg given over 3 – 5 minutes or a continuous intravenous infusion at the rate of 100 – 150 mg/24 hours. A small proportion of patients had a raised cell count in the CSF and the protein is frequently elevated. The latter elevation is thought to be due to increased capillary permeability. The exact aetiology of uraemic encephalopathy remains obscure; there is no exact correspondence between the biochemical findings in the serum and the cerebral disorder but it is probably due to an accumulation of toxic substances (? organic acids), which accumulate excessively and 'overwhelm the normal mechanism for excluding such compounds from the nervous system'.

Uraemic neuropathy

This is very frequent in severe uraemia. It often begins with abnormal sensations temporarily relieved by movement and therefore may give rise to what may be described as a syndrome of 'restless legs'. Continuous burning sensations are also quite common. It is indistinguishable symptomatically and on examination from other forms of mixed sensory and motor neuropathy. The symptoms of the neuropathy vary in their rate of progress, and the relationship between the course of the neuropathy and the severity of the uraemia is often uncertain. Treatment by dialysis or renal transplantation improves the condition. It seems established that the neuropathy is due to primary involvement of axons rather than affection of myelin, such as occurs in the Guillain – Barré syndrome. Demyelination is seen on histological preparations but this is considered to be secondary to the axonal damage.

Some neurological abnormalities are attributable to the treatment by dialysis itself. The clinical picture known as the 'dysequilibrium syndrome' is seen in about 8 per cent of all patients on dialysis and is likely to occur when dialysis is rapid. Headache, mental symptoms, convulsions and occasionally evidence of raised intracranial pressure are the important features of this state which is thought to be due to cerebral oedema. Subdural haematoma is also a well recognized complication and may be difficult to distinguish from the dysequilibrium syndrome on clinical grounds alone. Occasionally a progressive cerebral disorder may occur, initially related to periods of dialysis but later becoming continuous and irreversible. The neurological complications of renal transplantation are in part related to immunosuppressive agents although the incidence of cerebral tumour is higher in patients with renal transplants than in those receiving immunosuppressive agents for other reasons. The tumours are reticulum cell sarcomas of the brain. These are identical with the spontaneously occurring micro-gliomas. One important characteristic from the therapeutic point of view is their sensitivity to radiation treatment. Chronic opportunistic infection of the nervous system is fairly common. Fungal infections are the most frequently seen and are extremely difficult to diagnose, and they may easily be confused clinically and on CSF examination with reticulum cell tumours, although if malignant cells are carefully looked for this confusion might be avoided. Toxoplasmosis involving the nervous system has also been described. Cytomegalovirus infection of the brain (and of the lung) is found frequently in patients who have been treated with renal transplantation and the view has been put forward that this may be due to reactivation of a latent infection that has been present for many years.

REFERENCE
Raskin N. H. and Fishman R. A. (1976) Neurologic disorders in renal failure. *N. Engl. J. Med.* **294**, 143 – 148 and 204 – 210.

MULTIPLE SCLEROSIS

The clinical diagnosis of multiple sclerosis (MS) rests on the basis of the discovery of signs of an appropriate type involving the central nervous system, and disseminated 'in space and time'. It may be asked why the diagnosis of MS is important in the early stages of the disease, when in any case it is not possible to offer any specific form of treatment. The answer to this question must be that early diagnosis may spare the patient unpleasant and harmful investigations and mis-directed treatment. There are many situations in which this may be the case, although they are fortunately not very common. Perhaps the most extreme case is that in which an atypical and chronic retrobulbar neuritis is the presenting feature of the disease. In this situation, even in the absence of any suggestive evidence on radiological investigation, surgical exploration of the optic nerves and chiasm may be undertaken to exclude absolutely any possibility of optic nerve compression. A more common problem is that of the isolated cervical cord lesion in a middle-aged patient, without evidence of root involvement but with clear radiological evidence on myelography of cervical spondylosis with some cord compression. A number of such patients within the author's experience have been treated surgically and unsuccessfully for their spondylosis, only to later develop clear evidence of MS.

There have been improvements in recent years in our ability to demonstrate lesions in parts of the nervous system, other than those primarily affected, and in biochemical studies on the cerebrospinal fluid. It is important to remember, of course, that the demonstration of other lesions by refined electrophysiological techniques is of no more significance than demonstration by routine clinical examination and the advance lies in the fact that the evidence can be found when it is absent on routine testing.

Visual evoked responses

The first useful contribution of this sort is the study of visual evoked responses (VER) in patients with optic neuritis. The VER is the potential change that can be detected through scalp electrodes (as in the conventional EEG), placed over the occipital region, with the eyes stimulated by light (Halliday et al., 1972). The type of stimulus which was found to be most useful in this context was that provided by an illuminated black and white chequered board, the pattern of which could be instantly reversed. This reversal of pattern under standard conditions produced a wave form of constant pattern. When the patient with optic neuritis was studied it was found that in the affected eye there might be no response at all to the standard stimulus. Where a response was elicited the important finding in optic neuritis was a clear delay measured from the time of the stimulus to a peak in the wave form of the response.

The normal latency by this method was about 120 msec in patients and in patients with optic neuritis the mean latency was 155 msec. The amplitude of the response was also reduced by about 50 per cent. The interesting observation, however, was that this prolongation of the latency remained even when acuity had recovered and it was later shown that patients with a past history of retrobulbar neuritis, although their vision might have recovered and the disc might have remained normal in colour, never showed a normal latency of the visual evoked response. The abnormal VER, then, is a sign of past optic neuritis, which seems to be as reliable as a history of transient visual disturbance or the observation of a pathologically pale optic disc. Decisions about an abnormality of disc colour are sometimes extremely difficult and subject to serious error, from which measurement of the VER appears to be free. The original findings have been confirmed by other investigators such as Asselman et al. (1975). It should be remembered of course that the presence of the pale discs is not conclusive evidence of MS and may occur in other neurological disorders; as one might expect, therefore, Asselman et al. found delayed responses in patients with 'tropical spastic neuropathy' or spino-cerebellar degeneration. Both of these conditions are known sometimes to be associated with optic atrophy.

Auditory evoked potentials

Auditory evoked potentials may be recorded in response to 'clicks', by an electrode over the scalp. The resulting wave pattern of the response is more complex than that from the occipital region but part of it is known to depend on intact brainstem mechanisms. Robinson and Rudge (1977) have demonstrated that this part of the response pattern was abnormal in 90 per cent of patients with MS who had evidence on clinical examination of brainstem involvement. It was also abnormal in 60 per cent of patients with the disease without clinical evidence of brainstem lesions determined by other routine methods. The significance of this finding has yet to be fully assessed, but it seems likely that just as the VER has an importance equal to that of the pale optic disc in the diagnosis of MS, so the abnormal auditory evoked response will be equally significant with the presence of nystagmus.

CSF examination

Examination of CSF has been traditionally a part of the investigation of patients with MS or of patients suspected of suffering from it. The subject was reviewed recently by Thompson (1977). The cell count is usually normal, or there is a small excess of lymphocytes. The total protein is also usually either normal or slightly elevated but the type of protein found is often abnormal. Two empirical tests have been applied to the CSF of MS for many years. Positive results of these tests are now known to be due to the presence of excess gamma globulin in the CSF. Pandy's reaction and the Lange colloidal gold curve have in the past given useful and helpful diagnostic information, although it was known that they were not specific of MS. More specific tests are now available for the estimation of gamma globulin and of immunoglobulin, the level of which is often raised in patients with MS. The results of a further analysis of the immunoglobulin G, which are now available, may be even more significant (Thompson, 1977). In the appropriate clinical context the finding of a raised level of IgG in the CSF points to the diagnosis of MS, but it must be remembered that, like the classic Lange curve and Pandy test, these quantitative analyses of protein fractions are not specific tests for MS and similar patterns of protein abnormality may be found in other forms of central nervous inflammatory disease such as neurosyphilis and other forms of encephalitis.

Management and treatment

Liversedge (1977) has reviewed current views on the treatment and management of MS. He discusses treatment based on the unproved hypothesis of bacterial, rickettsial or viral infection, none of which have had any demonstrable effect. The importance of dietary factors was first emphasized by Swank (1953), who produced evidence suggesting that the incidence of disease was highest in communities consuming a high fat diet. Later interest was directed to the unsaturated fatty acid linoleate, the level of which was found to be low in the serum of patients with MS (Baker et al., 1964). A trial of the effect of an addition of linoleate, in the form of sunflower seed oil, to the diet was published by Millar et al. (1973). The results of this trial appeared to show a reduction in the severity, duration and frequency of relapses in the treated group, but the significance of this result has since been questioned and further trials are in progress. There has been no evidence that a gluten-free diet is of any benefit, although this form of treatment received considerable publicity a few years ago. Liversedge also discusses the use of transfer factor and anti-viral agents, neither of which has any certain effect. The possible value of immunosuppressive treatment is a more difficult problem to deal with. For many years it has been thought that cortisone or ACTH may modify the course of the disease in some patients and reports of a trial by Miller et al. (1962) suggested that ACTH might have some effect. Subsequent studies have given uncertain results. The most recent trial (Gould et al., 1977) concerns the use of triamcinolone injected behind the eye in patients with acute optic neuritis. Such a single injection of tramcinolone produces a high concentration of steroids within the optic nerve and the eye. Although there was 'a trend towards more rapid recovery of vision', in the treated group, there was no evidence that the final state of visual function was any better in those who were treated than in the controls. The authors suggest restricting the use of steroids to patients in whom speedy recovery is important, such as patients whose only useful eye is affected or those with bilateral acute optic neuritis. Millar et al. (1967) demonstrated clearly no useful effect from regular administration of corticotrophin in patients with the disease. More 'heroic' methods of immunosuppression have also been used with a combination of steroids, azothiaprine and anti-lymphocytic globulin, but as yet there is no proof of their effectiveness.

REFERENCES

Asselman P., Chadwick D. W. and Marsden C. D. (1975) Visual evoked responses in the diagnosis and management of patients suspected of multiple sclerosis. *Brain* **98**, 261 – 282.

Baker R. W. R., Thompson R. H. S. and Zilkha K. J. (1964) Serum fatty acids in multiple sclerosis. *J. Neurol. Neurosurg. Psychiatry* **27**, 408 – 414.

Gould E. S., Bird A. C., Leaver P. K. and McDonald W. I. (19777 Treatment of optic neuritis by retrobulbar injection of triamcinolone. *Br. Med J.* **1**, 1495 – 1497.

Halliday A. M., McDonald W. I. and Mushin J. (1972) Delayed visual evoked responses in optic neuritis. *Lancet* **1**, 982 – 985.

Liversedge L. A. (1977) Treatment and management of multiple sclerosis. *Br. Med. Bull.* **33**, 78 – 83.

Millar J. H. D., Vas C. J., Naronha M. J., Liversedge L. A. and Rawson M. D. (1967) Long term treatment of multiple sclerosis with corticotrophin. *Lancet* **2**, 429 – 431.

Millar J. H. D., Zilkha K. J., Langman M. J. S., Wright H. P., Smith A. D., Belin J. and Thompson R. H. S. (1973) Double blind trial of linoleate supplementation of the diet in multiple sclerosis. *Br. Med. J.* **1**, 765 – 768.

Miller H. G., Newell D. J., Ridley A. R. and Schapira K. (1962) Therapeutic trials in multiple sclerosis. *Br. Med. J.* **1**, 1726 – 1728.

Robinson K. and Rudge P. (1977) Abnormalities of auditory evoked potentials in patients with multiple sclerosis. *Brain* **100**, 19 – 40.

Swank R. S. (1953) Treatment of multiple sclerosis with low fat diet. *Arch. Neurol. Psychiatry* **69**, 91 – 103.

Thompson E. J. (1977) Laboratory diagnosis of multiple sclerosis: immunological and biochemical aspects. *Br. Med. Bull.* **33**, 28 – 33.

Surgical

HUW B. GRIFFITH MA, BM, BCh, MRCP(Lond), FRCS(Eng)

PITUITARY GLAND

One of the things about change in medicine which disturbs people is recurrent fashion. Rather like the length of the female skirt, but with a different periodicity, interest in the provision for roughage in the bowel has returned in recent years after half a century. Such a periodic swing has now occurred in pituitary surgery, but here the reason for the recurrent interest has been technical advance and new knowledge, and not simply the whim of man.

When neurosurgery inched its way into existence at the end of the nineteenth century its founder, Harvey Cushing, gave his name to one of the enduring syndromes of endocrinology. At that stage, because of the twin bugbears of haemorrhage and infection, neither of which could be adequately dealt with, the method of approach to the pituitary was via the sphenoidal sinus. The pituitary fossa was usually enlarged by the tumour, which was producing increasing blindness. The method of entry to the sphenoidal sinus was under the mucosa of the nasal septum. This had the theoretical advantage that once the mucosa of the septum had been incised, and the septum itself resected, the surgeon could be said to be working outside the potentially infected nose and air sinuses, being in a sterile tissue plane. The technique was to insert a bivalved speculum to provide the operating passage, and the operative manipulations were done through this. Electric lighting had been invented for only about 20 years and the difficulties of vision, instrumentation and lighting all combined to produce a long dark hole through which the surgeon had to operate. Nevertheless, Cushing persisted with this form of surgery until the 1920s. Then, with increasing experience of osteoplastic flap cranioplasty, and the fact that the tumours which demanded operation were invariably large and growing upwards to distort and displace the optic chiasm, the subfrontal route began to displace the transphenoidal. The distance involved was shorter, the operative aperture itself could be wider, although the frontal lobe had to be retracted to provide this extra room. The invention of diathermy had by now done something to give the neurosurgeon a weapon against the complications of bleeding. Cushing therefore switched over almost entirely to the subfrontal route for operating on pituitary adenomas. He retired in 1933, and six years later his last trainee, the late W. R. Henderson, of Leeds, went through his pituitary cases and published a unique document on the surgery of the pituitary at that stage (Henderson, 1939).

The conclusions that Henderson drew were derived from the series of 338 cases, made up of earlier transphenoidal operations, and later subfrontal ones. Henderson's analysis showed convincingly that the degree of measurable visual improvement obtained was superior with the frontal operation. Thus there seemed little doubt that for operating on pituitary tumours the intracranial route was best and the transphenoidal route virtually became defunct. In only a few centres in this country did transphenoidal surgery in the old style linger on, and the operation was then only invoked for frail patients who would not survive a frontal craniotomy. In a few other countries, notably in Sweden, in one hospital in the U.S.A. and in France the transphenoidal operation was still practised sporadically.

Paradoxically, in the very year in which Henderson's paper showed that the transphenoidal operation was less effective, a professor of E.N.T. surgery in Zurich visited London at the request of the Otolaryngological Society and gave the Semon Lecture on a different route of access to the sphenoidal air sinus and thence the pituitary fossa. F. R. Nager reported 39 cases operated by a route which went partly through the ethmoidal air sinuses, a direct anterior relation of the sphenoidal air sinus. This method had first of all been proposed by Chiari of Vienna, but Nager improved it, and produced evidence to show that rapid visual improvement in patients with optic nerve compression due to pituitary tumour could be achieved. Incidentally, he operated on at least 1 case of an unusual condition we now recognize under the term 'empty sella syndrome'. Nager's experience was not enlarged upon by neurosurgeons, but was taken up by the E.N.T. fraternity. J. Angell James (1967), of Bristol, began to exploit the possibilities of the operating microscope which was introduced at the end of the war, and turned his attention to the use of this instrument in reviving Nager's operation and extending its possibilities. This entailed a great deal of work, since suitable instruments had still to be devised and produced. This period in the 1950s was the time for the emergence of the concept of endocrine control of cancer, which produced an increasing demand for pituitary destruction in metastatic breast carcinoma. Angell James applied himself to the problem, and devised a means of getting over the main bugbear of the transphenoidal operation, namely cerebrospinal leak and infection. This done, he operated on some 500 cases over the next 15 years and taught many other E.N.T. surgeons to do so. At the same time neurosurgeons were persisting with the transfrontal method for the same disease, and the late Murray Falconer, at Guy's, and Gledhill, in Belfast, gained a great deal of experience with the intracranial operation in patients with metastatic breast disease. The demand was great and the results were on the whole encouraging.

It emerged that pituitary ablation was more effective than the adrenal operation for the same disease, and that bone pain was the prime indication.

However, interest had not ceased in the transeptal operation, and in particular Gerard Guiot of Paris persisted with this and also introduced the operating microscope to this operation. In a recent publication Guiot and Derome have outlined their experience of 613 cases of pituitary tumour, utilizing the transseptal transphenoidal operation to very good effect (Guiot and Derome, 1976).

It had by now become clear that with improvements in lighting, and stereo-scopic vision which the operating microscope had brought, transphenoidal operating was very much less difficult than it had previously been. The problems of instrumentation were overcome, and there were effective measures to protect the patients from the dangers of infection. For disease confined to the pituitary fossa, as opposed to the large tumours which grow outside it and impair vision, the transphenoidal operation was superior. There has arisen a demand for surgery on patients with endocrine syndromes such as acromegaly, Cushing's syndrome, and the newly defined syndrome of hyper-prolactinaemia. These became natural candidates for the transphenoidal operation.

Pituitary tumours are operated upon for two reasons, the first because of their bulk. In the past this was the sole reason. A tumour that exhibits exuberant growth characteristics most often expresses them by greatly enlarging the pituitary fossa, by growing upwards and compressing the optic nerves and chiasm, or, bypassing them, and growing into the frontal lobe or hypothalamus. Outpouchings of tumour less commonly grow into the temporal lobe. Again less commonly the tumour grows into one or both cavernous sinuses and produces ocular motor palsies. These bulky tumours are those which neurosurgeons have traditionally operated upon. Microscopically the tumour is greyish, can be soft, but frequently is fibrous and vascular. The dura may be infiltrated. These tumours are usually regarded as benign histologically. They are reported as 'chromophobe adenoma'. Some of these patients may have acromegaly, a condition which is traditionally associated with eosinophilic adenoma. Other large tumours are discovered to produce prolactin, but these too are indistinguishable macroscopically from tumours in which no form of secretory activity can be demonstrated. These prolactin secreting tumours are reported histologically as 'chromophobe adenomas'. The bulky tumours, whether they produce growth hormone or prolactin, or ACTH (as in Nelson's syndrome), tend to have this grey uniform macroscopic appearance, and a histological appearance associated with non-secreting tumours. When the tumour is soft, surgical evacuation can be virtually complete, and the usual response of the visual apparatus to decompression is prompt and gratifying. When the tumour is more fibrous and vascular the surgical task is more difficult. The tumour tends to infiltrate the dura despite its uniformly benign histological appearance. A complete removal in such cases is not easily achieved.

The majority of the tumours that are being offered for operation to correct endocrine hypersecretion are smaller than the traditional neurosurgical chromophobe adenomas. The tumour usually expands the sella modestly, and the adenoma tissue is macroscopically quite different from that of the large tumour. For instance, in acromegaly the adenoma is composed of soft diffluent white tissue quite clearly distinguishable from the normal pituitary tissue which usually surrounds it as the peel around an orange. These tumours show no tendency whatever to infiltrate either the rest of the pituitary fossa or the dura, and usually can be completely removed. The growth hormone level then drops to normal levels or below and the acromegalic features regress. In some of these cases there is a normalization of other endocrine aspects of pituitary function, such as the return of menstruation in the female and the return of long departed libido in the male. These discreet adenomas offer a perfect substratum for selective surgical removal which is a much more efficient method of treating acromegaly when compared with external radiation and certainly when compared to the implantation of radioactive seeds. Drug treatment of acromegaly with chlorpromazine or bromocriptine is vastly less effective than the complete removal of the tumour. Present information is that after complete removal, with normalization of growth hormone levels in the serum, the tumours very rarely regrow.

The second type of discreet adenoma is usually smaller than that found in acromegaly, namely the prolactinoma. By contrast with the whitish tumours found centrally in acromegaly, these small prolactinomas are dark brown in colour and again are quite clearly distinguishable from the yellow normal pituitary tissue, are usually soft, and are situated laterally in the pituitary fossa. Again they are completely removable. They usually come to attention in the female by the production of secondary amenorrhoea and galactorrhoea, but at present do not seem to be a common cause of lack of sexual drive or of infertility in the male. Sometimes these prolactin adenomas fail to enlarge the pituitary fossa at all, and in these circumstances have been termed 'micro-adenomas'. It would seem logical to extend this scheme of terminology to include those tumours which remain confined to the moderately enlarged pituitary fossa as 'mesoadenomas', and to call those large tumours which are often well outside the pituitary fossa 'macroadenomas'.

Curiously enough, when these discreet soft and secreting adenomas are removed the histological report is usually 'chromophobe adenoma'. Occasionally in acromegalics the discreet adenoma enlarges enough to transgress the pituitary fossa, and may then involve the optic chiasm, but this is uncommon. Equally curious, and something which to my knowledge has never been remarked upon, is the fact that no intermediate forms of the tumours mentioned have been encountered. A third surprising fact is that a surgeon at operation with the naked eye or through the operating microscope can distinguish between a discreet growth-hormone-secreting neoplasm, a discreet prolactin-secreting neoplasm, and the large diffuse traditional grey chromophobe adenoma. The histologist is unable to do this, all being reported as 'chromophobe adenoma'.

This new knowledge has come about because of the new interest in the transphenoidal operation. Hardy and Wigser (1965), of Montreal, were the first to describe the microadenomas, something which neurosurgeons were at first sceptical about. The reason for their scepticism was that surgeons whose task was to deal with bulky tumours never saw these quite different micro-adenomas.

What are the practical implications of all this? They are that neurosurgeons are now being called upon to offer to patients with acromegaly and hyperprolactinaemia operations which will have a high degree of success in normalizing the endocrine hypersecretion, provided that the appropriate pathology is present. However, if the pathology of the adenoma is that of the grey diffuse type the chances of normalizing the hypersecretion are not great. It is of first importance to recognize this as far as possible before operation, since all the patients with prolactin microadenomas, and most of the patients with acromegaly, will essentially be patients leading an asymptomatic life not overshadowed by the threat of visual damage, as in the big tumours. Equally, since bromocriptine is so efficient at producing pregnancy in patients with secondary amenorrhoea, it is of some importance to try to prevent occasional disastrous pituitary apoplexy in pregnancy due to the enlargement which pregnancy brings to the adenoma as well to the normal gland. In the past this has not been a consideration, since before the advent of bromocriptine patients with hyperprolactinaemia were virtually excluded from pregnancy.

Cushing's syndrome is recognized to be due frequently to a 'basophilic adenoma'. The surgeon who is called upon to operate transphenoidally on these so-called 'neoplastic' glands very rapidly learns that no neoplasm is anywhere to be seen. There is neither the diffuse grey tumour of the traditional chromophobe type, nor the discreet soft white or dark adenomas of growth hormone secretors or prolactin secretors respectively. There is some doubt whether a basophilic adenoma really exists. Certainly the surgeon attempting to normalize ACTH hypersecretion takes care to remove the whole of what looks like relatively normal or even atrophic pituitary gland. The histological report on the removed tissue is apt to be 'basophilic adenoma', but again can sometimes be 'chromophobe adenoma'. It is ironic that Harvey Cushing's name is assocated with the only pituitary syndrome not due to an adenoma! However, there is a circumstance whereby the pituitary in Cushing's syndrome may develop an adenoma and this is where the treatment of the syndrome has been by adrenalectomy. In a sizeable number of these patients the skin pigments darkly, the pituitary fossa enlarges, and, when operated upon, a grey adenoma of the diffuse type is discovered (Nelson's syndrome).

It seems to have taken three quarters of a century to realize that a whole new world of pituitary pathology has been revealed by the return of transphenoidal surgery. It may well be that new syndromes are still to be discovered in this secluded gland.

REFERENCES

Guiot G. and Derome P. (1976) Surgical problems of pituitary adenomas. *Advanced and Technical Standards in Neurosurgery,* Vol 3. Berlin, Springer-Verlag.

Hardy J. and Wigser S. M. (1965) Transphenoidal surgery of pituitary fossa tumours, with televised radio fluoroscopic control. *J. Neurosurg.* **23,** 612 – 619.

Henderson W. R. (1939) Pituitary adenomata. *Br. J. Surg.* **26,** 811 – 921.

James J. Angell (1967) *J. Laryngol. Otol.* **81,** 1283.

Nager F. R. (1939) The paranasal approach to intrasellar tumours. *J. Laryngol. Otol.* **55,** 361 – 381.

NUTRITION AND VITAMINS

IVAN M. SHARMAN PhD, FRIC

ALCOHOL CONSUMPTION: SOME EFFECTS

Influence on blood lipids

Consumption of alcohol is known to impinge on lipid metabolism and transport. Previous studies have mainly emphasized its influence on blood-triglycerides. In a recent investigation Castelli et al. (1977) have examined the data from five populations in the United States and have considered several other blood-lipids and their relation to reported alcohol intake. Alcohol consumption was found to be positively associated with high-density-lipoprotein (HDL) cholesterol level in all populations examined (r from $0 \cdot 16$ to $0 \cdot 30$), the lipid level appearing to be a graded response even over the low levels of alcohol consumption reported, viz. $1 - 3$ and $4 - 9$ oz alcohol per week. Less strong but consistently negative correlations were found with low-density-lipoprotein (LDL) cholesterol. Plasma triglycerides in this study showed a modest positive correlation with the amount of alcohol imbibed.

These observations suggest that moderate amounts of alcohol may shift the lipoprotein pattern in man with the result that there is less blood LDL cholesterol and more blood HDL cholesterol. It may be presumed that this lipid effect is a metabolic response to alcohol since alcohol is known to influence lipid metabolism and transport. These new findings require considerable follow-up before they can be fully understood and before the improved understanding can be implemented.

Alleged influence on blood pressure

In another study in the States the relationship between alcohol consumption and blood pressure has been investigated (Klatsky et al., 1977). The drinking history over the previous year was investigated in over 100 000 individuals. They were divided into non-drinkers, those taking $0 - 2$ drinks each day, $3 - 5$, and more than 6 alcoholic drinks each day. Because of the very large number of subjects investigated it was possible to evaluate the relation of drinking to age, sex, race, cigarette and coffee use, education level and adiposity.

When compared with non-drinkers, those taking 6 or more drinks a day had significantly higher systolic (mean $10 \cdot 9$ mm Hg higher), and diastolic blood pressure (mean $4 \cdot 5$ mm Hg higher) in all the groups examined. Significant hypertension was defined as a blood pressure in excess of 160 systolic or 95 diastolic. The percentages of drinkers and non-drinkers with both systolic and diastolic 'hypertension' were found to be: $11 \cdot 21$ for drinking white men v. $4 \cdot 7$, $1 \cdot 3$ v. $6 \cdot 3$ in white women, $15 \cdot 1$ v. $10 \cdot 2$ in black men, and $24 \cdot 2$ v. $14 \cdot 7$ in black women.

As the effect did not become significant in all the sex and racial groups until more than two drinks were taken each day there seemed to be a threshold effect. Furthermore the effect was independent of age, sex, race, smoking, drinking of more than 6 cups of coffee per day or of educational attainment. The authors noted that these findings were similar to those of three other epidemiological studies.

However, in comparison with other studies the increase of blood pressure in drinkers does seem greater in the present study. These studies reinforce the contention that a heavy intake of alcohol may contribute to the development of hypertension.

REFERENCES
Castelli W. P., Doyle J. T., Gordon T., Hames C. G., Hjortland M. C., Hulley S. B., Kagan A. and Zukel W. J. (1977) Alcohol and blood lipids. The cooperative lipoprotein phenotyping study. *Lancet* **2**, 153.
Klatsky A. L., Friedman G. D., Siegelaub A. B. and Gerard M. J. (1977) Alcohol consumption and blood pressure. *N. Engl. J. Med.* **296**, 1194.

FOOD AND FIBRE

The role of fibre in man's diet continues to receive considerable attention. Since the nutritional significance of dietary fibre was last reviewed (Sharman, 1975) an international symposium on the subject has been held at Marabou in Sweden. The proceedings of this meeting have been fully reported in *Nutrition Reviews* (1977).

The bran hypothesis

In a recent book Burkett and Trowell (1975) have amplified their hypothesis of the aetiology of the so-called 'Western diseases'. These include appendicitis, diverticular disease of the colon, other diseases of the large intestine, ischaemic heart disease, diabetes, and diseases associated with constipation and straining at stool. The incidence of all these diseases is believed by them to relate to a reduction in the consumption of dietary fibre resulting from modern methods of refining foods. The changes that have taken place in the milling of cereals and the refinement of sugar during recent years have resulted in a drastic reduction in the fibre content of the diet. Burkett and Trowell also consider in their book the relationship of gastrointestinal transit times, and stool weights and consistency, with the fibre content of the diet.

In later chapters the authors contrast the prevalence, in Western and developing countries, of the diseases of the large intestine, of varicose veins and haemorrhoids, of gallstones, obesity and other diseases. They show that the incidence of these diseases in countries where cereals are refined is much greater than in those where the whole grain is still consumed. The book may be criticized for giving relatively imprecise information, but the authors take care to point out that such information can be of epidemiological value and that much of the evidence set out in the book may be considered in that category.

Definition of fibre

Agreement has still not been reached concerning the precise definition and terminology of fibre, nor are the details for its determination by analysis regularized. Although the word 'fibre' has been in use for about 200 years there are many objections to the term, though most authors deprecate the use of synonyms such as 'roughage'. The term 'dietary fibre' was defined in 1953 by Hipsley to include 'lignin, cellulose and hemicelluloses'. Trowell (1974) introduced a new definition based on physiological considerations, viz. 'as the remnants of plant cells resistant to hydrolysis by the alimentary enzymes of man'. Dietary fibre has, however, recently been redefined to include undigested storage polysaccharides, present within the contents of the cell, as well as the undigested polysaccharides and lignin present in the cell wall (Trowell et al., 1976). Alongside these definitions Hegsted (1977) has suggested that the correct definition should be based on functional terms, i.e. dietary fibre should be regarded as the material in foods which decreases the transit time, and increases the faecal volume, faecal water content, etc. Other aspects of defining 'dietary fibre' have been considered by Trowell (1977).

Analysis of dietary fibre

Southgate (1977) has pointed out that the analysis of 'dietary fibre' will depend upon what definition is adopted for this material. Thus if the extended definition, proposed by Trowell et al. (1976), is accepted then the term 'dietary fibre' will include the algal polysaccharides, such as alginates and carrageenan; gums, such as guar and locust ben; mucilages such as ispaghula and all other polysaccharides which are not digested by the endogenous secretions of the human digestive tract. The inclusion of these polysaccharides is justified, Southgate contends, on three main grounds: 1, Many of them are structurally related, chemically, to the polysaccharides present in the plant cell wall; 2, because they behave physiologically in the same way by increasing faecal bulk and retention of water in stools; and 3, because it is virtually impossible to distinguish, analytically, some components derived from the plant cell walls in the diet from those derived from other sources.

The range of polysaccharides present in the cell wall and therefore in any plant food or diets containing plant foods, together with the wide range of polysaccharide additives now implicated, means that the complete analyses of all the components in a mixed diet, for example, would be a major undertaking. Therefore any analytical procedure for dietary fibre must be a compromise between the complete separation and measurement of all the constituents, and a more simplified, empirical approach. Actual methods of analysis employed will depend upon what is of particular interest in individual cases. Methods are available for determining (1) the constituents of plant cell walls, (2) crude fibre, (3) unavailable carbohydrates, and (4) indigestible residues. However, few detailed comparisons of the different methods are available and more work is needed to assess the relative merits of the different approaches. For a full discussion of the analytical methods available see Southgate (1976).

As we do not know at present which components of dietary fibre are important in influencing such physiological properties as faecal bulking and retention of water in stools, Southgate (1977) suggests it is important not to seek for rapid methods for total dietary fibre evaluation as such values may well conceal the types of polysaccharide present. Southgate further proposes that it may well be time to consider the relationship of specific classes of polysaccharide in the diet, rather than the all embracing term 'dietary fibre', to health and disease.

Fibre and enterohepatic circulation

Eastwood (1977) has reviewed the characteristics of vegetable dietary fibre, the most basic being its ability to alter stool weight. In the plant, polysaccharides and lignins are interwoven for various anatomical reasons and physiological functions. During cooking and subsequent digestion this anatomy is lost and a heterogeneous mixture, retaining the physical properties which were of importance to the plant, results. These physical properties, which include gel formation, water and organic acid adsorption and cation exchange capacity, are translated into the gut. They may well be influenced by bacterial degradation in the colon. Plant fibre may be regarded as an entity which will have physico-chemical properties dependent both on its chemical constituents and on the age and possibly the anatomy of the plant that is eaten.

Certain absolute functions of vegetable dietary fibre are known in terms of human nutrition; this is particularly true with regard to its ability to increase stool weight. This function varies with different plant sources and depends on the water-holding capacity of vegetable dietary fibre, as well as the amount of fibre in the plant. The wide variations that are encountered may be illustrated by considering the differences between bran and carrot fibre. Thus bran which is 80 – 90 per cent dry material holds five times its weight in water. Carrot fibre, on the other hand, which forms only 9 per cent of the fresh weight, holds 20 – 30 times its own weight of water. 50 g of bran is capable of holding 200 g of water and is functionally equivalent to 100 g of raw carrot, 150 g of apple or 200 g of orange.

Fibre is thus a complex which is probably best defined in terms of its physico-chemical properties, the full biological implications of which are now being unravelled.

Carbohydrate tolerance after pectin administration

Administration of dietary fibre as wheat bran is known to improve carbohydrate tolerance in patients with diverticular disease, and the insulin requirements of diabetics can be reduced by other high-fibre diets. Pectin is known to reduce postprandial glucose and insulin levels when consumed with a carbohydrate meal, and is hypocholesterolaemic. Jenkins et al. (1977) have studied carbohydrate tolerance and cholesterol levels in normal subjects before and after 36 g pectin were added daily to metabolically controlled diets for 6 weeks. Three weeks after a control metabolic diet a breakfast containing 102 g carbohydrate, without pectin, was eaten after fasting overnight. Blood glucose and serum insulin levels were found to be similar after control and pectin diets, but there was 13 per cent fall in serum cholesterol after 6 weeks of pectin administration. It is therefore concluded that pectin does not exert a long term effect on carbohydrate tolerance when added in sufficient quantity to lower serum cholesterol levels. As pectin may have therapeutic applications, this finding that it does not impair insulin output after long term administration in healthy subjects is regarded as important.

REFERENCES

Burkitt D. P. and Trowell H. C. (1975) *Refined Carbohydrate Foods and Disease.* London, Academic.
Eastwood M. A. (1977) Fibre and enterohepatic circulation. *Nutr. Rev.* **35**, No. 3, 42.
Hegsted D. M. (1977) Food and fibre: evidence from experimental animals. *Nutr. Rev.* **35**, No. 3, 45.
Jenkins D. J. A., Leeds A. R., Houston H., Hinks L., Alberti K. G. M. M. and Cummings J. H. (1977) Carbohydrate tolerance in man after six weeks of pectin administration. *Proc. Nutr. Soc.* **36**, 60A.
Nutrition Reviews (1977). Fifth Annual Marabou Symposium, 'Food and Fibre'. *Nutr. Rev.* **35**, No. 3, 1 et seq.
Sharman I. M. (1975) Nutritional connotations of dietary fibre. In: Scott R. Bodley and Fraser J. (ed.), *Medical Annual,* 93rd Issue. Bristol, Wright, p. 240.

Southgate D. A. T. (1976) The analysis of dietary fiber In: Spiller and Amen (ed.) *Fiber in Human Nutrition.* New York, Plenum.
Southgate D. A. T. (1977) The definition and analysis of dietary fibre. *Nutr. Rev.* **35,** No. 3, 31.
Trowell H. (1974) Definitions of fibre. *Lancet* **1,** 503.
Trowell H. (1977) Food and dietary fibre. *Nutr. Rev.* **35,** No. 3, 6.
Trowell H., Southgate D. A. T., Wolever T. M. S., Leeds A. R., Gassull M. A. and Jenkins D. J. A. (1976) Dietary fibre redefined. *Lancet* **1,** 967.

HIGH-DENSITY LIPOPROTEIN LEVELS AND CORONARY HEART DISEASE

Interest in a possible relationship between plasma high-density lipoprotein and the pathogenesis of coronary heart disease has been stimulated by the hypothesis that such lipoprotein retards the progression of atherosclerosis by transporting cholesterol out of the arterial wall (Miller and Miller, 1975). The pool size of body cholesterol was found to be negatively correlated with the plasma high-density lipoprotein cholesterol concentration, and low concentrations of high-density lipoprotein were found in patients with clinical coronary heart disease. Subsequent investigations showed that the prevalence of coronary heart disease in middle-aged and elderly North Americans is independently and inversely related to the plasma high-density lipoprotein concentration. Other studies have shown that the plasma from patients with clinical coronary heart disease has lower concentrations of high-density lipoprotein peptides and a reduced capacity to bind additional exogenous cholesterol compared with the plasma from healthy controls. Another mechanism for a possible antiatherogenic effect of high-density lipoprotein has been suggested by Carew et al. (1976) from tissue culture studies. These have shown that high-density lipoprotein inhibits the uptake of the cholesterol-rich low-density lipoprotein by arterial smooth muscle.

However, it remains to be determined whether a low plasma high-density lipoprotein concentration precedes the onset of clinical coronary heart disease independently of other coronary risk factors, and is not merely a consequence of subsequent changes in diet or physical activity, both of which influence the concentration of high-density lipoprotein. This question has now been investigated, as part of the Tromsø Heart Study, in a cohort of young men living in the municipality of Tromsø in Norway. The large number of subjects participating in this investigation has allowed a prospective case-control comparison to be made two years after the initial cross-sectional survey made in 1974. Miller et al. (1977) have reported the details of this further study in which they examined over 6000 men aged 20 – 49 years. Measurements were made of high-density lipoprotein cholesterol concentrations in the plasma and these were examined in relation to the incidence of future clinical heart disease. Measurements were also made of the cholesterol concentration in lower-density, i.e. less than 1·063 g/ml, lipoproteins; plasma triglycerides; systolic and diastolic blood pressures; relative body weight; and cigarette consumption. Discriminant function analysis showed that coronary risk was inversely related to high-density lipoprotein cholesterol concentration and directly related to density less than 1·063 cholesterol. These relationships were independent of each other and of the other variables measured, which showed no significant differences between the cases and controls. High-density lipoprotein cholesterol levels were shown to make a threefold greater contribution to the prediction of future coronary heart disease than did density less than 1·063 cholesterol.

These findings therefore support the proposition that a low concentration of high-density lipoprotein is a frequent antecedent of clinical heart disease and is an important contributing factor in accelerating the progression of coronary atherosclerosis.

Differences in high-density lipoprotein cholesterol in adolescents

Ischaemic heart disease is a major cause of mortality in New Zealand, particularly among the Maori population, the relationship being more marked in males than females in both Maoris and non-Maoris. However, the prevalence of coronary heart disease in New Zealand does not seem to relate to the major risk factors, viz. cigarette smoking, blood pressure, and serum cholesterol concentration in Maori females, and only blood pressure seemed related in Maori males. An incidence study has shown that only blood pressure has a predictive value in Maoris of both sexes. In an endeavour to establish other ways of forecasting liability to heart disease attention has been directed to other risk factors and to a more detailed examination of serum lipids. Stanhope et al. (1977) have now explored lipid patterns in New Zealand adolescents in more detail and have measured cholesterol in serum high-density and low-density lipoprotein fractions in both girls and boys of Maori and non-Maori extraction. Low concentrations of HDL cholesterol and higher serum triglyceride levels were found in Maoris than in non-Maoris. Boys had lower HDLC and TG levels than girls. LDL cholesterol levels did not show any sex or racial differences. Stanhope and his colleagues suggest there may be a relation between these lipid distributions and the higher mortality, especially amongst females, from ischaemic heart disease. It will be interesting to see whether this suggestion can be supported in future studies.

REFERENCES

Carew T. E., Koschinsky T., Hayes S. B. and Steinberg D. (1976) A mechanism by which high-density lipoproteins may slow the atherogenic process. *Lancet* **1**, 1315.
Miller G. J. and Miller N. E. (1975) Plasma high-density lipoprotein concentration and development of ischaemic heart disease. *Lancet* **1**, 16.
Miller N. E., Forde O. H., Thelle D. S. and Mjos O. D. (1977) The Tromso heart study. High-density lipoprotein and coronary heart disease: a prospective case control study. *Lancet,* **1**, 965.
Stanhope J. M., Sampson V. M. and Clarkson P. M. (1977) High-density lipoprotein cholesterol and other serum lipids in a New Zealand biracial adolescent sample. The Wairoa College survey. *Lancet* **1**, 968.

NUTRITION: GENERAL

The booklet *Manual of Nutrition,* originally written by Dr Magnus Pyke when in the Ministry of Food during World War II, has recently been again revised and reprinted (Ministry of Agriculture, Fisheries and Food, 1976). This publication is designed to provide the reader with a basic understanding of nutrition. Thus it describes the main types of nutrients: carbohydrates, fats, proteins; it discusses energy needs and how these are obtained from foods by digestion and absorption into the body. Later it covers the necessary minerals and vitamins and continues with a discussion of all the main foods and the many factors which effect their nutritional value. There is also a guide to meal planning and a description of how to meet the requirements of special groups of subjects. In this eighth edition the booklet has been extensively revised by the Ministry's Nutrition Section to include a number of new items. The volume provides up-to-date information on the fundamentals for providing adequate nutrition for the varying needs of different individuals, including babies, children, pregnant and nursing mothers, old people, slimmers, vegetarians and immigrants. New features of this latest edition include sections on nutritional value for money; texturized vegetable protein; the so-called 'health foods'; dietary fibre; and the legislation relating to the nutritional value of food. Much of the information provided on the nutrient content of food is based on the recently revised edition of McCance and Widdowson's (1977) *The Composition of Foods*.

Another recent publication of general nutritional interest is Bingham's (1977) *Dictionary of Nutrition*. In this book detailed information is provided for over 200 entries of food, nutrition, and allied topics. Each of the main food groups is described, and at the end of every such entry there is a table showing the nutrient contents of each individual food in the group. For example, in the case of fruit, values are given for energy, protein, iron and other minerals, and for the relevant vitamins. Particulars are also provided to show the differences in the nutritional values of cooked and processed foods. Other sections deal with vitamin deficiency diseases, the reasons why specific nutrients are essential for health and the treatment of disease by special diets. Another section describes food additives and the reasons for their inclusion in certain commodities. The principles behind slimming regimes are explained and practical details are given for diets in cases of obesity.

REFERENCES

Bingham S. (1977) *Dictionary of Nutrition*. London, Barrie & Jenkins.
McCance R. A. and Widdowson E. M. (1977) *The Composition of Foods,* 4th edition revised and extended by Paul A. and Southgate D. A. T. (4th revised edition of M.R.C. Special Report No. 297). London, H.M.S.O.
Ministry of Agriculture, Fisheries and Food (1976) *Manual of Nutrition,* 8th ed. London, H.M.S.O.

SAFETY IN MAN'S FOOD

The provision of adequate nutrition for the human subject depends ultimately on the availability of clean and wholesome food. The food industry has made great strides in the manufacture, packaging, and marketing of foods today, but there are still a number of risks incurred in eating them.

Risk and benefit in food and additives

McLean (1977) has emphasized that food is 'dangerous stuff'. Obesity is a major disease, and the high fat diet eaten in many developed countries has been linked both to coronary artery disease and also to cancers of breast and colon. We accept the risks of unwise eating on the grounds that it is both voluntary and pleasurable, but this does not absolve us from informing the public of the consequences of some patterns of food choice.

For certain contaminants, McLean points out, there is an apparent anomaly in our attitude. Thus nitrate in drinking water is present at a level of about 50 mg/l, which leaves a safety margin of less than 2 before methaemoglobinaemia is likely to become a problem for infants. For most substances added intentionally to food we demand a safety margin of 100 between the dose that causes any adverse effect—or perhaps any physiological effect in animals—and the dose used by man. However, such margins are, of course, impossible for common salt, or dietary protein, fats, or modified starches.

The wide range of food additives includes the antioxidants, preservatives, flavourings, many substances such as modified starches, and colours. The additive is often chemically very close to natural and known food components, such as ascorbic acid. However, acetylated and phosphated starches are really new molecules that can form a high proportion of the carbohydrate intake of infants, and this for a benefit that is essentially one of marketing. Thus the canned baby foods containing these starches do not settle into a lump requiring re-mixing after storage.

The benefits of food additives are largely that they make processed convenience foods possible. Thus the storage of biscuits, crisps and most fat-containing manufactured foods would not be possible without antioxidants. Food colours in this country, when permitted, are free of control in respect of how much is added and to what food. As a result an increasing concentration and total intake of colours comes about as competitive marketing leads to deeper coloured soft drinks, sweets and confectionery.

Elton (1977) suggests that it is always necessary to keep a sense of proportion about the risks to health arising from the consumption of these foods. There is a risk associated with every human activity, and the number of deaths known to be caused by food poisoning every year is very small compared with deaths from road accidents or from accidents in the home. However, food does have a special place in our minds and the public understandably tends to view hazards from food with more emotion than those from other human activities. Many of the toxic hazards that plagued the national food supply a century ago have been eliminated, and the regular surveillance of food for potentially hazardous substances is part of the continuing work to improve the situation still further.

Assessing the safety of novel protein-rich foods

Synge (1977) considers the recommendations on safety of protein-rich foods made in the M.A.F.F. (1974) report is likely to shape developments for many years to come. In this report a first distinction is made between familiar, e.g. soya and conventional food-legume seeds, and unfamiliar starting materials. It may well be a long time before processed-protein manufacturers need to use unfamiliar starting materials and even if they eventually do it will be after many years experience of their use in animal feedingstuffs. A second distinction made by the Food Standards Committee is between processing procedures. Those involving mainly mechanical or physical treatments will require little or no surveillance, whereas those involving chemical treatments, including the use of solvents, will need to obtain some kind of official approval.

Toxic materials can and do occur in familiar foods. Extraneously arising mycotoxins, etc., need surveillance. Some low-molecular toxic substances—e.g. the substances of *Vicia faba,* responsible for favism in susceptible subjects, and the potato glycoalkaloids—may be largely eliminated in the course of processing. Furthermore toxic proteins, in particular the lectins or phytohaemagglutinins, which represent a substantial fraction of the proteins of many foods, e.g. legume seeds, lose their toxicity on suitable heating. Yet heating does not destroy the toxicity of wheat protein to which coeliac patients react adversely, so it would be unwise to allow wheat gluten to be used as a general additive to a wide range of processed protein foods.

Toxicity can also arise during some processing procedures. Thus sulphite, which is used very extensively in the food industry, can give rise to the destruction of thiamine. It can also form a variety of coupling products with reducing carbohydrates, some of which might be toxic.

Synge concludes by urging conservatism on food processors in their choice of both protein sources and in their choice of processes. With this conservative approach, there should be ample scope for palatable and nutritious innovations. Such conservatism is urged because when dealing with man the effects of a new dietary constituent may not be manifested as disease until 50 years or more after beginning to eat it. Any danger may also elude detection in the course of animal testing and in the practical feeding of farm livestock that is comparatively short-lived.

Food surveillance and food safety

Surveillance of food can be defined as the systematic determination of amounts of selected potentially toxic substances present in samples representative of individual foods or of total diets, either naturally or locally. Food surveillance is normally undertaken to provide a factual basis for the assessment, by expert committees, of any possible hazard to the consumers' health from the consumption of such foods.

Elton (1977) considers that the practical value of surveillance procedures depends largely on the type of contaminant present. As a generalization, total diet studies and routine monitoring of food samples for chemical contaminants have often proved valuable in the past and are continuing to do so; in some cases, however, our ability to detect minute traces of some chemical contaminants has outstripped our ability to interpret the significance, if any, of the resultant findings on human health. The problems facing the Toxicity Sub-Committee of the Committee on Medical Aspects of Chemicals in Food and the Environment and the Food Additives and Contaminants Committee of the Ministry of Agriculture, Fisheries and Food, are not easy ones, but these committees do play an important part in the safeguarding of public health in this country.

Methods for the assessment of contamination of foods by pathogenic micro-organisms are often less satisfactory than those for chemical contaminants. Nonetheless, monitoring as practised by Health Authorities, and epidemiological surveys carried out by the Public Health Laboratory Service and by research microbiologists have identified particularly troublesome sources of food poisoning. Elton points out that the most effective control in the interests of consumer protection is exercised, however, not by the use of legal standards and end-product sampling, but by the legal requirements or codes of practice for adequate processing and regular quality control checks by the processor.

REFERENCES
Elton G. A. H. (1977) Food surveillance and food safety. *Proc. Nutr. Soc.* **36,** 113.

M.A.F.F. (Ministry of Agriculture, Fisheries and Food) (1974) Food Standards
    Committee Report on Novel Protein Foods (FSC/REP/62). London, H.M.S.O.
McLean A. E. M. (1977) Risk and benefit in food and additives. *Proc. Nutr. Soc.*
    36, 85.
Synge R. L. M. (1977) The problem of assessing the safety of novel protein-rich foods.
    Proc. Nutr. Soc. **36**, 107.

VITAMIN A AND CANCER

It has long been known that there is a direct relationship between the role of
vitamin A when controlling epithelial cell differentiation and the development
of malignancy in epithelial tissues. Recently efforts have been made to apply
this relationship for the express purpose of preventing epithelial cancer. Since
vitamin A is required in the normal pathway of epithelial cell differentiation in
practically all of the epithelial target sites of origin of cancer, and because
epithelial cancers account for the majority of new cancer cases, and of cancer
deaths, it is understandable that this approach to cancer control is receiving
considerable attention.

Dietary deficiency of vitamin A and susceptability to carcinogenesis

Several recent studies have indicated that deficiency of vitamin A enhances
susceptibility to carcinogenesis in both experimental animals and man. Thus in
an extensive 5-year study of over 50 cases of lung cancer Bjelke (1975) reported
a lower prevalence of the disease in subjects who had received for some years a
relatively larger intake of vitamin A-containing foods. Furthermore this
protection could not be attributed to any association between ingested vitamin
A and smoking because the effect persisted when the statistical analysis was
repeated for each category of smokers. Even so, this finding might be
attributable to chance except for the fact that animal experimental work points
in the same direction.

These results suggest that vitamin A active compounds, or some closely
associated dietary factors, may modify the expression of pulmonary
carcinogens or cocarcinogens in man. In view of the difficulties of influencing
smoking behaviour in some confirmed subjects Bjelke suggests that the use of
ingested agents, that may be potent prophylactics against the effect of
smoking, should be of more than theoretical interest.

Pharmacological prevention of cancer with vitamin A

It is evident that many people whose diets meet all the known recommended
nutritional requirements develop invasive epithelial cancer. But can the
administration of large amounts of vitamin A, or vitamin A-active
compounds, prevent cancer? The first attempts at cancer prevention by
vitamin A used the common forms of the vitamin such as retinyl acetate and
retinyl palmitate. Although in some studies these retinyl esters were reported
to be beneficial, results in general have been conflicting. These varying effects
are, no doubt, partly due to the fact that even though high levels may be
included in the diet, these esters may not be available at specific epithelial
target sites because of the special mechanisms for transport of retinol in the
blood and the storage of retinyl esters in the liver. Furthermore, the resultant
excessive deposition in the liver may lead to damage by toxicity. Such readily
available vitamin A compounds are therefore not particularly effective agents

for pharmacological use for attempting to prevent cancer. For this purpose it has therefore been necessary to synthesize other retinoids that have different patterns of tissue distribution, metabolism, and storage in the body and which are less toxic to the liver.

A very wide range of retinoids, with modifications of the ring, side chain, and polar terminal group, have been developed. Such compounds, although structural analogues of vitamin A, have biological and pharmacological properties that are distinctly different from those of retinol, retinyl acetate and retinyl palmitate. Many of these synthetic retinoids have been found to be highly active in controlling normal differentiation of epithelial cells though they do not support growth when fed to animals deficient in vitamin A.

The availability of such compounds has led to the development by Sporn et al. (1976) of an approach to 'chemoprevention' of common forms of epithelial cancer during the period of preneoplasia. This approach is in contrast to 'chemotherapy' which is used for the treatment of invasive, malignant cells. In contrast to the cytotoxic approach of chemotherapy of invasive cancer, in which a deliberate attempt is made to destroy cancer cells by blocking key metabolic pathways, in chemoprevention during the period of preneoplasia an attempt is made to arrest or reverse premalignant cells during their progression to invasive malignancy, using physiological mechanisms that are not cytotoxic. There is good reason to believe that such mechanisms are usually operative in man during the period of preneoplasia, but that they are relatively ineffective if the exposure to carcinogens or cocarcinogens is excessive. A nutritional, physiological, or pharmacological enhancement of these protective mechanisms is thus required if the goal of the prevention of invasive cancer is to be achieved. The potential future usefulness of this new approach to cancer prevention in man may also depend on further synthetic modifications of the retinol molecule.

REFERENCES

Bjelke E. (1975) Dietary vitamin A and human lung cancer. *Int. J. Cancer* **15**, 561.
Sporn M. B., Dunlop N. M., Newton D. L. and Smith J. M. (1976) Prevention of chemical carcinogenesis by vitamin A and its synthetic analogs (retinoids). *Fed. Proc.* **35**, 1332.

OCCUPATIONAL HEALTH

G. KAZANTZIS MB, BS, PhD,
FRCS, MRCP, MFCM

THE ROLE OF HYPERSENSITIVITY IN INFLUENCING RESPONSE TO METAL TOXICITY

The reactivity of the host has to be taken into account in any consideration of factors influencing susceptibility to a toxic agent. An untoward, or idiosyncratic effect may result from a variety of causes, as for example from a genetically determined enzyme deficiency or as a result of allergy or increased reactivity, dependent on prior exposure. The term 'hypersensitivity' is used here to describe such an increased reactivity, resulting from the immune response. A simple molecule, such as a metal, requires complexing with protein or with some other complex molecule in order to become capable of stimulating an immune response, which involves the formation of covalent bonds to form a hapten-carrier conjugate. Immune responses harmful to the tissues have been classified by Coombs and Gell (1968) into four basic types: anaphylactic or immediate hypersensitivity (type I); cytotoxic hypersensitivity (type II); immune complex hypersensitivity (Arthus or type III); and cell mediated or delayed hypersensitivity (type IV). Only certain metals have been shown to provoke an immune response, but the hypersensitive states to which they can give rise are in some cases common and therefore important. Platinum, mercury, gold, nickel, chromium and beryllium have been chosen to illustrate the variety of hypersensitive reactions which can be produced (Kazantzis, 1978).

Platinum

Exposure to certain complex salts of platinum gives rise to an allergic reaction involving skin or respiratory tract even in persons with no atopic tendency after a variable period of exposure. Sensitized subjects may present with conjunctivitis, rhinitis, asthma, urticaria or contact dermatitis. Anaphylactic reactions have also been reported following the use of complex platinum salts as chemotherapeutic agents (Van Hoff et al., 1976). Typical type I skin, nasal and bronchial reactions have been elicited with platinum halide complexes, indicating the presence of mast-cell sensitizing antibody. Immediate, late and dual bronchial reactions were demonstrated by Pepys (1973) in sensitized subjects exposed to complex salts of platinum mixed with lactose. An Arthus Type III reaction indicative of the additional presence of precipitating antibody has also been demonstrated.

Mercury

Hypersensitive reactions following exposure to inorganic or organic mercurials involve the kidney or the skin and are not uncommon. Both proteinuria and the nephrotic syndrome have followed occupational and therapeutic exposure to mercury (Kazantzis et al., 1962). Electron microscopy of the kidney in mercury-induced nephrotic syndrome has shown basement membrane thickening with fusion of epithelial cell foot processes. Immunofluorescence has demonstrated deposits indicative of a membranous glomerulonephritis with a likely immune complex pathogenesis, the lesions being caused by the deposition of antigen-antibody complexes.

Thiomersal and ammoniated mercury are common skin sensitizers, and skin sensitization to amalgam dental fillings has also been reported (Feuerman, 1975). Cutaneous hypersensitivity to mercury, as demonstrated by a standard patch test technique, has been investigated in dental students and found to increase with length of exposure to mercury on the course (White and Brandt, 1976).

Gold

Both proteinuria and the nephrotic syndrome have followed exposure to gold compounds, but only after therapeutic administration in organic form. Renal biopsy with electron microscopic and immunofluorescent studies has indicated that complexes of immunoglobulin and of complement were involved, with appearances similar to those seen in idiopathic membranous glomerulonephritis (Morel-Maroger and Verroust, 1975). Bone-marrow depression with thrombocytopenia, granulocytopenia and aplastic anaemia are further examples of a hypersensitivity reaction to gold, and lymphocyte transformation in patients with bone-marrow depression following gold therapy has been demonstrated. Pulmonary fibrosis in some rheumatoid patients may also have been induced by gold, for exacerbation and remission has been noted to coincide with courses of therapy (Geddes and Brostoff, 1976). While contact dermatitis may occur from metallic gold, allergic dermatitis following organogold therapy is much more common. In one investigated series, the rash was preceded by eosinophilia and raised IgE levels (Davis and Hughes, 1975). The evidence presented shows that gold may give rise, under appropriate circumstances, to Types I, III or IV hypersensitivity reactions.

Nickel

Nickel was found to be the most common skin sensitizer in patch testing studies (Epidemiology of Contact Dermatitis, 1973), both occupational and general environmental exposure being responsible. The type of immune reaction involved, as with most other forms of contact dermatitis, is Type IV, T-cell mediated or delayed hypersensitivity. Both lymphocyte transformation and leukocyte migration inhibition have been demonstrated in subjects with a history of nickel dermatitis. Jordan and Dvorak (1976), using nickel sulphate without prior coupling to a carrier protein, were able to distinguish subjects with nickel dermatitis from controls by inhibition of migration of polymorphonuclear leukocytes, and they detailed the technical requirements for the test.

Chromium

Hypersensitivity to chromium as shown by the patch test using potassium dichromate was found to be second only to nickel as the most common form of skin sensitization in the studies quoted above, both occupational and general environmental contact being responsible. It is likely to be the most frequently occurring occupational dermatosis. Again Type IV, delayed hypersensitivity, is involved, hypersensitivity occurring to chromium acting as a hapten conjugated to protein rather than to any specific chromium compound (Polak et al., 1973). Hexavalent chromium is a more potent sensitizer than the trivalent form, probably because of its greater skin penetration. However, it has poor protein binding capacity in contrast to trivalent compounds. Polak et al. have proposed that following skin penetration hexavalent chromium is converted to the trivalent form by sulphur containing amino acids in the skin followed by conjugation with protein to produce the full antigen. All chromium compounds give a positive response in the macrophage migration inhibition test.

Beryllium

Exposure to beryllium, most often occupational, may give rise to acute tracheobronchitis, pneumonitis, contact dermatitis or to chronic beryllium disease, this latter being a multisystem disorder principally affecting the lungs. Contact dermatitis following exposure to beryllium compounds is of the delayed form and likely to be due to T-cell mediated hypersensitivity. Both lymphocyte transformation and leukocyte migration inhibition have been demonstrated in beryllium-sensitive subjects and in animal models. The evidence suggests that chronic berylliosis is an autoimmune disorder (Reeves, 1976). Reeves found an apparent immunity in guineapigs to pulmonary berylliosis following previous skin sensitization, and furthermore cutaneous hypersensitivity was suppressed following inhalation exposure. He postulated that the cellular response following cutaneous hypersensitivity may help to destroy an auto-antigen formed in the lungs. The beryllium-induced macrophage migration inhibition test was found to be positive in 2 patients with chronic beryllium disease but not in others on steroid suppressive therapy. Some beryllium workers also gave a positive response, while all controls tested, both normal and patients with sarcoidosis, were negative (Price et al., 1977). The significance of sensitization in such workers, with regard to a disease which may first develop many years after exposure, is unknown.

REFERENCES

Davis P. and Hughes G. R. V. (1975) *Ann. Rheum. Dis.* **34**, 203 – 204.
Epidemiology of Contact Dermatitis in North America, 1972 (1973) *Arch. Dermatol.* **108**, 537 – 540.
Feuerman E. J. (1975) *Int. J. Dermatol.* **14**, 657 – 660.
Geddes D. M. and Brostoff J. (1976) *Br. Med. J.* **1**, 1444 – 1445.
Gell P. G. H. and Coombs R. R. A. (ed.) (1975) *Clinical Aspects of Immunology*, 3rd ed. Oxford, Blackwell, p. 761.
Jordan W. P. and Dvorak J. (1976) *Arch. Dermatol.* **112**, 1741 – 1744.
Kazantzis G. (1978) Environmental health perspectives. To be published.
Kazantzis G., Schiller K. F. R., Asscher A. W. and Drew R. G. (1962) *Q. J. Med.* **31**, 403 – 418.
Morel-Maroger L. J. and Verroust P. J. (1975) Clinicopathological Correlations in glomerular diseases. In: *Recent Advances in Renal Disease* (ed. Jones N. F.). London, Churchill Livingstone, pp. 48 – 89.
Pepys J. (1973) *Clin. Allergy* **3**, 1 – 22.
Polak L., Turk J. L. and Frey J. R. (1973) *Prog. Allergy* **17**, 145 – 226.
Price C. D., Jones Williams W., Pugh A. and Joynson D. H. (1977) *J. Clin. Path.* **30**, 24 – 28.
Reeves A. L. (1976) *Ann. Clin. Lab. Sci.* **6**, 256 – 262.
Van Hoff D. D. Slavik M. and Muggia F. M. (1976) *Lancet* **1**, 90.
White R. R. and Brandt R. L. (1976) *J. Am. Dent. Assoc.* **92**, 1204 – 1207.

TESTING INDUSTRIAL CHEMICALS FOR TOXICITY

Some four million new chemicals have been identified over the last ten years, providing a formidable problem in screening for hazard. Only a small proportion of these will have been handled in significant quantities by people at work, possibly with lower environmental exposures at a population level. In the past, effective action in safeguarding the health of the worker was often hampered by a paucity of information on the hazard associated with many of the chemicals used. The need for an effective monitoring system was given impetus by the realization, in 1973, of the hazard associated with exposure to vinyl chloride monomer in the manufacture of PVC, as recorded in this *Annual* in 1974 (p. 303) and in 1975 (p. 251). The Health and Safety at Work Act 1974 requires manufacturers and suppliers to provide information on the toxic properties of substances intended for use at work. A scheme has now been proposed for their statutory notification to the Advisory Committee on Toxic Substances of the Health and Safety Commission. This scheme, which accords with a directive from the Council of the European Communities, is outlined in a discussion document (Proposed Scheme for the Notification of the Toxic Properties of Substances, 1977).

It is hoped that the proposed scheme will help to safeguard the health of persons at work and to protect the community from work activities. Notification will assist the earlier detection of hazards so that they may be controlled, and information collected may in the long term be of value when linked with the epidemiology of occupational diseases. Initially, only new substances will come under the scheme and, of these, only those introduced in quantities greater than 1 tonne per annum. It was not thought practicable to include the large number of chemicals synthesized for research and development purposes and handled only by small numbers of experienced personnel. The scheme will not provide for clearance or approval of chemicals submitted. The information given on each chemical should give a reasonable assessment of its toxic hazard and of the appropriate precautions to be taken for its safe handling and use. While additional data may be required for some chemicals, guidance is given on the minimum, basic information which should be made available. The various screening tests proposed are costed at 1976 financial levels, and are summarized as follows:

1. Chemical and physical information relevant to the toxicity hazard: This should include nomenclature, formulas, degree of purity, respirable fraction, hazardous thermal decomposition products etc.
2. Acute effects: Under this heading is included the LD_{50} or LC_{50} in appropriate groups of 6 rats observed for 14 days, also dermal toxicity studies, skin and eye irritation and skin sensitization.
3. Chronic effects: While standard tests are usually performed on a daily exposure basis for 90 days, a 30-day test on groups of 10 animals is recommended on the grounds that the great majority of adverse effects are seen during this period.
4. Carcinogenicity tests: Life time animal studies are accepted as the best available test, but on the grounds of expense and time two short term tests are proposed. These are, the observation of mutagenic changes in bacteria (Ames Test) and the in vitro transformation of cultured cells.
5. Mutagenicity tests: Again, the Ames test and in vitro cell transformation are recommended, as these tests measure both carcinogenic and mutagenic potential. Three generation studies – dominant lethal assay,

specific locus assay for detecting point mutations and other tests—are not recommended on the grounds of cost.

6. Teratogenicity tests: Fetal toxicity is proposed as an indicator of teratogenic potential. In this test fetal death is measured by counting resorptions in the pregnant animal or litter size after delivery, and it is recommended that the results be interpreted in conjunction with the other tests described above.

7. Tests for environmental effects: Two screening tests are recommended as initial requirements in the assessment of environmental hazard: These are (a) toxicity to one or two species of fish, and (b) susceptibility of the chemical to biodegradation.

These proposals, amended in the light of comments received, will form the basis of draft regulations.

McLean (1977), commenting on the proposals, pointed to the multiplicity of organizations that will be monitoring chemicals. In addition to the Health and Safety Executive Scheme there will be the Pesticide Safety precautions Scheme and the DHSS committee on the safety of chemicals in Food and Environment. Four essential steps have been defined in the decision-making process on the fitness of a chemical for use. These are the measurement of toxicity, the assessment of hazard, the evaluation of risk and the epidemiological follow-up. The new scheme, says McLean, introduces a 'mini toxicity' test without reference to the intended use of the new chemical, so that the wrong test may be done. Furthermore, the scheme does not make it clear to industry that the evaluation of hazard can only be made as a series of steps culminating in careful observation and recording of the health of exposed workers. Inadequate toxicological testing may give false negatives·which may harm the workers, whilst false positives may harm society in preventing the use of a potentially valuable chemical.

REFERENCES
Proposed scheme for the notification of the toxic properties of substances (1977) Health and Safety Commission Discussion Document. London, H.M.S.O.
McLean A. E. M. (1977) *Lancet* 2, 1070 – 1071.

HEALTH AND SAFETY IN MEDICAL LABORATORIES

The provisions of the Health and Safety at Work Act 1974 now apply to hospital and other medical laboratories in the same way as they do to all other workplaces. The lack of earlier legislative cover, together with a certain disregard for preventive principles by some members of the medical profession, may be in part responsible for working conditions in some laboratories which have not been noted for their safety. Lunch has often been taken at the workbench and smoking permitted in the laboratory, and the author has seen food and beverages stored in fume cupboards. Yet medical laboratories harbour a wide variety of potential hazards—biological, chemical and physical. Few studies have been carried out on the health of laboratory staff, who are often not covered by the provision of an occupational health service.

A retrospective postal survey of over 20 000 medical laboratory workers in Great Britain has confirmed some suspected hazards and shown the need for more stringent control of laboratory procedures by an approved code of practice or regulations under the Act (Harrington and Shannon, 1976, 1977). The study, performed in 1971, showed 18 new cases of pulmonary tuberculosis, a fivefold increased risk compared with the general population. Technicians were at greatest risk, in particular those working in departments of morbid anatomy. Technicians were also found to have an increased risk of developing hepatitis, 35 cases being reported in the survey. However, verification of the diagnosis was not obtained. The risk of infection may be particularly high in research laboratories. Marburg disease was first described in laboratory workers and has been seen again recently, and the last outbreak of smallpox in this country originated in a research laboratory. The Report of the Working Party on the Laboratory Use of Dangerous Pathogens (D.H.S.S., 1975) recommended that general guidance on safety in laboratories should be drawn up and applied.

Laboratory safety procedures and the standard of occupational health care in the National Health Service, Public Health Laboratory Service and the National Blood Transfusion Service was assessed in the postal survey of laboratory workers referred to above. The dangerous procedure of mouth pipetting was practised in 65 per cent of laboratories in England and Wales. The wearing of protective clothing for hazardous tasks was not compulsory in an equal number of establishments. Two per cent of medical and technical staff had handled the carcinogen β-naphthylamine during the preceding year, and a larger proportion had handled benzidine. Six per cent of the laboratories allowed eating and 30 per cent allowed smoking while at work. Centrifuges were inadequately serviced and many safety cabinets had no check on the adequacy of their air flow. Safety training was more likely to be provided by the larger laboratories and in particular by the Public Health Laboratory Service. Less than half the laboratory population had any form of pre-employment examination and only a minority had been offered BCG or other vaccinations. Thus, this survey showed a great lack of uniformity in health and safety practice in British Laboratories.

Inspection of laboratories in four hospitals in the Hull area revealed deficiencies in health and safety practice which would have been unacceptable in a factory environment (Brown and Souter, 1977). While all laboratory workers took steps to avoid contact with material potentially infected with hepatitis virus, centrifuges were being used without their protective covers in some laboratories, so that aerosol spraying of blood took place. Fume cupboards were used without adequate checks on air flow rates, and laboratory ventilation procedures where toxic fumes were evolved were often makeshift. Furthermore, lack of consideration of health and safety factors in architectural design in one of the newer buildings meant that toxic fumes from a laboratory could contaminate higher floors in the building.

Histopathology laboratories often use mercuric chloride as a tissue fixative and the possibility of mercury absorption by technicians has been investigated by Stewart et al. (1977). Atmospheric concentrations of mercury vapour up to 0·5 nmol/l and of mercury compounds up to 1·0 nmol/l were found. Technicians exposed to this environment showed increased urinary mercury excretion levels, ranging from 119 to 443 nmol/24 hours, with a median value of 266 nmol/24 hour. While mercurialism was not seen, urinary protein excretion in the mercury-exposed workers as a group was at least twice that seen in a control group, and, furthermore, when control measures were instituted the proteinuria cleared.

Nursing personnel and technicians who use formalin to sterilize artificial kidney machines may develop respiratory hypersensitivity with wheezing and productive cough. In a study of 28 staff members of a renal dialysis unit, 8 had experienced attacks described as 'bronchitic' since becoming exposed to formalin (Hendrick and Lane, 1977). Inhalation provocation tests with formalin gave late asthmatic responses in two nurses similar to those seen with toluene diisocyanate, with reactions to single exposures lasting for several days or even weeks.

New regulations are being introduced covering exposure to ionizing radiation, with more stringent environmental monitoring where unsealed sources are used, as in radioisotope laboratories. Stringent regulations will also be applied to safeguard against possible hazards resulting from genetic engineering.

REFERENCES

Brown P. M. and Souter R. V. (1977) *J. Soc. Occup. Med.* **27**, 148 – 150.
D.H.S.S. (1975) Report of Working Party on the Laboratory Use of Dangerous Pathogens. Cmnd. 6054.
Harrington J. M. and Shannon H. S. (1976) *Br. Med. J.* **1**, 759 – 762.
Harrington J. M. and Shannon H. S. (1977) *Br. Med. J.* **1**, 626 – 628.
Hendrick D. J. and Lane D. J. (1977) *Br. J. Indust. Med.* **34**, 11 – 18.
Stewart W. K., Guirgis H. A., Sanderson J. and Taylor W. (1977) *Br. J. Indust. Med.* **34**, 26 – 31.

ORTHOPAEDICS AND TRAUMATOLOGY

C. J. E. MONK MChOrth,
FRCS(Edin), FRCS(Eng)

BASIC RESEARCH

The arterial supply of the head of the femur during early development

For many years now the disposition of the arteries supplying the head and neck of the femur has been the subject of intense study. Most of the papers published to date have reported experiments done in two planes, i.e. the upper end of the femur was sectioned and then the arteries studied. This tends to give an erroneous impression of the blood supply of this area. In October, 1976, Dr Stanley Chung of Philadelphia published the findings in a study of 150 specimens which had been subjected to injection moulding and then clearance of the specimen by the Spalteholz technique. In this way, the three-dimensional model of the arterial tree surrounding the upper end of the femur is obtained. Two other techniques were used, particularly for specimens from older children: rubber latex perfusion was done in 17 specimens; and perfusion with Batson compound in 28 specimens, of which only 9 provided sufficient filling for assessment. The results of this study can be summarized as follows.

The main blood supply to the proximal femur comes from the medial and lateral circumflex femoral vessels. These arise either from the femoral artery or from the profunda artery. The medial and lateral circumflex femoral arteries form an extracapsular arterial ring around the base of the neck of the femur. There is some additional arterial input to this ring from the superior gluteal vessel filling it from above. From this arterial ring branches pierce the capsule at the level of the capsular attachment to the femur and then pass up the neck of the femur to form another intracapsular ring at the edge of the articular surface of the femoral head. The branches from the extra-articular ring passing through the capsule comprise an anterior, a posterior, a lateral and a medial branch.

Most of the blood supply to the upper neck and head of the femur arises from the large lateral branch. The lateral, medial, anterior and posterior branches are referred to as ascending branches or ascending cervical arteries. As they pass deep to the synovium on the surface of the neck of the femur these arteries give off branches which penetrate the bone to supply the metaphysis. From the fine intra-articular ring branches pass into the epiphysis. There are no arteries penetrating the growth plate cartilage. The deep intra-articular ring is usually complete, but in some specimens examined there was a gap, which was most commonly seen in the anterior part of the ring, and less commonly in the posterior, or in the anterior and posterior parts combined. Two other interesting findings occurred:

1. The lateral ascending cervical artery appeared to supply most of the upper neck and head of the femur, and this artery lies in a constricted area in the growing child. It lies in the angle between the greater trochanter and the neck of the femur. This would make it more than usually liable to compression by intracapsular pressure.

2. The other interesting finding was that if the capital epiphysis was ossified from several ossific nuclei, these each had an artery of supply. The author suggests that when the separate ossific centres combine, the blood supply to each still remains separate. This would account for the segmental occurrence of necrosis in some cases of Perthes disease.

The pathogenesis of Perthe's disease

Between the years 1963 and 1969, 56 children suffering from Perthe's disease of the hip were investigated by bone biopsy at Osaka University, Japan. The results of these biopsies were available for a comparative study made during the last few years and reported in November, 1976, by Inoue et al. (1976). This study is a comparison between the findings in human subjects in Japan and findings in dog experiments carried out in this country.

The basic thesis presented is that the changes are identical in the two groups, and that since these histological changes in the dog cannot be produced unless the femoral head is infarcted twice, the assumption is made that Perthe's disease in the human subject is only evident if there has been more than one interruption of the blood supply of the capital epiphysis. The authors describe various degrees of changes in the capital epiphyses depending on whether there have been one or more infarcts and whether the repair is partially or fully complete. This article adds extra weight to the thesis that Perthe's disease is totally due to interruption of the arterial supply of the capital epiphysis.

Investigation of disc disease

The diagnosis of the cause of low back pain and sciatica remains a difficult problem to the orthopaedic surgeon. In recent years new techniques have been devised for identifying the level and size of encroachments into the spinal canal. The common causes of these encroachments are prolapse of the intervertebral discs and increase in the size of the posterior articulations of the vertebrae due to osteoarthrosis.

The introduction of radiculography using a water-soluble dye has increased the precision with which nerve root compression can be identified; but the older method of oil-soluble myelography had the advantage that the patient could be examined and X-rayed in the prone position, and the size of the 'bulge' of the disc backwards into the vertebral canal could be assessed.

There have been two important papers recently on the use of venography in the assessment of disc disease. The technique used in this examination is to pass a radio-opaque dye into the lumbar veins and allow it to flow into the spinal canal and demonstrate or outline particularly the veins lying on the posterior surface of the lumbar vertebrae. Normally these veins drain downwards into the internal iliac veins, but pressure on the inferior vena cava either by pressing on the abdominal wall or the Valsalva procedure will reverse the flow in the veins in the lumbar area. The veins within the spinal canal contain no valves, and reversal of flow can be easily produced.

MacNab and his associates (1976), in Toronto and Boston, present the results in 50 cases who had not had prior disc surgery and in whom the venographic findings were confirmed by operation. They record a 98 per cent accuracy as against a 90 per cent accuracy after myelography. In 29 patients who did not have an exploratory operation both the venograms and the myelograms were normal. The results of venography in patients who have had prior operations are less impressive.

O'Dell and his colleagues (1977), from San Diego, California, use both the anteroposterior and the lateral views of the spine as against the MacNab series in which anteroposterior views only were used. O'Dell and his colleagues report an 82 per cent accuracy of surgically proved cases. Both groups of workers pay tribute to Gargano and his associates for establishing the technique and for originally describing the positive findings (Gargano et al., 1974).

The treatment of unstable fractures of the spine by fusion and Harrington rod immobilization

Flech and his colleagues report a series of 40 patients from Minneapolis and St Paul who had unstable fracture dislocations of the spine treated by Harrington instrumentation and fusion (Flech et al., 1977). The types of cases were 34 rotary fracture dislocations; 2 bursting fractures, which were initially stable but became unstable after posterolateral decompression; and 4 compression fractures, of which 2 also became unstable, one after posterolateral decompression and the other following laminectomy. The 2 compression fractures were noticed to be unstable on serial radiography, which showed an increase in the deformity. The interesting point that immerges from the results is that there was some improvement in the neurological state of the lower limbs if the patient initially had an incomplete lesion and was subjected to decompression. In those in whom the initial response resulted in a total neurological loss, the decompression and fusion did not cause any improvement. It is also noted that more than half of the patients subjected to this operative procedure required some corrective second operation because of mechanical failure or failure of the spinal fusion.

REFERENCES

Chung S. M. K. (1976) The arterial supply of the developing proximal end of the human femur. *J. Bone Joint Surg.* **58A**, 961 – 970.
Flech J. R., Leider L. L., Erickson D. L., Chou S. N. and Bradford D. S. (1977) Harrington instrumentation and spine fusion for unstable fractures and fracture dislocations of the thoracic and lumbar spine. *J. Bone Joint Surg.* **58A**, 143 – 153.
Gargano F. P., Meyer J. D. and Sheldon J. J. (1974) Transfemoral ascending lumbar catheterization of the epidural vein in lumbar disc disease. *Radiology* **111**, 329 – 336.
Inoue A., Freeman M. A. R., Vernon-Jones B. and Mizuno S. (1976) The pathogenesis of Perthe's disease. *J. Bone Joint Surg.* **58B**, 453 – 461.
MacNab I., St. Louis E. L., Grabias S. L. and Jacob R. (1976) Selective ascending lumbosacral venography in assessment of lumbar disc herniation. *J. Bone Joint Surg.* **58A**, 1093 – 1098.
O'Dell C. W. jun., Coel M. N. and Ignelzi R. J. (1977) Ascending lumbar venography in lumbar-disk disease. *J. Bone Joint Surg.* **59A**, 159 – 163.

THE KNEE

Lesions of the menisci

Many individuals can be shown to have lesions of the menisci which do not cause symptoms. These lesions are found when the knees are examined or operated on for some other condition, e.g. chondromalacia patellae.

In order to ascertain the incidence of these lesions in clinically normal knees, Noble has examined menisci in postmortem studies on 70 individuals who had not had operations on their knees and who had apparently not complained of knee symptoms (Noble, 1977). All the subjects were less than 55 years old.

Of these subjects 18·6 per cent had a demonstrable horizontal cleavage tear. The actual occurrence of the lesion was 18 tears in 280 menisci; 11 cleavage tears were in the medial and 7 in the lateral meniscus. Only 1 subject was less than 40 years old. Five of the subjects had discoid menisci.

This series compares favourably with an earlier series by the same author in which the selection was random and the average age was 65. In that series 60 per cent of the individuals showed a horizontal cleavage lesion in at least one meniscus.

The author also studied the dimensions of the medial meniscus and found that it is always wider and thicker at its posterior end. The author puts forward the suggestion that the thickness of the medial meniscus means that its deeper fibres are remote from the synovial fluid. Their nutrition, therefore, is defective, and they are more likely to undergo degeneration and splitting.

The histological appearance of 80 menisci from 20 of the younger individuals was also studied, and it was found that 76 per cent of the medial and 54 per cent of the lateral menisci showed varying degrees of degenerative change.

Contractures of the knee extensor mechanism

Orthopaedic surgeons working in children's hospitals in which there are large open-heart surgery departments can rely on seeing several cases of quadriceps fibrosis each year. The accepted explanation of this phenomenon is that it follows multiple intramuscular injections into the thigh in the early months of life.

Classically the condition affects the more laterally placed muscles and, if left untreated, leads to progressive loss of knee flexion range and later to lateral dislocation of the patella.

In the Far East, the ability to squat is essential for a normal social life, and therefore it is not surprising that the condition of quadriceps contracture has been extensively studied there and reported in a series of cases collected in Singapore.

Bose and Chong (1976) report a series of 50 knees in 38 patients, all children or adolescents.

The authors divide the knees into 2 groups:

Group 1. 'Stiff knees' with loss of flexion range. This group includes those patients with genu recurvatum.

Group 2. Habitual dislocation of the patella (i.e. lateral dislocation on flexion). Included in this group were 2 cases of 'congenital dislocation of the patella' in which the patella remained in the dislocated position at all angles of flexion of the knee

There were 33 knees in the first group and 17 in the second group.

In the first group exploratory operation revealed that the fibrotic contracture was mainly in the rectus femoris or vastus medialis. In the second group the fibrosis was mainly in the vastus lateralis and iliotibial tract.

TREATMENT

The first group were treated by releasing the vastus medialis. If this did not allow adequate knee flexion, the rectus femoris tendon was lengthened by a Z-plasty.

In the second group, release of the vastus lateralis, fascia lata and some fibres of vastus intermedius and rectus femoris was necessary. Medical plication of the knee capsule added to the stability of the patella.

In the cases of congenitally dislocated patella, there was an additional valgus deformity of the knee which had to be corrected by varus osteotomy.

In some of the severe cases of genu recurvatum there was bony deformity and anterior subluxation of the tibia. These had to be corrected by osteotomy.

Satisfactory results were obtained in the majority of cases, but some of the releases had to be repeated. The cases of genu recurvatum regained a substantial range of flexion, but some were left with a considerable extension lag. The function of these knees was satisfactory.

REFERENCES
Bose K. and Chong K. C. (1976) The clinical manifestations and pathomechanics of contracture of the extensor mechanism of the knee. *J. Bone Joint Surg.* **58B**, 478 – 484.
Noble J. (1977) Lesions of the menisci. *J. Bone Joint Surg.* **59A**, 480 – 482.

THE USE OF ANTIBIOTICS IN CEMENT

The problem of the infected prosthesis remains one of the most important in the field of joint replacement. Various measures have been adopted to reduce the incidence of infection arising during the operation; for example, the use of the 'clean-air' theatre and the administering of antibiotics before, during and after the operation.

In 1970, Buchholz and Engelbrecht, working in Hamburg, reported the results of a trial of antibiotics mixed with the cement used to hold the components of hip prostheses in position. The infection rate was lowered.

During the subsequent years several experiments have been carried out to attempt to measure the rate of diffusion of antibiotics from cement and to decide which antibiotic and which cement to use.

Laboratory studies carried out by Picknell et al. (1977) show that antibiotics diffuse rapidly, but for a disappointingly short time, from impregnated cement plugs tested in vitro; 70 – 90 per cent of the antibiotic released had appeared within 3 hours, and the concentration then fell over the next 4 days. All the antibiotics tested inhibited the growth of organism on day 1, but by day 4 only flucloxacillin and clindamycin were active, and their activity ceased on day 5.

The amount of antibiotic released was of the order of 10 per cent of that used (lowest, methicillin—2·3 per cent; highest, cloxacillin—11·0 per cent). This suggests that only that part of the antibiotic near the surface of the cement is able to diffuse out.

The antibiotics were not damaged by the exothermic reaction during the hardening of the cement.

Hill et al. (1977) report a similar series of experiments and conclude that better antibiotic activity can be obtained at the operation site by topical application of antibiotics at operation or intravenous administration before, during and after operation.

Elson et al. (1977) confirm Buchholz and Engelbrecht's findings, including the unexplained higher diffusion from Palacos R cement than from other types, and include some results of a clinical trial.

The level of antibiotic activity of the fluid from the wound drain, the urine and the serum has been measured and shows a rapid fall in the first 24 – 48 hours and then a gradual decline over the following days.

The mechanical effects of antibiotic powder on cement is uncertain, and there are contradictory reports published, Watts and Elson (1976) reporting that the strength of the cement is diminished and Weinstein et al. (1976) suggesting that the antibiotic inclusion does not alter the strength of the cement.

Further clinical studies will no doubt be forthcoming to help in the assessment of this method of combating infection in joint replacement.

Buchholz H. W. and Engelbrecht H. (1970) Über die Depotwirking einiger Antibiotica be Vermischung mit dem Kinstharz Palacos. *Chirurg* **41**, 515 – 551.

Elson R. A, Jephcott A. E., McGechie D. B. and Verettas D. (1977) Antibiotic-loaded acrylic cement. *J. Bone Joint Surg.* **59B**, 200 – 205.

Hill J., Klenerman L., Trustey S. and Blowers R. (1977) Diffusion of antibiotics from acrylic bone cement in vitro. *J. Bone Joint Surg.* **59B**, 197 – 199.

Picknell B., Mizen L. and Sutherland R. (1977) Antibacterial activity of antibiotics in acrylic bone cement. *J. Bone Joint Surg.* **59B**, 302 – 307.

Watts N. H. and Elson R. A. (1976) The mechanical properties of antibiotic-loaded acrylic cement. In: *Proceedings of the International Biomaterials Symposium,* Philadelphia, USA, 1976.

Weinstein A. M., Bingham D. N., Sauer B. W. and Lunceford E. M. (1976) The effect of high pressure insertion and antibiotic inclusions upon the mechanical properties of polymethylmethacrylate. *Clin. Orthop.* **121**, 67 – 73.

PHARMACOLOGY AND TOXICOLOGY

H. SCHNIEDEN MD, MSc

LABETALOL

Since the blood vessels of the skin and splanchnic area are under sympathetic control and since the adrenoceptors on such vessels have been characterized as α receptors it may be though that α-blocking agents would produce a profound fall in blood pressure in vivo and that therefore they might be of value in the treatment of hypertension. Whilst, experimentally, such drugs can be shown to lower blood pressure acutely their effects in long term therapy have been less dramatic. This is because of the homeostatic mechanisms of the body. A fall in blood pressure will elicit stimulation of carotid and aortic arch reflexes which in turn can result in an increase in sympathetic drive to the heart, followed by a rise in cardiac output to negate the fall in blood pressure produced by the fall in total peripheral resistance. Since the adrenoceptors in the heart are $\beta 1$ receptors, a drug which blocks both α and β receptors might be expected to be a useful antihypertensive agent. Labetalol (*Fig.* 1) is such a compound and is now being used clinically.

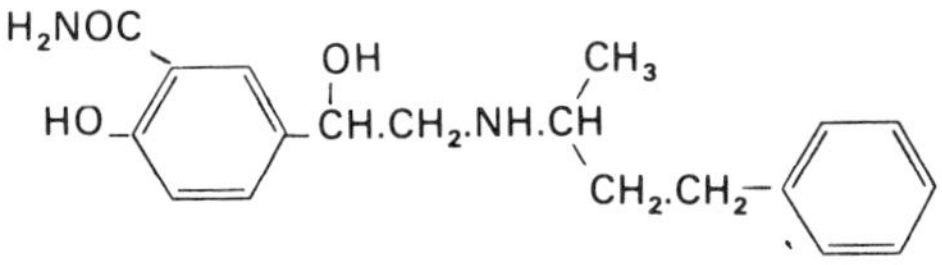

Fig. 1. Chemical structure of labetalol, 5-{-I-hydroxy-2-[(1-methyl-3-phenylpropyl)amino]ethyl} salicylamide. (*Figs.* 1 – 4 by kind permission of the *British Journal of Clinical Pharmacology*).

Brittain and Levy (1976) reported on the pharmacology of the compound. It is a competitive antagonist blocking both α and β-adrenoceptors. On isolated tissues, such as aortic strips, it was 6 – 10 times less potent than phentolamine in blocking α-adrenoceptors and on preparations, such as guineapig isolated left atrium, it was approximately half as potent as propranolol in blocking β-adrenoceptors.

Further work by these authors on anaesthetized dogs showed that labetalol blocked the increase in blood pressure induced by phenylephrine and diminished the increase in heart rate induced by isoprenaline (*Fig.* 2), suggesting that in vivo it had α and β-blocking activities.

Of potential therapeutic importance is the effect of labetalol on hypertensive animals: both in the conscious renal hypertensive dog (*Fig.* 3) and in the conscious doca-induced hypertensive rat, the drug caused a fall in systolic blood pressure.

The investigators also reported that, like propranolol, labetalol also has local anaesthetic and membrane stabilizing actions, but that the latter effect appears at doses much higher than those needed to achieve α and β-blockade.

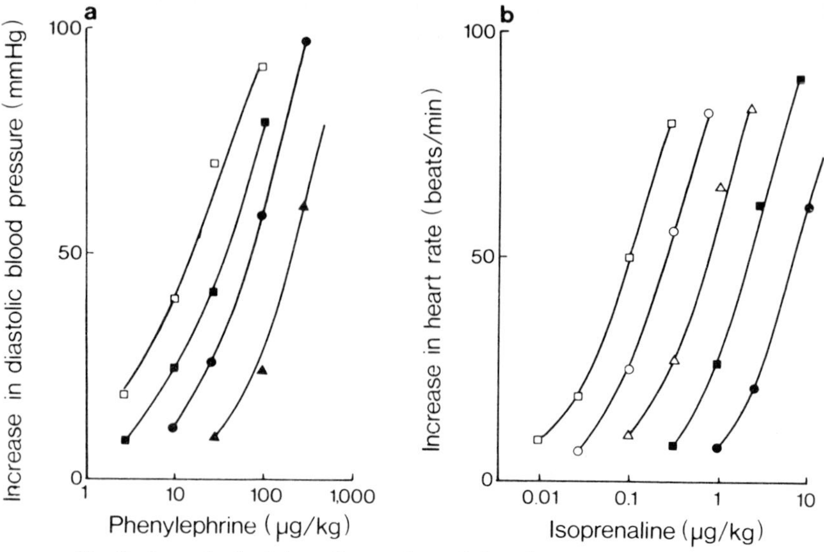

Fig. 2. Anaesthetized dog. Comparison of the adrenoceptor-blocking actions of labetalol (*a*) against phenylephrine-induced vasopressor responses; and (*b*) against isoprenaline-induced positive chronotropic responses. □, Controls; ○, after labetalol 0.1 mg/kg; Δ,0.3 mg/kg; ■, 1 mg/kg; ●, 3 mg/kg; ▲, 10 mg/kg. All drugs given intravenously.

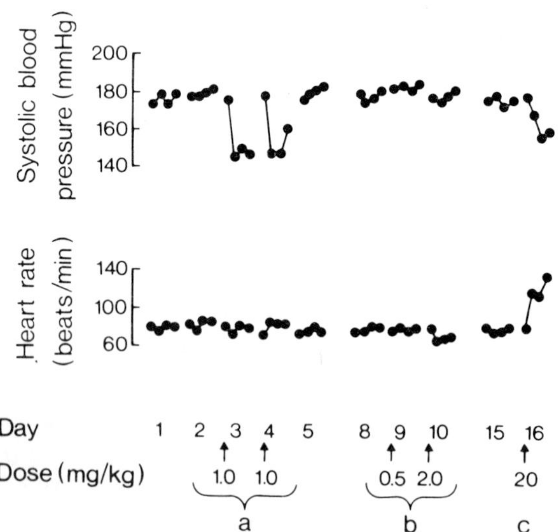

Fig. 3. Effects of orally administered labetalol (*a*), propranolol (*b*) and phenoxybenzamine (*c*) on blood pressure and heart rate in the conscious renal hypertensive dog ($n = 4$).

Using radioactive-labelled labetalol, Martin et al. (1976) noted that, in man, the drug was about 50 per cent bound to plasma proteins. Dose-dependent rises in plasma labetalol levels occurred following administration of 100, 200 and 400 mg labetalol orally to human subjects (*Fig.* 4). In man about 5 per cent of the drug dose is excreted unchanged.

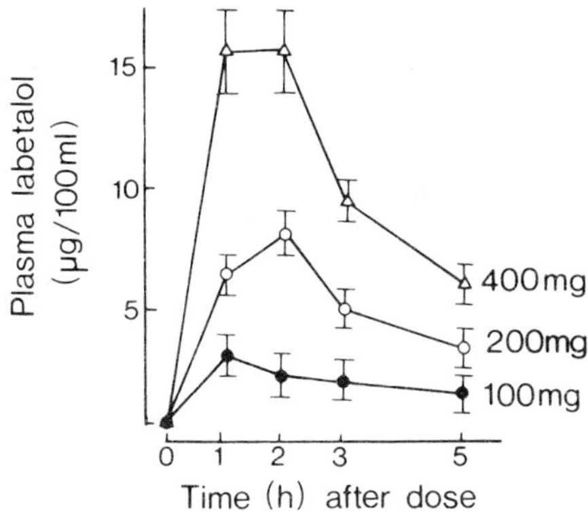

Fig. 4. Human plasma labetalol concentration after oral doses of 100 (●), 200 (○) and 400 mg labetalol (Δ). Mean of 5 subjects ±s.e.

Studies have also been conducted on potential toxicity of labetalol (Poynter et al., 1976). Of interest was the finding that radioactive labetalol bound to the melanin pigment of the eye. However, when oral doses of 20 mg labetalol per day were given to cats for 7 months no oculotoxic effects were seen. Many drugs bind to melanin without producing toxic effects in man; others, such as the β-blocking drug practalol, do so. Thus, though labetalol appears on animal evidence to be unlikely to produce adverse effects in the eye, careful monitoring of the drug clinically for this potential toxic hazard is advisable.

Clinically, the drug has been shown to be effective in hypertensive patients. Koch (1976) has reported on 12 patients who had been treated with oral labetalol for between 8 and 16 months. Significant lowering of blood pressure occurred and plasma renin levels had fallen. Kane et al. (1976) noted that after 4 weeks of treatment with a dose of 800 mg/day orally, mean falls in blood pressure of 36 – 24 mm Hg respectively for systolic and diastolic blood pressure occurred.

Side effects reported have been a posture-related dizzyness, headache and, in male patients, decreased potency, the latter presumably related to the α-blocking effect of the drug. Dargie et al. (1976) have also noted postural hypotension as a side effect of treatment and also drug-related urinary retention occurred in 1 patient. They quote that some patients have vivid dreams or are sedated on labetalol, suggesting that the drug has an effect centrally. In rabbits central injection of the drug can lower blood pressure.

In summary, labetalol is a clinically useful antihypertensive agent which appears to have a similar potency to methyl dopa (Pritchard and Boakes, 1976). Built into the molecule is a fixed ratio of α to β-blocking activity. More flexibility could be achieved by using a combination of two drugs: (1) an α-blocking agent, e.g. phentolamine, and (2) a β-blocking drug, e.g.

oxprenolol. Such a combination has been tried clinically (Johnson et al., 1976).

REFERENCES

Brittain R. T. and Levy G. P. (1976) A review of the animal pharmacology of labetalol, a combined α and β-adrenoceptor-blocking drug. *Br. J. Clin. Pharmacol.* **3**, 681 – 694 S.

Dargie H. J., Dollery C. T. and Daniel J. (1976) Labetalol in resistant hypertension. *Br. J. Clin. Pharmacol.* **3**, 751 – 755 S.

Johnson B. F., LaBrooy J. and Munro-Faure A. D. (1976) Comparative antihypertensive effects of labetalol and the combination of oxprenolol and phentolamine. *Br. J. Clin. Pharmacol.* **3**, 783 – 787 S.

Kane J., Gregg I. and Richards D. A. (1976) A double-blind trial of labetalol. *Br. J. Clin. Pharmacol.* **3**, 737 – 741 S.

Koch G. (1976) Combined α and β-adrenoceptor blockade with oral labetalol in hypertensive patients with reference to haemodynamic effects of rest and exercise. *Br. J. Clin. Pharmacol.* **3**, 729 – 732 S.

Martin L. E., Hopkins R. and Bland R. (1976) Metabolism of labetalol by animals and man. *Br. J. Clin. Pharmacol.* **3**, 695 – 710 S.

Poynter D., Martin L. E., Harrison C. and Cook J. (1976) Affinity of labetalol for ocular melanin. *Br. J. Clin. Pharmacol.* **3**, 711 – 721 S.

Pritchard B. N. C. and Boakes A. J. (1976) Labetalol in long-term treatment of hypertension. *Br. J. Clin. Pharmacol.* **3**, 743 – 750 S.

DIFLUNISAL

This compound is a modified aspirin derivative (*see Fig.* 5) which was synthesized in an endeavour to overcome the disadvantages of aspirin. It was hoped that the new compound would be better tolerated by the patient and have a longer duration of action.

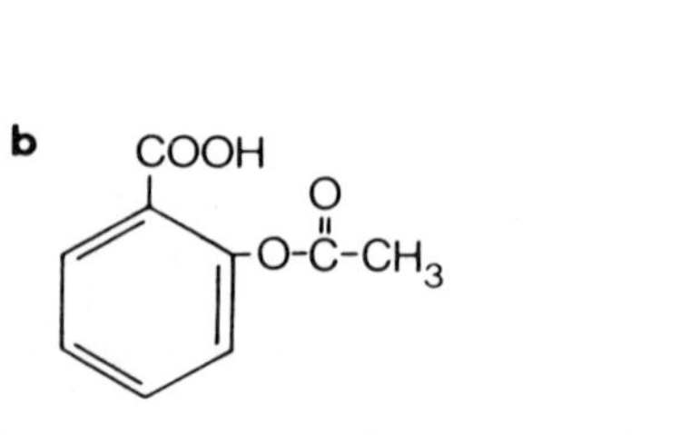

Fig. 5. Structure of diflunisal (*a*) and aspirin (*b*). (*Figs.* 5 and 6 by kind permission of the *British Journal of Clinical Pharmacology*).

Aspirin is known to inhibit prostaglandin synthesis (Ferreira and Vane, 1974). Majerus and Stanford (1977) reported that diflunisal also inhibits prostaglandin synthetase. However, in platelets aspirin covalently and irreversibly binds to the enzyme whilst diflunisal does not, and the inhibition produced by this drug appears to be reversible.

Stone et al. (1977) have studied the pharmacology and toxicology of diflunisal. They observed that the drug was effective in adjuvant arthritis in the rat (about nine times as potent as aspirin) and that whilst in vitro it inhibited thrombin-induced aggregation of human platelets it was less effective than aspirin.

Both diflunisal and aspirin induced gastric haemorrhages in starved rats, and diflunisal but not aspirin produced perforation of the small intestine in the rat. The dose level required for this latter effect was greater than that necessary to show anti-inflammatory and analgesic action in this species and appears to be associated with the biliary excretion of the drug in the rat. Whether diflunisal is excreted in the bile in man is an open question (Tempero et al., 1977).

Tempero et al. have reported that diflunisal is highly protein-bound (approximately 98 per cent and that the drug is almost wholly excreted in the urine as unchanged or conjugated drug. As might be expected a drug interaction has been reported with at least one orally acting anticoagulant. Diflunisal, in doses of 375 mg 12-hourly, had a uricosuric effect. Of interest is the effect of 'equianalgesic' doses of aspirin (ASA) and diflunisal. Diflunisal produced less gastrointestinal blood loss than aspirin (*Fig.* 6). Alcohol administered with either drug did not appear to significantly increase rate of blood loss.

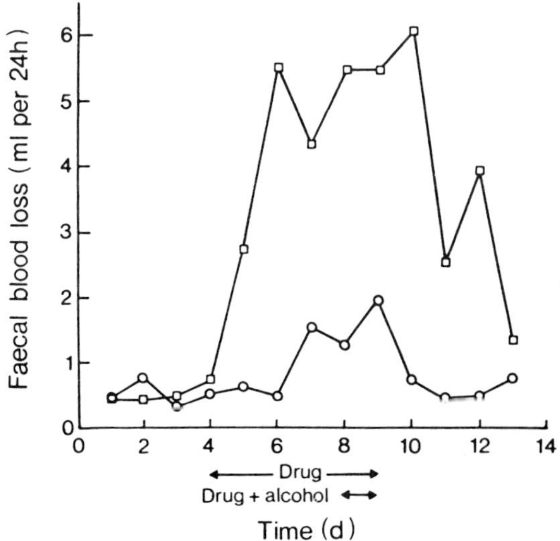

Fig. 6. Mean gastrointestinal blood loss experienced by 12 normal male subjects after administration of equianalgesic doses of ASA 2.4 g/day (□) and diflunisal 500 mg/day (○).

Clinically the drug has proved effective (though not in all patients) in postoperative pain in doses of 250 – 375 mg twice daily (Van Winzum and Rodda, 1977). It has also proved effective in relieving the symptoms of osteoarthritis. In one clinical trial in which patients were initially randomly assigned to diflunisal (250 mg, twice daily) or aspirin (500 mg, four times a day) 685 patients entered the study. Approximately 25 per cent discontinued the study due to adverse reactions from either drug, lack of therapeutic effect or loss of follow-up. Of the remainder, after 12 weeks of treatment, both the aspirin and the diflunisal group showed significant improvements from baseline in some parameters measured. In some respects, e.g. performance of a specific function in the patient's normal activity, diflunisal was more effective (Andrew et al., 1977). Whether the latter is a specific advantage of diflunisal or merely a reflection of the dosages used remains to be determined.

To summarize, diflunisal is a drug, chemically related to aspirin, undergoing clinical evaluation at present. It is an effective non-narcotic analgesic and may produce less gastrointestinal bleeding than aspirin in equianalgesic doses. However, its full spectrum of toxicity has still to be evaluated clinically.

REFERENCES

Andrew A., Rodda B., Verhaest L. and Van Winzum C. (1977) Diflunisal: 6-month experience in osteoarthritis. *Br. J. Clin. Pharmacol.* **4**, 45S – 52S.

Ferreira S. H. and Vane J. R. (1974) New aspects of the mode of action of non-steroidal anti-inflammatory drugs. *Annu. Rev. Pharmacol.* **14**, 57 – 73.

Majerus P. W. and Stanford N. (1977) Comparative effects of aspirin and diflunisal on prostaglandin synthetase from human platelets and sheep seminal vesicles. *Br. J. Clin. Pharmacol.* **4**, 15S – 18S.

Stone C. A., Van Arman C. G., Lottin V. J. et al. (1977) Pharmacology and toxicology of diflunisal. *Br. J. Clin. Pharmacol.* **4**, 19S – 29S.

Tempero K. F., Cirillo U. J. and Steelman S. C. (1977) Diflunisal: A review of pharmacokinetic and pharmacodynamic properties, drug interactions and special tolerability studies in humans. *Br. J. Clin. Pharmacol.* **4**, 31S – 36S.

Van Winzum C. and Rodda B. (1977) Diflunisal: efficacy in postoperative pain. *Br. J. Clin. Pharmacol.* **4**, 39S – 43S.

MALE CONTRACEPTION

The recent Royal College of General Practitioner's study of the dangers of oral contraceptive therapy in women aged 35 and over (Beral and Kay, 1977) will again focus attention on possible substitutes for the 'pill', and the question of whether an orally acting compound which can inhibit male fertility can be developed will again be discussed. The criteria for a male contraceptive could be as stated in *Table* 1.

Table 1. CRITERIA FOR A MALE ORAL CONTRACEPTIVE

a.	Rapid onset of action
b.	Predictable duration
c.	Completely reversible
d.	No effect on libido
e.	Non-toxic to the recipient and non-mutagenic
f.	Stable

α-chlorohydrin (*Fig.* 7) fulfills many of these criteria. It can be given orally to animals, acts only on spermatozoa and is therefore effective in a few days of starting adequate treatment. It is reversible and there is no evidence of mutagenicity in animal tests since sperm are prevented from fertilizing eggs. However, it produced bonemarrow damage in primates (Kirton et al., 1970) and probably for that reason its possible trial in man was properly excluded.

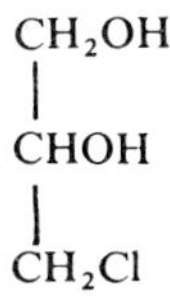

$$CH_2OH$$
$$|$$
$$CHOH$$
$$|$$
$$CH_2Cl$$

Fig. 7. Structure of 3-chloro-1, 2-propanediol. (By kind permission of *Nature.*)

However, recent work by Jackson (1977) suggests that it might be worth while to study the toxicity of this compound in greater depth. Firstly α-chlorohydrin is a liquid and therefore very difficult to get free of contamination. Commercially obtained α-chlorohydrin certainly contains impurities, some of which can be removed by redistillation. Most of the toxicological studies on α-chlorohydrin do not list if the commercial material was purified, and certainly redistilled α-chlorohydrin is well tolerated on chronic administration to the rat and dog, i.e. there appears to be no cumulative toxic action.

In addition, the commercial preparation of α-chlorohydrin is a racaemic (50:50) mixture. Recently Jackson and his colleagues (Jackson and Robinson, 1976; Jackson et al., 1977) have succeeded in separating the two isomers. One isomer only shows the antifertility effect in rats, and is several times less toxic than the biologically inactive isomer. The intriguing question is whether this isomer is also less toxic in other species, e.g. does it cause blood changes in primates. If not, the possibility for a male contraceptive is much improved.

REFERENCES

Beral V. and Kay C. R. (1977) Mortality among oral-contraceptive users. Royal College of General Practitioners Oral Contraception Study. *Lancet* **2**, 727 – 731.

Jackson H. (1977) Toxicological aspects of male antifertility α-chlorohydrins. *Br. J. Pharmacol.* **61**, 455 P.

Jackson H. and Robinson B. (1976) The antifertility effects of α-chlorohydrins and their sterio-isomers in male rats. *Chem. Biol. Interact.* **13**, 193 – 197.

Jackson H., Rooney F. R. and Fitzpatrick R. W. (1977) Characterization and antifertility activity in rats of S(+) α-chlorohydrin. *Chem. Biol. Interact.* **17**, 117 – 120.

Kirton K. T., Ericsson R. J., Ray J. A. et al. (1970) Male antifertility compounds: efficacy of U-5897 in primates. *J. Reprod. Fertil.* **21**, 275 – 8.

PLASTIC SURGERY

D. O. MAISELS FRCS(Edin)

OMENTAL FLAPS

For most medical students the greater omentum has only nuisance value in presenting them with difficulties in understanding the complexities of the form and development of the greater and lesser sacs. Later one comes to appreciate some of the more useful roles of the omentum in acting as the 'policeman of the abdomen'. Its great vascularity has been employed in many situations. Thus it has been used to transport blood to the ischaemic myocardium in cases of angina, an omental flap being transposed extra-abdominally, and Goldsmith and Beattie of New York have used it to protect major vessels or prostheses after radical resections (1969, 1970). Being rich in lymphatics it has also been used in the treatment of lymphoedema by the same group of workers as well as others (Goldsmith et al., 1968).

In the early 1960s Kiricuta (1963, 1965) of Rumania reported his use of omental flaps in a variety of conditions ranging from bronchial, bladder and vesico-vaginal fistulas associated with radiotherapy to the treatment of carcinoma of the breast, including postmastectomy reconstruction. Since then there has been an increasing interest in the use of the omentum in reconstructive surgery.

Recognizing the value of the omentum both in terms of its great vascularity and also the ability of the peritoneum to accept split-skin grafts, and based on Kiricuta's work, Dupont and Menard of Montreal reported its use in the reconstruction of postradiation necrosis of the chest wall (1972). The omentum is approached through a paramedian incision and freed from the transverse colon and mesocolon. It is then separated from the greater curve of the stomach, care being taken to protect the integrity of the gastro-epiploic arch. The omental flap may be based on either the right or left gastro-epiploic vessels, depending upon the site of the chest wall defect (*Fig.* 1). It is then brought out of the abdomen through the main wound or a separate incision, ensuring that the vascular pedicle is neither kinked nor constricted (*Fig.* 2). The omental flap is secured over the chest wall defect and covered with a split-skin graft. If the chest wall defect is large and full-thickness in depth, Marlex mesh is placed beneath the omentum.

The next stage in the development of this technique has been its application to postmastectomy breast reconstruction. Arnold and his colleagues from Atlanta (1976) have shown how a large custom-made prosthesis for the resected muscle and breast can be covered by the remaining chest wall skin augmented by a skin-grafted omental flap (*Figs.* 3 – 6). A similar and equally gratifying result has been reported by Woods and his colleagues of the Mayo Clinic (1977).

The repair of large, full-thickness defects of the scalp including the periosteum can prove a formidable challenge in reconstruction involving a fairly prolonged series of staged procedures. In 1972, however, McLean and Buncke of California were able to treat such a case by a one-stage operation. They were able to repair a large scalp defect by a free graft of omentum covered by a meshed split-skin graft. The omental graft was revascularized by micro-vascular anastomoses between the gastro-epiploic and superficial

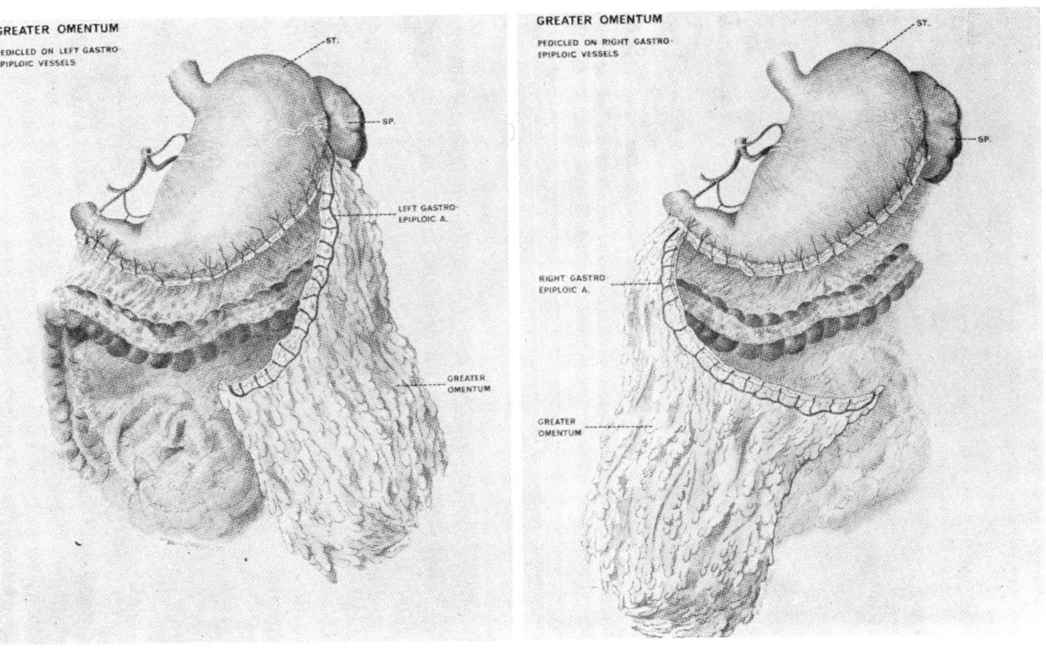

Fig. 1. Preparing the greater omentum as a direct flap based on the left or right gastroepiploic vessels. (*Figs.* 1 – 2 reproduced from *Plastic and Reconstructive Surgery.*)

temporal arteries and veins. The success of this technique has been confirmed by reports of similar cases from Japan (Harii and Ohmori, 1973; Ikuta, 1975) and elsewhere.

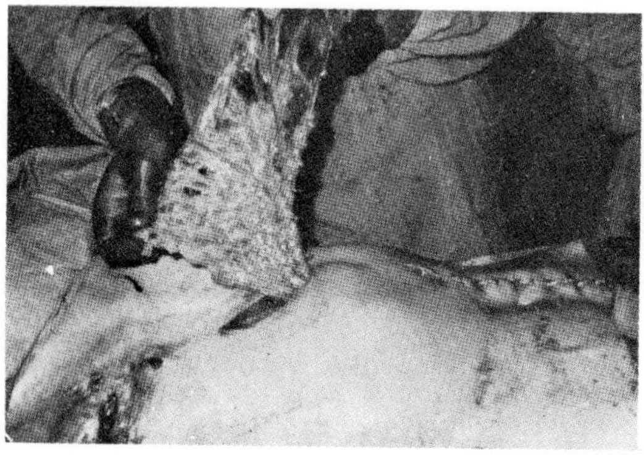

Fig. 2. A patient, in whom the omentum has been prepared as a direct flap, based on the right gastroepiploic vessels (to repair a radiation defect of the right chest wall). The omentum has been brought through a subcutaneous tunnel in the lower anterior chest wall, and is now ready to swing into position in the right axilla.

Casten and Alday (1971) of New York used the omentum in an attempt to increase the vascularity of ischaemic lower limbs and Kiricuta and Popescu recommend omental flaps in selected cases of hand surgery (1976).

Stimulated by the increasing use of the omentum in reconstructive surgery, Das of Bristol (1976) set out to establish if possible the size of the omentum to be expected in any patient and whether it will reach the recipient area. His work included the studies of two hundred cadavers as well as measurements made at one hundred laparotomies. In his paper he discusses the various ways of lengthening the omentum (*Fig.* 7) and surprisingly has shown that the tip will always reach the vault of the skull and mid-leg. In 5 per cent of subjects it even reached the big toe! Das stressed however that where extreme lengthening was obtained, width was sacrificed so that in practice the more distal transfers must be done as free transplants with microvascular anastomoses.

There are two other interesting facts in the omental story. Harii and Ohmori in 1973 found they could lead the gastro-epiploic vessels as an extraperitoneal cord to the subcutaneous region to act as recipient vessels for a free composite flap. Two workers from New York have recently reported some interesting experimental work towards the reconstruction of mucosal defects in the head and neck region using gastric flaps or patches carried on an omental pedicle (Papachristou and Fortner, 1977). Using dogs, they were able to transfer segments of the greater curve of the stomach to the neck (*Fig.* 8).

Needless to say, all these omental procedures entail the addition of an intra-abdominal operation with all its attendant risks and complications. In carefully selected cases, however, the advantages of the new techniques will doubtless prove justifiable.

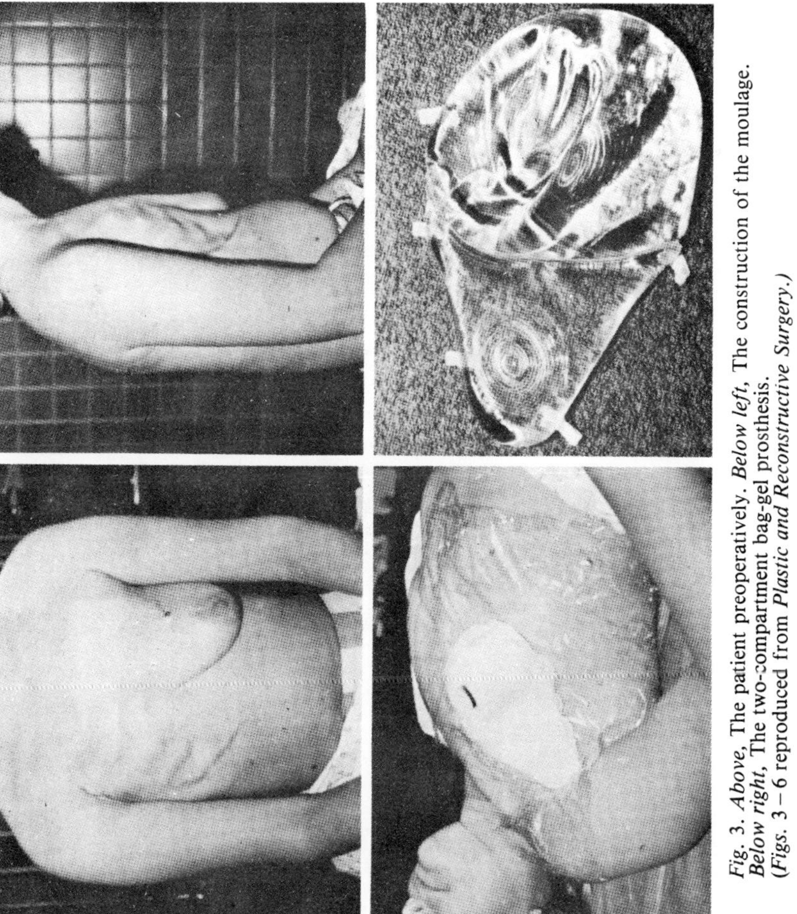

Fig. 3. Above, The patient preoperatively. *Below left,* The construction of the moulage. *Below right,* The two-compartment bag-gel prosthesis. (*Figs.* 3 – 6 reproduced from *Plastic and Reconstructive Surgery.*)

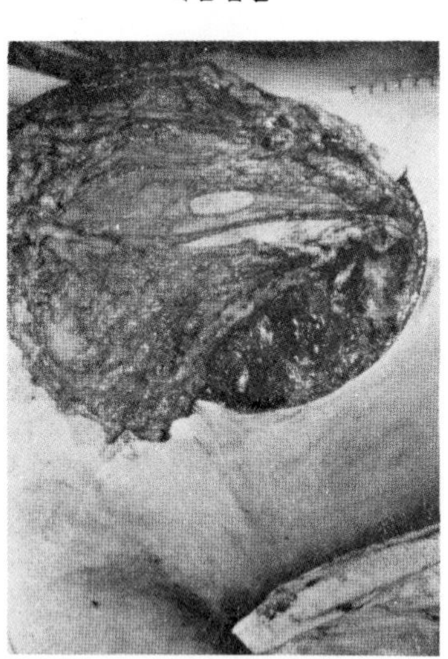

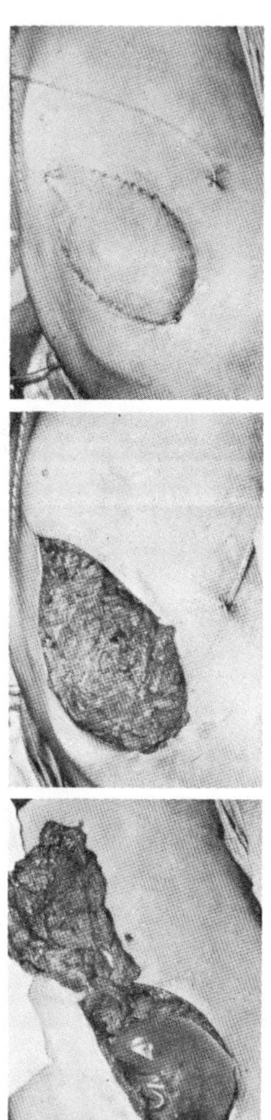

Fig. 4. The mobilized omentum has been passed through a subcutaneous tunnel into the old mastectomy wound. (Note the size of the wound after the incision has been reopened.)

Fig. 5. Left, The old flaps have been elevated again and the prosthesis has been aligned anatomically. *Centre,* The omentum is now placed over the exposed prosthesis, and a suction drain is placed in the axilla. *Right,* A split-skin graft is over the exposed omentum. (*See also* Fig. 6).

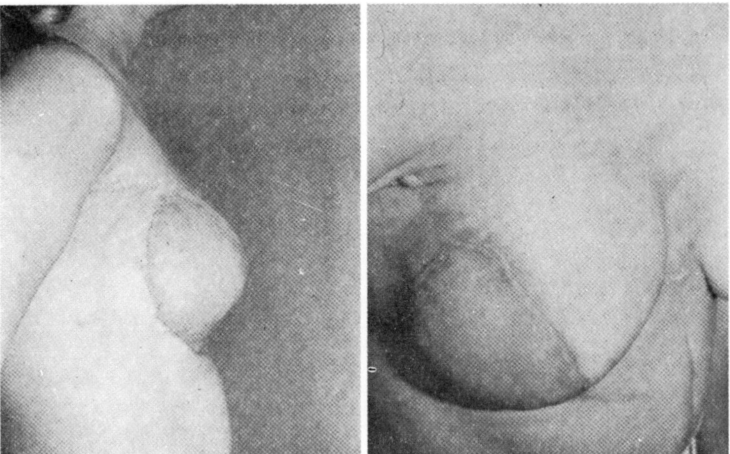

Fig. 6. The patient standing, 6 months after surgery.

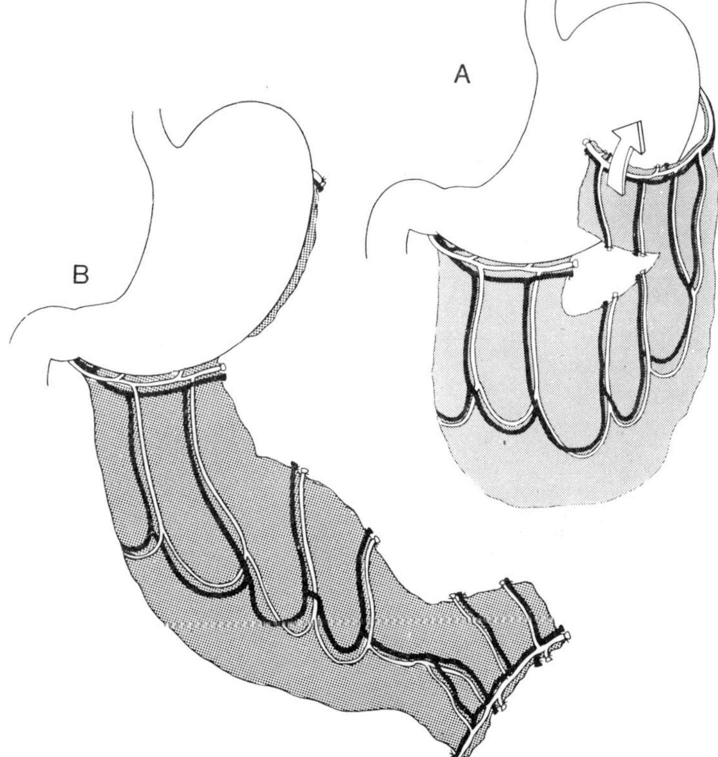

Fig. 7. Dividing the omentum to permit extension while preserving the blood supply. (By kind permission of the *British Journal of Plastic Surgery.*)

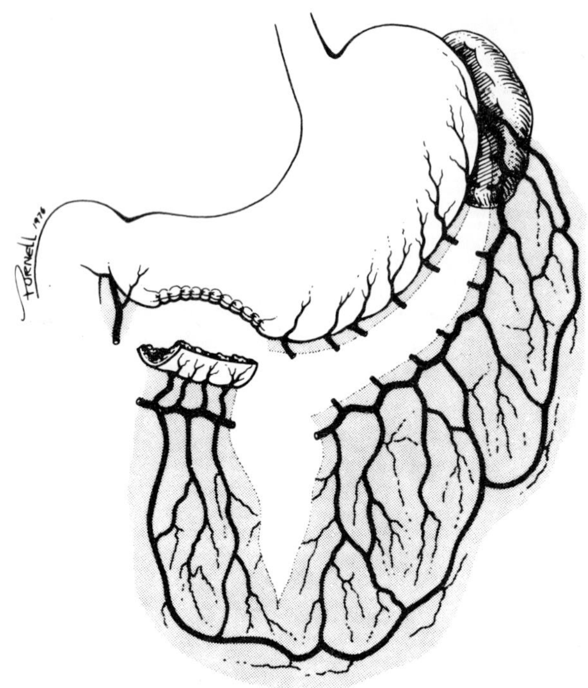

Fig. 8. A gastric antral flap, based on the left gastroepiploic vessels, is shown.
The distal omental arcade carries the blood supply. (Reproduced from
Plastic and Reconstructive Surgery).

REFERENCES

Arnold P. G., Hartrampf C. R. and Jurkiewicz M. J. (1976) One stage reconstruction
of the breast, using the transposed greater omentum. Case report. *Plastic Reconstr.
Surg.* **57**, 520.
Casten F. D. and Alday E. S. (1971) Omental transfer for revascularisation of the
extremities. *Surgery, Gynecol. Obstet.* **132**, 301.
Das S. K. (1976) The size of the human omentum and methods of lengthening it for
transplantation. *Br. J. Plast. Surg.* **29**, 170.
Dupont C. and Menard Y. (1972) Transposition of the greater omentum for
reconstruction of the chest wall. *Plastic Reconstr. Surg.* **49**, 263.
Goldsmith H. S. and Beattie E. J. (1969) Protection of vascular prosthesis following
radical inguinal excision. *Surg. Clin. North Am.* **49**, 413.
Goldsmith H. S. and Beattie E. J. (1970) Carotid artery protection by pedicled
omental wrapping. *Surg. Gynecol. Obstet.* **130**, 57.
Goldsmith H. S., de los Santos and Beattie E. J. (1968) Omental transposition in the
control of chronic lymphoedema. *J.A.M.A.* **203**, 1119.
Harii K. and Ohmori S. (1973) Use of the gastroepiploic vessels as recipient or donor
vessels in the free transfer of composite flaps by microvascular anastomoses. *Plastic
Reconstr. Surg.* **52**, 541.
Ikuta Y. (1975) Autotransplant of omentum to cover large denudation of the scalp.
Case report. *Plastic Reconstr. Surg.* **55**, 490.
Kiricuta I. and Goldstein M. B. (1961) Das omentum als Ersatzmaterial der
Blasenwand bei durch Straklen verursachten. *Krebsarzt* **16**, 202.

Kiricuta I. (1963) L'emploi du grand épiploon dans la chirurgie du sein cancéreux. *Presse Med.* **71**, 15.
Kiricuta I. (1965) L'utilisation du grand épiploon dans la traitement des fistules postradiothérapeutiques vesico-vaginales, recto-vesico-vaginales et dans les cysto-plasties. *J. Chirurg.* **89**, 477.
Kiricuta I. and Popescu V. (1976) The uses of omentum for the management of burns and trauma of the hands. *Ann. Chir. Plast.* **21**, 147.
McLean D. H. and Buncke H. J. (1972) Autotransplant of omentum to a large scalp defect with microsurgical revascularisation. *Plastic Reconstr. Surg.* **49**, 268.
Papachristou D. and Fortner J. G. (1977) Experimental use of a gastric flap on an omental pedicle to close defects in the trachea, pharynx or cervical oesophagus. *Plastic Reconstr. Surg.* **59**, 382.
Woods J. E., Irons G. B. and Masson J. K. (1977) Use of muscular, musculo-cutaneous and omental flaps to reconstruct difficult defects. *Plastic Reconstr. Surg.* **59**, 191.

BURNS

Plasma protein fraction

Since the withdrawal of freeze dried human plasma by the National Blood Transfusion Service in 1975 those Burns Units employing plasma as their colloid solution in the resuscitation of patients have had to switch to human plasma protein fraction (PPF). PPF is a solution made from pooled human blood from which the cells and the bulk of the globulin have been removed. The main differences between dried plasma and PPF are, first, that while plasma contains more total protein than PPF the albumin content is much lower and therefore PPF exerts a much higher osmotic pressure. Second, PPF contains less than 1 g/l of globulin as compared with 22 g/l in dried plasma. The sodium content of both solutions is about equal and somewhat higher than that of circulating plasma and whereas dried plasma has a high potassium and low calcium content, both plasma and PPF have low potassium and calcium content.

The switch to PPF resulted in the development of a clinical impression, among many surgeons treating burns, that larger quantities of PPF were required to resuscitate patients than had been their experience when using freeze dried plasma. This clinical impression was tested by Watson and his colleagues at the Rainsford Mowlem Burns Centre in London (Watson et al., 1977). They studied 30 patients treated with dried plasma and 51 treated with PPF, and using the same criteria for both groups they measured the amount of fluid required for resuscitation. Their results have confirmed the clinical impression that larger volumes of PPF are required. In adults roughly 30 per cent more PPF than plasma was required in the course of the first 48 hours post burn, while in children 60 per cent more was required. In the second 24 hours only, the figures for burns of over 40 per cent body surface area were as high as 80 per cent more PPF in adults and 40 per cent more PPF in children.

This confirmation of the clinical impression will be of interest to all who treat burns. Provided the increased volumes of PPF are employed there is no suggestion that it is less effective than dried plasma and when Sanders presented this paper at a meeting of the British Burn Association his findings were confirmed by others in the discussion which followed. One additional point raised was whether the reduction in the globulin fraction would have any influence on immunity and the ability of the patients to combat infection. This, of course, could be of great importance but there does not appear to be any firm evidence for this side effect at present.

REFERENCE
Watson J. S., Walker C. C. and Sanders R. (1977) A comparison between dried plasma
and plasma protein fraction in the resuscitation of burn patients. *Burns* **3**, 108.

FLAPS

Surviving length

Success in flap surgery is, of course, absolutely dependent upon correct
assessment of whether or not a proposed flap will survive in its whole length.
As a result, the constant length-to-breadth ratio of 1:1 for random flaps on the
trunk and limbs, particularly the breadth of the base, is among the first lessons
an aspiring plastic surgeon must learn. All was well and apparently simple until
Milton, of Oxford, published a series of papers which seemed to contradict the
classic concepts. When, however, it was appreciated that his work was done
on axial rather than random flaps it seemed we could revert to the old teaching
learned in the hard school of clinical experience.

Milton's concept that the area-to-base ratio of a flap was constant would
suggest that a triangular flap would survive to a greater length than a
rectangular flap with a base of the same width. This theory was tested by Stell
of Liverpool (1975) in a carefully designed experiment on pigs. His results
showed that triangular and rectangular random flaps with bases of equal
widths survived to the same length. The area-to-base ratio was also calculated
and it was shown that the surviving area of a triangular flap is less than that of
a control rectangular flap. In other words, the surviving length of both
rectangular and triangular random flaps is governed by the 'pumping load' of
the blood supply to its base.

Stell has extended his work on flaps and his conclusions form the basis for
his Hunterian Lecture (1976). Milton's suggestion that flaps survive to the
same length regardless of width has led to considerable controversy because it
is in conflict with classic teaching and clinical experience. As Stell points out,
Milton's flaps were axial and not random flaps and also they were large flaps.
This latter fact is of paramount importance since in Stell's flaps it was shown
that increasing width of base led to increasing surviving length up to a point
where a maximum length is reached. As he points out, most random flaps
employed in clinical practice would lie on the rising part of the curve and he
suggests that the upper limit, beyond which increasing the size of the base will
not increase the surviving length, is of the order of 12·5 cm in the adult
human. This suggestion is further supported by clinical work done by others
whose work is quoted in his lecture.

REFERENCES
Stell P. M. (1975) The viability of triangular skin flaps. *Br. J. Plast. Surg.* **28**, 247.
Stell P. M. (1976) The viability of skin flaps. *Ann. R. Coll. Surg. Engl.* **59**, 236.

COMPLICATIONS OF BLEPHAROPLASTY

The demands for cosmetic surgery are increasing apace, not only from the
younger members of society who simply wish to improve their appearance but
also from those of middle age and above who wish to look younger. This
desire to turn back the clock may stem from vanity or pride, but in many cases

is dictated by society's present youth cult so that the patient's request for surgery is prompted by the need to retain or obtain employment. One of the most rewarding operations in this type of surgery is the blepharoplasty or baggy lid reduction and it seems appropriate to remind oneself that every surgical procedure has its complications. What then are those specific to this operation?

Perhaps the commonest complication of all is patient dissatisfaction with the result. This may be because of poor doctor – patient relationship and failure to explain preoperatively the limited degree of improvement possible. Patients who seek cosmetic surgery are usually hypercritical or they would not be prepared to submit themselves to what many would regard as 'unnecessary' operations. It is therefore only to be expected that they will be hypercritical of the results obtained, so that it is a bold and foolish surgeon who promises a better result than he can obtain. On the other hand, it may well be that the amount of skin and/or fat removed is inadequate and this is usually due to over-caution on the part of the surgeon. Removal of excess fat gives the 'hollow eye' appearance, while removal of excess skin on the lower lids to ectropion, and on the uppers to exposure, both of which can be disastrous. Little wonder then that the cautious surgeon prefers to come back another day rather than take too much.

Another trap for the unwary or the inexperienced is damage to the inferior oblique muscle where it forms the boundary between the middle and medial fat compartments. If it is cut or damaged in the course of removal of fat hernias in the lower lid, diplopia can result.

The 'dry eye' or keratoconjunctivitis sicca is a feature of Sjorgen's syndrome but it is also a fairly common and often asymptomatic disorder of middle life. Any operative procedure on or around the eye may precipitate symptoms of irritation, 'tightness', photophobia, itching and dryness of the eyes, for which the patient blames the surgeon. It is therefore essential to be aware of this condition and to seek for signs or symptoms of it preoperatively, and to warn the patient of possible postoperative exacerbation for periods of up to eighteen months. A series of recent papers, mainly from the United States (Swartz et al., 1974; Rees, 1975; and Graham et al., 1976), have drawn attention to the 'dry eye' complications which may follow blepharoplasty, and to their treatment which is founded upon wetting agents or 'artificial tears'. As Rees has emphasized the sheet-anchor of treatment is recognition of the syndrome, preoperative warning of the patient and postoperative support and sympathetic understanding of the patient's problem.

The worst possible complication following a blepharoplasty is, of course, blindness, and although Moser et al., of Pennsylvania, could find no reports in the literature in 1973, Hueston and Heinze of Melbourne did find two papers in French (1974). Clearly it is a very rare complication indeed, De Mere et al. (1974), of Tennessee, estimating the incidence of 0·04 per cent on the basis of an extensive national survey in the United States. It is, of course, true that patients presenting themselves for blepharoplasty are usually in the age group in which blindness may develop at any time from other causes such as optic neuritis, glaucoma, retinal detachment, etc., and many people are quite unaware of defective vision in one eye until something happens which draws their attention to it, so that it behoves the surgeon to exclude these conditions in so far as it is reasonably possible.

A survey of the literature would seem to suggest that blindness occurring immediately or soon after a blepharoplasty is due to two main causes. The first is acute closed-angle glaucoma which developed in twenty-four hours in a case reported from Leeds by Green and Kadri (1974). They point to a number of factors in blepharoplasty which may predispose to acute closed-angle glaucoma which in their case was not diagnosed until the second postoperative day and responded inadequately to medical treatment, but successfully to a drainage operation.

The second main cause is retrobulbar haemorrhage, either from damage to a vessel in the course of injecting local anaesthetic or from persistent bleeding of a vessel after removal of fatty herniae, despite careful coagulation of the stump after excision. Such a haemorrhage rapidly infiltrates the tissues and does not form a localized haematoma that can be drained. Because the orbit is for practical purposes a closed space, bounded anteriorly by the orbital septum, bleeding into the orbital contents will continue until it reaches arterial pressure. At this point the retinal artery will be occluded and ischaemic blindness develops. This process is further complicated by the fact that rising pressure tends to produce closed-angle glaucoma.

The presence of acute retrobulbar haemorrhage is recognized by increasing tension in the eye which feels wooden, by proptosis, and by a fixed dilated pupil and of course decreasing vision. There is a good deal of argument as to how best to deal with the condition should it arise. Hartley and his colleagues, of Atlanta, Georgia, (1973) performed and recommend paracentesis of the anterior chamber combined with medical measures such as the infusion of hyperosmolar solutions and diuretics. This view was criticised by two distinguished ophthalmologists and a plastic surgeon who pointed to the great dangers associated with paracentesis, especially in the hands of a plastic surgeon. The consensus of opinion seems to be that conservative medical measures should be instituted at once. Should these fail to produce any improvement, surgical decompression of the orbit should be carried out. Hueston and Heinze (1974) did this by incisions in the lids and in a second case by removing the sutures (1977), but Kraufhar et al. (1974) and Jafek et al. (1973) recommend lateral canthotomy as did Barclay, of Wakefield, when discussing decompression of the orbit in cases of acute retrobulbar haemorrhage resulting from trauma (1963). Paracentesis should be left for the ophthalmologist, who doubtless will have been summoned to the assistance of the plastic surgeon, and by the time he arrives in the theatre it will be obvious whether or not this final measure should be embarked upon.

REFERENCES

Barclay T. L. (1963) Some aspects of treatment of traumatic diplopia. *Br. J. Plast. Surg.* **16**, 214.

De Mere McC., Wood T. and Austin W. (1974) Eye complications with blepharoplasty or other eyelid surgery: Anatomical survey. *Plast. Reconstr. Surg.* **53**, 634.

Graham W. P., Messner K. H. and Miller S. H. (1976) Keratoconjunctivitis sicca symptoms appearing after blepharoplasty: The 'dry eye' syndrome. *Plast. Reconstr. Surg.* **57**, 57.

Green M. F. and Kadri S. W. M. (1974) Acute closed-angle glaucoma, a complication of blepharoplasty: report of a case. *Br. J. Plast. Surg.* **27**, 25.

Hartley J. H., Lester J. C. and Schatten W. E. (1973) Acute retrobulbar haemorrhage during elective blepharoplasty. Its pathophysiology and management. *Plast. Reconstr. Surg.* **52**, 8.

Hueston J. T. (1977) A second case of relief of blindness following blepharoplasty. *Plast. Reconstr. Surg.* **59**, 430.

Hueston J. T. and Heinze J. B. (1974) Successful early relief of blindness occurring after blepharoplasty: Case report. *Plast. Reconstr. Surg.* **53**, 588.

Jafek B. W., Kreiger A. E. and Morledge D. (1973) Blindness following blepharoplasty. *Arch. Otolaryngol.* **98**, 366.

Kraufhar M. F., Seelenfreund M. H. and Froelich D. B. (1974) Central retinal artery closure during orbital haemorrhage from retrobulbar injection. *Trans. Am. Acad. Ophthalmol.* **78**, 65.

Moser M. J., DiPirro E. and McCoy F. J. (1973) Sudden blindness following blepharoplasty: Report of several cases. *Plast. Reconstr. Surg.* **51**, 364.

Rees T. D. (1975) The 'dry eye' complication after a blepharoplasty. *Plast. Reconstr. Surg.* **56**, 375.

Swartz R. M., Schultz R. C. and Seaton J. R. (1974) 'Dry eye' following blepharoplasty. *Plast. Reconstr. Surg.* **54**, 644.

RADIODIAGNOSIS

J. H. MIDDLEMISS CMG, MD,
FRCP, FRCR

IS YOUR X-RAY EXAMINATION REALLY NECESSARY?

Medical diagnosis and treatment may be regarded as an example of decision-making under uncertainty. Medical decision-making is often more dramatic than business decision-making because issues of health are involved. Medical decision-making has increasingly come to rely on sophisticated and expensive diagnostic procedures.

Choices as to appropriate diagnostic procedures must be made by doctors. The possibility that these choices may not always be wise ones is reflected in the widespread view that many of the procedures requested cannot be justified by cost-benefit analysis, and that large amounts of money are being wasted. Yet there is scarcely any evidence available as to which procedures in which circumstances are effective or ineffective. Forty million units (a report on a chest radiograph represents one unit) of radiological investigation were undertaken in the National Health Service in 1974 (DHE, 1976). Demands on diagnostic radiology are growing at the rate of 5 – 10 per cent per annum (Evans, 1977). In 1970 two-thirds of the total population of the United States underwent medical radiographic examination (U.S. Public Health Service, 1970). Yet very little is known about how diagnostic radiological procedures influence the subsequent management of patients.

A recent retrospective survey of 100 consecutive patients admitted to hospital in Bristol with a clinical diagnosis of left ventricular failure showed that 95 of them had a chest radiograph taken, 50 of them died (28 with 7 days of admission, including those not X-rayed), and of those who survived the radiographic examination did not appear to have influenced the management of their condition (McLean, 1978). Though 61 of the patients were X-rayed a second or even a third time, there did not appear to be any specific event or course of treatment which influenced the timing of these repeat examinations nor were regimes altered as a result of them.

In 1971 Bell and Loop studied the use of radiographic skull examinations following trauma (Bell and Loop, 1971). Their main conclusion was that unless certain signs and symptoms were present the probability was low that an X-ray examination of the skull following trauma would show a skull fracture and that the probability was even lower that the radiographic findings would affect patient management or the final outcome for the patient. They estimated that society in the United States was paying $7,650 per skull fracture found in patients X-rayed for medico-legal reasons, and they questioned whether the benefits were worth the costs. It is well recognized that the most expensive department in any hospital is the department of Diagnostic Radiology. It is essential, therefore, that optimum use should be made of available resources and that expensive and 'unnecessary' examinations should not be requested or carried out.

The Royal College of Radiologists in this country and the American College in the United States have set up working parties to look into the problems of clinical audit in diagnostic radiology (Editorial, 1977), and more recently the World Health Organisation set up a committee to consider the possibility of instigating retrospective and prospective studies of the efficacy of radiological investigations. Efficacy, of course, is a notoriously difficult condition to assess, as in some respects it is bound to be subjective. In the long term, however, the factor which will probably have most effect will be education—education of the referring doctor. Most radiological examinations are carried out in hospital, and most requests for such examinations are probably written and signed by junior doctors.

It is important that when such requests are made there should be a clear tentative 'first' (likely) diagnosis in the mind of the referring doctor; there should also be a clear knowledge on the part of the referring doctor that the problem being investigated is one that is amenable to radiological examination, and preferably there should be the implication that, if the diagnosis is confirmed and thus established, this will lead to a particular course of action and so influence management of the clinical problem. In this context must be considered the 'negative' diagnostic examination. By definition the negative diagnostic test has zero yield. Yet it can spare the patient unneeded treatment, rule out the need for further examinations or better direct the subsequent diagnostic process. An X-ray examination that shows no kidney abnormality in a patient with haematuria contributes to efficacy just as does one that shows a stone or a tumour.

Thus in the education of the referring doctor it is important that the scope and limitations of radiological investigations, as well as the interpretation of simple abnormalities, should be emphasized rather than attempting to make each medical student or junior doctor into a minor radiologist. Such radiological teaching needs to be integrated into a clinical context, and ideally in hospital practice high yield criteria should be established for the request for radiological examinations. High yield criteria for examinations could for educational purposes be drawn up as lists of clinical events or signs. For example, in one hospital a 'policy on skull radiography' has been drawn up which reads as follows (Philips, 1977):

All patients presenting with complaints or symptoms referring to the cranium or its contents, or with a history of trauma to the same, should receive a careful and complete clinical evaluation. If any of the following criteria are present, skull radiography should be requested.

1. Non-alcohol related unconsciousness at the time of admission, or documented decreasing level of consciousness.
2. Skull depression palpable or identified by a probe through a laceration.
3. Haemotympanum or fluid discharge from the ear.
4. Cerebrospinal fluid discharge from the nose.
5. Bilateral orbital ecchymoses.
6. Unexplained focal neurological signs.
7. History of previous craniotomy.

If none of these criteria are present and you believe that skull radiography is needed, you must seek consultation with a neurology house officer or a full-time Accident Surgeon.

It must be emphasized that all decision-making cannot be reduced to lists of high yield criteria, and that what would be acceptable as criteria in one hospital might not be acceptable in another. A doctor must be able to exercise his judgement. Nevertheless, the preparation of lists of criteria for the undertaking of certain examinations does help to clarify unclear thinking and does help to crystallize a doctor's approach to a clinical problem, his diagnostic thinking and his further intentions dependent on confirmation or otherwise of his diagnosis. However, in the preparation of high yield criteria lists, room must be made for the judging of true positive and false positive results, and for judging the efficacy or usefulness of negative results.

In the setting up of efficacy studies the Royal College, the American College and the World Health Organisation have had to try to define terms, if they are in any way to attempt quantification in this field. Some degree of success has attended their deliberations and WHO have agreed to adopt a modification of the codified definition of 'efficacy' proposed by the American College (Lusted, 1968). The code thus produced defined the 'efficacy' of a radiological examination as:

> Efficacy 1 is the measure of the ability of a diagnostic test to influence the physician's diagnostic thinking.
>
> Efficacy 2 is the measure of the ability of a diagnostic test to influence the proposed patient management and treatment.
>
> Efficacy 3 is the measure of the ability of a diagnostic test to influence the health outcome of a patient.
>
> Efficacy 4 is the measure of the ability of a diagnostic test to influence the health of the population.

With these problems in mind, and ever mindful of the need to make optimum use of all available resources to the maximum benefit of individual patients and to populations as a whole, WHO (1978) has recommended to member nations that both retrospective and prospective studies in certain specific fields, and in countries with widely differing economies and widely differing methods of delivering health care and of providing health services, should be undertaken.

REFERENCES

Bell R. S. and Loop J. W. (1971) The utility and futility of skull examination for trauma. *N. Engl. J. Med.* **284**, 236 – 239.
Editorial (1977) *Br. Med. J.* **2**, 479 – 480.
Evans K. T. (1977) Radiology now; the radiologist's dilemma. *Br. J. Radiol.* **50**, 299 – 301.
Lusted Lee (1965) *Introduction to Medical Decision Making.* Springfield, Ill., Thomas.
McLean C. (1978) A study of patients with a clinical diagnosis of acute left ventricular failure. In the press.
Office of Health Economics (1976) Information Sheet No. 28, London, OHE.
Philips L. A. (1977) *Comparative Evaluation of a High Yield Criteria List upon Skull Radiograph Utilisation in Emergency Rooms.* WHO Working Paper. Geneva, WHO.
U.S. Public Health Service (1970) Population Exposure to X-rays U.S. Publication (HSM) 8047. Department of Health, Education and Welfare, Washington.
World Health Organisation Report. In the press (1978).

RADIOTHERAPY

W. DUNCAN FRCPE, FRCSE, FRCR
S. J. ARNOTT FRCSE, FRCR

TOTAL BODY IRRADIATION

The therapeutic use of whole-body irradiation (TBI) is a most interesting concept. The low doses which are normally employed (e.g. 15 rads twice weekly for 5 weeks) are such that it is surprising that regression of tumour is observed. Nevertheless, the efficacy of this treatment is no longer in doubt in the management of the generalized lymphomas and its use in the treatment of a variety of disseminated solid cancers is being widely investigated.

Total body radiotherapy is not new. Only a few years after the discovery of X-rays the principles of this type of treatment were described by Dessauer (1907). Technical difficulties, however, prevented its application until 1927, when Teschendorf described this method of treatment in patients with leukaemia (Teschendorf, 1927). Further reports appeared over the years (Chaoul and Lange, 1923; Scott, 1940) but it was not until Medinger and Craver (1942) published the results of a 10-year experience of whole-body irradiation in 270 patients that some idea of the potential of this therapy was appreciated. This study described a doubling of the average survival time in patients with disseminated lymphosarcoma following TBI compared to those receiving radiotherapy confined to areas of known disease. It was about this time that Nitrogen Mustard was first used as a cancer chemotherapeutic agent, and its successful application in a variety of malignancies led to virtual abandonment of further investigation of whole-body X-ray therapy. More recently, however, the severe toxicity often associated with chemotherapy using multiple cytotoxic drugs, together with the disappointing responses in most solid tumours, has led to a reappraisal of the use of TBI in patients with disseminated cancers.

The first encouraging recent report of TBI again described its value in the treatment of disseminated lymphosarcoma (Johnson et al., 1970). This was a pilot study in which radiotherapy was used as the primary treatment for patients with advanced lymphosarcoma. The aim of treatment was the production of complete resolution of disease using either TBI or total nodal irradiation. Although the number of patients investigated was small, a feature of note was that 7 out of 8 patients with Stage IV disease, treated by TBI, obtained remission of their disease for periods varying from 7 to 43 months at the time of reporting.

Similar results have been reported more recently by Chaffey et al. (1975). They describe the effectiveness of TBI as the primary treatment in a group of 25 patients with advanced (Stage III and IV) lymphosarcoma. The patients were all treated twice weekly for 5 weeks giving a total dose of 150 rad. The toxicity experienced was perfectly acceptable, certainly being much less than that produced by chemotherapeutic agents. All the patients responded to the treatment and a complete remission of disease was produced in 80 per cent. So far 64 per cent have remained in remission for periods of up to 39 months without maintenance therapy of any kind. The actuarial survival of this group of patients is 87 per cent at two years which would compare favourably with that which could be achieved by drug therapy.

In order to try to determine further the place of TBI in patients with non-

Hodgkin's lymphoma, several clinical trials have been established. Preliminary results have been reported from one of these (Canellos et al., 1975). At the time of reporting 65 patients had been included in the study all of whom had Stage III or IV disease. The follow-up period of this investigation is short and therefore it is too early to derive definitive results, but those patients treated by TBI have shown an 84 per cent response rate compared to 81 per cent in patients receiving chemotherapy. The response of patients with the diffuse form of the disease has been particularly good when treated by TBI. Further reports from this particular trial are awaited eagerly.

TBI has also been investigated in chronic lymphatic leukaemia (Johnson, 1970), a disease which currently is managed principally by chemotherapy. This form of radiotherapy, however, has been found to be extremely effective in producing clinical and haematological remission in leukaemia patients. In the series reported by Johnson one-third of patients with chronic lymphatic leukaemia obtained complete symptomatic remission, a return of the white blood count and differential count to normal, associated with significant improvement in the bone marrow picture. These patients also survived significantly longer than those treated by other forms of therapy. Results such as these suggest that the role of radiotherapy in the management of chronic lymphatic leukaemia deserves reappraisal.

The promising results that have been obtained from TBI in the non-Hodgkin's lymphomas and chronic lymphatic leukaemia have led to its investigation in the treatment of solid tumours. Huys and co-workers (1977) have described an experience of treating 26 patients with a variety of disseminated malignant diseases. The majority of these patients were suffering from breast cancer, the remainder having other forms of generalized malignant disease which included Hodgkin's disease and non-Hodgkin's lymphoma. It was found that the best responses occurred in patients with Hodgkin's and non-Hodgkin's lymphoma, but worth while palliation was achieved in patients with solid tumours.

A larger group of patients, all of whom had metastatic solid tumours, has been reported by Saenger et al. (1973). A total of 85 patients with metastatic colo-rectal, bronchial, breast and other carcinomas were treated with TBI. Many were known to have liver metastases at the time of treatment. The survival of these patients was compared to that of historic controls, some of whom had not had any form of treatment and others who had had chemotherapy. Patients with colo-rectal cancer showed the most promising response to TBI in that their average survival was 391 days, compared to 255 days in similar patients treated by chemotherapy and 146 days in untreated patients. Less dramatic improvements were seen in the other groups of patients.

An important modification of the technique of TBI has been described for the treatment of patients with advanced cancer (Fitzpatrick and Rider, 1976). This treatment involves the giving of large single doses of radiotherapy, in the region of 800 rads to the upper or lower half of the body (Half Body Irradiation or HBI). The interval between the two treatments is not less than five weeks. The treatment by HBI of 139 patients is described, all of whom had advanced cancers which had not been controlled by other methods of treatment. The majority had cancers of the breast, lung or prostate, and were referred for treatment most commonly because of severe, generalized pain. Significant palliation was achieved in 97 of the 139 patients which lasted for varying periods up to one year. Side effects experienced were mainly nausea and vomiting especially following treatment to the upper half of the body. These symptoms generally were short-lived. Surprisingly bone marrow toxicity was not a problem. The results of this treatment have proved so encouraging that further studies are now taking place in order to evaluate which patients are most likely to benefit from HBI. This new technique could have an important role as a form of adjuvant therapy in patients with lung and breast cancers known to have a high probability of metastases.

Much further study is required into the role of TBI and HBI in the treatment of patients with disseminated cancer, but these preliminary studies suggest that it may be as effective as cytotoxic chemotherapy. If this is confirmed to be the case and the responses obtained prove to be as long lived as those with chemotherapy, the implications are obvious. TBI and HBI is much less toxic than drug therapy, and is administered over a short period often without the need for hospital admission. In addition, TBI is much less expensive than most chemotherapeutic regimes with which it might be compared in the management of patients with generalized malignant disease.

REFERENCES
Canellos G. P., DeVita V. T., Young R. C. et al. (1975) Therapy of advanced lymphocytic lymphoma: A preliminary report of a randomized trial between combination chemotherapy (CVP) and intensive radiotherapy. *Br. J. Cancer* Suppl. 31, 474 – 480.
Chaffey J. T., Rosenthal D. S., Pinkus G. et al. (1975) Advanced lymphosarcoma treated by total body irradiation. *Br. J. Cancer* Suppl. 31, 441 – 449.
Chaoul H. and Lange K. (1923) Über Lymphogranulomatose und ihre behandlung mit röntgenstrahlen. *Münch. Med. Wochenschr.* 70, 725 – 727.
Dessauer F. (1907) Eine neue Anordnung zur röntgenbestrahlung. *Arch. Phys. Med. Techn.* 2, 218 – 223.
Fitzpatrick P. J. and Rider W. D. (1976) Half-body radiotherapy of advanced cancer. *J. Can. Assoc. Radiol.* 27, 75 – 79.
Huys J. V., Simons M. J., Dewulf L. M. et al. (1977) Total body irradiation with 8 MeV X-rays in generalised malignant disease. *Cancer* 1435 – 1438.
Johnson R. E. (1970) Total body irradiation of chronic lymphatic leukaemia. *Cancer* 25, 523 – 530.
Johnson R. E., O'Connor G. T. and Levin D. (1970) Primary management of advanced lymphosarcoma with radiotherapy. *Cancer* 25, 787 – 791.
Medinger F. G. and Craver L. F. (1942) Total body irradiation. *Am. J. Roentgenol.* 48, 651 – 671.
Saenger E. L., Silberstein E. B., Aron B. et al. (1973) Whole-body and partial body radiotherapy of advanced cancer. *Am. J. Roentgenol.* 117, 670 – 685.
Scott G. S. (1940) Clinical investigations (1920 – 1938) *Am. J. Roentgenol.* 43, 1.
Teschendorf W. (1927) Über bestrahlungen des ganzen menschlichen korpers bei blutkrankheiten. *Strahlentherapie* 26, 720 – 728.

FAST NEUTRON THERAPY

Fast neutron therapy continues to be one of the most promising fields of development in modern radiotherapy. The rationale for the use of fast neutrons in preference to conventional X-ray or gamma ray beams is based on the evidence that neutron irradiation is more effective, by a factor of about 3, in the destruction of hypoxic tumour cells which may comprise 10 – 15 per cent of most solid tumours. The relative radio-resistance of these cells is believed to be a major cause of local failure in the treatment of many cancers. A further factor accounting for radio-resistance of cancer cells is their ability to recover from some of the damage inflicted by each dose fraction of X-rays. This ability is also much reduced following neutron irradiation. Thus it would appear that fast neutrons are able to overcome two major factors accounting for radio-resistance encountered during courses of X-ray therapy.

In 1975 the first results of a randomized clinical trial investigating neutron therapy in patients with advanced head and neck cancers were reported from the M.R.C. Cyclotron Unit at the Hammersmith Hospital, London (Catterall et al., 1975). Complete regression of tumour was seen in 37 out of 52 patients receiving neutron therapy compared to 16 in the control group of 50 patients treated by conventional photon (X or gamma ray) therapy. There was, however, a greater spread of dose delivered to the tumours treated by X-rays and the average dose was higher in the neutron-treated group. It was considered that the large difference in results did represent, at least in part, a qualitative difference in the response to neutrons compared to X-rays.

An updated report has recently been published (Catterall et al., 1977). A greater number of patients has now been included in the study and follow-up is longer. The benefit demonstrated in the earlier report has been maintained and patients receiving neutron therapy have obtained a significantly greater degree of local tumour control than those treated by X-rays. In this latest report 53 (76 per cent) of 70 patients treated with fast neutrons had complete· tumour regression compared with only 12 (19 per cent) of 63 patients in the X-ray therapy group. Survival at two years was also better in the neutron treated group of patients (28 per cent) compared to those treated with X-rays (15 per cent), but these differences are not statistically significant. However, patients included in this trial had such very advanced cancers that it was difficult to assess definitively the qualitative advantage of fast neutrons. Further trials have now begun both at the Hammersmith Hospital and at the new M.R.C. unit in Edinburgh in which patients with earlier tumours will be studied which will help to evaluate in greater detail to what extent the therapeutic ratio is increased with fast neutron therapy.

Berry et al. (1976) in America have described similarly encouraging results of the treatment of secondary cervical lymph nodes. They report that 58 per cent of patients obtained complete clinical resolution of large cervical lymph node masses and that in 52 per cent of patients with fixed masses in the neck complete tumour resolution was achieved. This is greatly in excess of what might be expected from conventional radiotherapy treatment of similar disease. On the other hand, results of a pilot study of advanced cerebral tumours carried out by the same group (Parker et al., 1977) has failed to show any improvement in survival after neutron therapy, in spite of the fact that some striking examples of tumour regression were obtained. Some of these patients did show evidence of brain necrosis and diffuse demyelinization and further investigation is required on the response to neutron radiation of normal brain, in the hope that an optimal treatment schedule may be found.

An alternative to using neutron irradiation alone in cancer therapy has been reported from the M.D. Anderson Hospital in Houston, Texas (Caderao et al., 1976). This centre has been investigating the use of combined neutron and X-ray treatments. The results of using this technique have been described in the treatment of 79 patients with advanced gynaecological, prostatic and rectal tumours. Patients received one of three possible regimes of treatment: neutron therapy alone, mainly X-ray therapy with a short boost of neutron radiation at the end, or both neutrons and photons in the course of treatment. In this regime patients were given neutron treatment on two days and X-ray treatments on three days per week for 6 – 7 weeks. They report that patients receiving the mixed beam therapy responded best and had the lowest incidence of complications. Although the three groups of patients are not strictly comparable, this experience does indicate that there may be advantages in combining neutrons with X-ray therapy regimes.

With several centres throughout the world beginning further trials of fast neutron therapy, the assessment of this important development in radiotherapy will be the subject of increasing attention.

REFERENCES
Berry H. C., Parker R. G. and Gerdes A. J. (1976) Preliminary results of fast neutron teletherapy of metastatic cervical adenopathy. *Cancer* **37**, 2613 – 2619.
Caderao J. B., Hussey D. H. and Fletcher G. H. (1976) Fast neutron radiotherapy for locally advanced pelvic cancer. *Cancer* **37**, 2620 – 2629.
Catterall M., Bewley D. K. and Sutherland I. (1977) Second report on results of a randomized clinical trial of fast neutrons compared with X- or gamma rays in treatment of advanced tumours of the head and neck. *Br. Med. J.* **1**, 1642.
Catterall M., Sutherland I. and Bewley D. K. (1975) First results of a randomized clinical trial of fast neutrons compared with X- or gamma rays in treatment of advanced tumours of the head and neck. *Br. Med. J.* **2**, 653 – 656.
Parker R. G., Berry H. C., Gerdes A. J., Soronen M. D. and Shaw C. M. (1976) Fast neutron beam radiotherapy of glioblastoma multiforme. *Am. J. Roentgenol.* **127**, 331 – 335.

SOFT TISSUE SARCOMAS

Many problems are encountered in the management of patients with soft tissue sarcomas. Surgical excision is frequently followed by local tumour recurrence and the addition of chemotherapy has, as yet, made little difference to the overall survival results. A factor which has not always been appreciated is the significant contribution which is made by radiotherapy both in terms of local tumour control and overall survival. One of the first reports indicating the efficacy of X-ray therapy in these tumours was by Cade (1951). He showed that of 22 patients with fibrosarcomas, treated solely by irradiation, in 6 there was complete tumour regression, which was of long duration. Similar encouraging results were described by Windeyer et al. (1966) in the treatment of 22 patients with very advanced fibrosarcomas: 11 of these patients had massive inoperable tumours and a further 11 were treated for tumour recurrences after previous surgical excision. No fewer than 9 of the 22 patients were alive at the time of reporting without evidence of either local or metastatic disease from between 28 and 75 months after irradiation. A more recent report from the M.D. Anderson Hospital in Houston, Texas, describes the efficacy of combining surgical excision with postoperative radiotherapy (Suit et al., 1975). The extent of surgical removal varied from simple excisional biopsy to radical en bloc resection. All patients were free from any evidence of metastatic disease at the time of referral for radiotherapy. A total of 57 patients was treated by this method which achieved complete local tumour control in no less than 87 per cent of cases. A particularly important feature of this approach to management is that it avoids amputation of limbs and in others makes unnecessary extensive and possibly mutilating excision. The functional results achieved in patients with tumours of the limbs treated in this way was extremely good.

In the hope of improving results even further an investigation was carried out at the same centre giving the radiotherapy treatments under conditions of tourniquet-induced hypoxia (Suit and Russell, 1977). The rationale for attempting to give treatments in this way is based on the concept that a proportion of the local treatment failures is due to the presence during irradiation of viable, hypoxic tumour cells which are relatively radio-resistant. The use of the tourniquet produces hypoxia in the normal tissues also and this reduces the differential radio-sensitivity between the tumour and normal cells, therefore hopefully improving the therapeutic ratio. Initially a group of 21 patients with sarcomas of the extremities was treated. Most patients had had some surgical excision but 4 patients had local disease which was either inoperable or grossly recurrent. Only 1 patient developed local recurrence after irradiation but 7 patients required amputation for severe late normal tissue damage produced by the course of X-ray treatment. A probable explanation of this effect is that extremely large treatment fields were used in this pilot study and thus large volumes of normal tissues were irradiated, obviously to dose levels that were unacceptably high. The local tumour control rates which were observed led to the establishment of a clinical trial comparing the irradiation of patients using tourniquet-induced hypoxia and those treated by orthodox techniques. This demonstrated that there was no statistically significant difference between the results of the two forms of treatment but the study did confirm the effectiveness of postoperative radiotherapy in the control of soft tissue sarcomas (Suit and Russell, 1977).

Investigation of other methods of improving the results of treatment are continuing, and already there is some evidence that fast neutron radiation may be more effective than X-rays in treating these tumours. It would seem, however, that at the present time combined local surgical excision followed by postoperative radiotherapy is the treatment of choice in the management of soft tissue sarcomas.

REFERENCES
Cade S. (1951) Soft tissue tumours: their natural history and treatment. *Proc. R. Soc. Med.* **44**, 19 – 36.
Suit H. D. and Russell W. O. (1977) Soft-part tumours. *Cancer* **39**, 830—836.
Suit H. D., Russell W. O. and Martin R. G. (1975) Sarcoma of soft tissue: clinical and histopathologic parameters and response to treatment. *Cancer* **35**, 1478 – 1483.
Windeyer B., Dische S. and Mansfield C. M. (1966) The place of radiotherapy in the management of fibrosarcoma of the soft tissues. *Clin. Radiol.* **17**, 32 – 40.

RESPIRATORY TRACT

JOHN COLLINS MD, MRCP
and
RICHARD E. LEA FRCS

Medical

JOHN COLLINS MD, MRCP

ASTHMA

The past year has not seen the introduction of new types of treatment or major
advances in understanding of the physiological and biochemical mechanisms
in asthma, but three important new books about asthma have recently been
published drawing upon the many scientific and therapeutic advances that
have taken place in the last decade (Jones, 1976; Weiss and Segal, 1976; Clark
and Godfrey, 1977). The time-honoured division of patients into intrinsic and
extrinsic groups according to the apparent relevance of recognizable atopic
factors in relationship to asthma has not proved of great importance for
treatment in that many of the drugs available are equally effective in both
types of patient. In addition, it has been recognized that factors which
provoke airways obstruction, such as respiratory infections, climatic changes
and exercise, may affect patients with seemingly different types of asthma.
Surprisingly, too, in spite of a large literature relating the effectiveness of
sympathomimetic bronchodilators, disodium cromoglycate and corticosteroids, there is little published information to suggest means by which future
response to treatment in asthma may be predicted from short-term studies of
their effects such as the ability of disodium cromoglycate to protect from
exercise-induced airways obstruction (B.T.A. Committee, 1977). It seems
unlikely that there will be major therapeutic advances in the near future and
much current interest centres on attempts to define clinical subgroups of
patients in order that present drugs may be used to better effect. In this respect
the United States is at some disadvantage compared to Europe as many of the
well tried newer medicines for asthma are not yet licensed for use in America.

Recently attempts have been made to delineate patterns of chronic asthma
as a step to rationalizing treatment and in one such attempt patients have been
classified as 'brittle', 'irreversible' and 'morning dippers', with suggestions for
further definable subdivisions (Turner-Warwick, 1977). The 'brittle' asthmatic
is recognized to have intractable persistent asthma resistant to all forms of
therapy. The important feature is responsibeness to sympathomimetic drugs
but failure to stabilize with these and cromoglycate or corticosteroids. This
short-lived responsiveness to sympathomimetic drugs often leads to a
diagnosis of 'addiction' to aerosols. The 'irreversible' group includes at least
three recognizable patterns, one in which persistent airways obstruction
results in measurements of airflow always being below predicted levels but
with temporary improvements either occurring spontaneously or as a result of
treatment. A second pattern in this group is one in which improvement in
forced vital capacity (FVC) occurs with treatment without comparable change
in forced expired volume in one second (FEV_1) or peak expiratory flow rate

(PEFR): in some instances this may be accompanied by deflation of the lungs with reduction in the amount of air trapping. The third 'irreversible' group, referred to as 'dippers', show apparently irreversible airways obstruction which improves very gradually after weeks of intensive treatment. Many patients with asthma have long known that their symptoms are worse early in the day but the interest of the medical profession in these 'morning dips' is relatively recent (Soutar et al., 1975; Hetzel et al., 1977; Clark and Hetzel, 1977). In many patients measurements of lung function taken during the day may show normal results and unless repeated early in the morning this feature of asthma may pass unrecognized.

Measurements of airflow in children have been found to reach lowest levels at about 2·00 a.m. (Kales et al., 1970) but in adults the timing of the lowest readings is more variable with some developing slowly from about midnight (Soutar et al., 1975) while others happen rapidly towards morning (Clark and Hetzel, 1977). This circadian rhythm of airflow obstruction is not due to recumbency in bed but is directly related to sleep and in shift workers it has been found to be independent of solar time (Clark and Hetzel, 1977). Except in a minority of patients exposure to house dust mites in bedding seems unlikely to be the cause of these nocturnal exacerbations of airways obstructions. The changes in diurnal variations of airflow in shift workers on changing shift are more rapid and seemingly unrelated to known changes in other circadian rhythms of body temperature and catecholamine secretion. A relationship with circadian cortisol rhythms seemed possible but when this is abolished by cortisol infusions the changes in airways obstruction persist (Soutar et al., 1975). For some patients there may be a connection with: irregularities in the timing of medication and some success has been obtained by more careful spacing of doses to ensure continued effective treatment of asthma during the night. Slow-release bronchodilator preparations taken last thing before sleep may be helpful in abolishing or reducing the severity of 'morning dips'. When patients convalescing from exacerbations of asthma were studied marked falls of PEFR at 6·00 a.m. were associated with temporary increases in static lung volumes and airways resistance similar to those described in acute attacks of asthma (Woolcock and Read, 1966).

Mild hypoxaemia and a widened alveolar-arterial oxygen tension gradient persisted throughout the study in these patients and these were little influenced by variations in the degree of airways obstruction. The results of the studies suggested that the calibre of both small and large airways was reduced at night and that improvement during the day was more marked in the larger airways. Most of the patients showed a marked improvement in airways obstruction early in the morning after inhalation of a bronchodilator aerosol. A further study from the same group of sudden deaths in patients in hospital with asthma showed that most deaths occurred in the early hours of the morning in patients who still showed marked diurnal variations in PEFR (Hetzel et al., 1977), thus providing one example where careful observation of clinical patterns of asthma may perhaps be used to influence the choice and intensity of treatment. Further refinements of observation are needed but these initial attempts to differentiate between various clinical patterns of asthma seem to provide a means by which the limited number of treatments available may be adjusted to the requirements of individual patients.

REFERENCES

B.T.T.A. Committee (1977) Clinical trials methods in asthma. Ed. Start J. E. and Collins J. V. *Br. J. Dis. Chest* **71.**

Clark T. J. H. and Godfrey S. (1977) *Asthma.* London, Chapman & Hall.

Clark T. J. H. and Hetzel M. R. (1977) Diurnal variation of asthma. *Br. J. Dis. Chest* **71,** 87.

Hetzel M. R., Clark T. J. H. and Branthwaite M. A. (1977) Asthma: Analysis of sudden deaths and ventilatory arrests in hospital. *Br. Med. J.* **1,** 808.

Hetzel M. R., Clark T. J. H. and Houston K. (1977) Physiological patterns in early morning asthma. *Thorax* **32,** 418.

Jones R. S. (1976) *Asthma in Children,* London, Arnold.

Kales A., Kales J., Sly R. M. et al. (1970) Sleep patterns of asthmatic children. *J. Allergy* **46,** 300.

Spoutar C. A., Costello J., Ijaducha O. et al. (1975) Nocturnal and morning asthma: relationship to plasma corticosteroid and response to cortisol infusion. *Thorax* **30,** 436.

Turner-Warwick M. (1977). On observing patterns of airflow obstruction in chronic asthma. *Br. J. Dis. Chest* **71,** 73.

Weiss E. B. and Segal M. S. (1976) Bronchial asthma: mechanisms and therapeutics. Boston, Mass., Little, Brown.

Woolcock A. J. and Read J. (1966) Lung volumes in exacerbations of asthma. *Am. J. Med.* **41,** 259.

CHRONIC BRONCHITIS

Mention of chronic bronchitis can usually be counted upon to produce sighs of boredom and loss of attention in most medical audiences, yet this puzzling disorder remains a major medical, social and economic problem requiring further research and elucidation. Systematic study of chronic bronchitis and emphysema did not begin until the second half of this century and initial attempts foundered for lack of a consensus on definitions for the two diseases. Subsequently a morbid anatomical definition of emphysema as an increase in the size of the airspaces distal to the terminal bronchioles, with destruction of tissue but excluding simple overdistension (CIBA Foundation, 1959), has been widely accepted. Earlier failures to agree upon the definition or diagnosis of chronic bronchitis seemed to have been overcome when the Medical Research Council's Committee on research into chronic bronchitis (1965) proposed a classification into three stages: simple, mucopurulent and obstructive. At that time the received opinion amongst British doctors, apparently supported by pathological studies (Reid, 1954), was that the disease initiated as mucus hypersecretion by cigarette smoking and progressed through scarring in small bronchi, bronchioles and acini from repeated or persistent bacterial infection. In spite of reports showing that prophylactic or early intensive treatment of bacterial infections did not affect the rate of deterioration of ventilatory function (MRC Working Party, 1966), the view that infection was a major factor in the causation of chronic bronchitis persisted.

An alternative view of the pathogenesis of chronic bronchitis (Orie et al., 1961; Van der Lende, 1969) held that the major mechanism leading to airways obstruction was bronchial hyperreactivity to allergic and environmental stimuli and implied a closer relationship between chronic bronchitis and asthma. In this view bacterial infections were thought to be of secondary importance in the pathogenesis. However, retrospective studies have so far only incriminated cigarette smoking (Doll and Hill, 1964; Doll and Peto, 1976; Fletcher et al., 1959) and to a lesser extent high atmospheric pollution (Holland et al., 1965) as important factors contributing to morbidity and mortality rates in chronic bronchitis. Many patients with severe airflow obstruction have no obvious emphysema and in such cases widespread anatomical changes have been recognized in small airways (Thurlbeck, 1976). Increasingly it has seemed possible that airways obstruction, emphysema and mucus hypersecretion may be products of independent processes which occur in response to one or more of the same group of stimulants, their presence or absence in individuals being controlled by factors as yet unidentified. In this context a detailed study of fundamental importance and interest has recently been published (Fletcher et al., 1976). It is the result of eight years painstaking research and a similar period of analysis by a team of clinical scientists and epidemiologists. Much thought has been given to the manner of presentation so that the study is readily accessible to specialist and general readers alike. The findings are of great interest: in answering some questions many more are posed and directions for future research are indicated.

A preliminary survey for this study of the prevalance of respiratory symptoms in men aged 30 – 59 years working in an office block and an engineering works in West London showed that it would be possible to examine the associations of mucus hypersecretion, smoking habits, bronchial infections and ventilatory function. Of 1136 men who entered the study in 1961, 792 attended regularly for 6-monthly assessment until 1969. The sample was weighted at the outset to increase the proportions of those with symptoms and of non-smokers. At each attendance mucus hypersecretion was assessed by questionnaire and measurements of specimens of early morning sputum. Infection was assessed by the presence of pus in the sputum specimens and records of illnesses assumed to be chest infections. Current smoking habits were recorded and airflow obstruction was assessed by measurements of forced expired volume in one second (FEV_1) and at some visits by forced vital capacity (FVC).

The main conclusions of the study are that smoking causes two distinct but independent disorders, mucus hypersecretion and airflow obstruction, and that chest infections are associated with mucus hypersecretion but do not cause permanent increase in airflow obstruction. Many men showed mucus hypersecretion alone, others had mucus hypersecretion with airflow obstruction and a third group had airway obstruction with little or no mucus hypersecretion.

Fletcher et al. believe that their results show that there is no evidence that the presence of either mucus hypersecretion or airflow obstruction predisposes to the development of the other condition. In their study men with mucus hypersecretion were predisposed to chest infections resulting in temporary increase of expectoration, and in those men with airflow obstruction this was also increased temporarily but returned to previous levels on recovery. Airflow obstruction, of itself, did not predispose to infection. Those men with clinical evidence of asthma showed more rapid progression of airflow obstruction but a personal or family history of hay fever or allergy was not well correlated with the rate of deterioration of FEV_1. The rate of progress of airflow obstruction was greater in those men with sputum eosinophilia but this was not well correlated with clinical asthma as recorded by questionnaire. When the acute response of FEV_1 to smoking a single cigarette was measured it was not well correlated with the overall rate of progress of airflow obstruction. This would seem to indicate that progressive airflow obstruction and episodic asthma may be caused by different factors and does not support the hyperreactive hypothesis for the basis of chronic bronchitis.

From these results there seem to be at least three detectable injuries resulting from cigarette smoking: mucus hypersecretion in larger bronchi, for which the older term 'bronchial catarrh' might usefully be revived, changes in small airways leading to widespread obstruction, and emphysema in acini.

There are clearly individual differences in susceptibility which are probably in part due to genetic factors, the link between alpha-1 antitrypsin deficiency and rapidly-progressive emphysema being but one example presently recognizable. Exposure to environmental hazards such as atmospheric pollution and dust at work seem likely to be factors weighting individual susceptibilities. What is needed is a means for early detection of the minority of smokers at risk of developing progressive airflow obstruction. This study has shown that mucus hypersecretion, previously thought to be a good marker of susceptibility, will not do. So far, of the newer tests of airway function which are thought to reflect early changes in small airways (Macklem, 1974), none has yet been shown to provide a practicable, reliable screening test for large scale studies and the value of such programmes is questionable (Macklem, 1972). All at present suffer from the same defect as FEV_1, in that the range of normal values is rather wide. Fletcher et al. suggest that a low FEV_1 in middle life is still the most reliable indicator that a smoker may develop progressive airflow obstruction, but how much loss has been sustained since early life in those showing FEV_1 results at the lower limit of normal in middle age cannot be judged without a previous measurement made in youth. it seems that for preventive medicine a health profile at the outset of adult life should include a record of FEV_1 and FVC, in addition to such things as blood pressure measurements.

Further studies of the value of the newer 'sensitive' tests of airway function in following subjects from early adult life will be important, especially if they can be shown to detect at an early stage individuals who later develop progressive airway obstruction. New hypotheses for differential susceptibilities to the effects of smoking and atmospheric pollution and the propensity to develop airflow obstruction and mucus hypersecretion are needed. At present we have no alternative but to advise the public to stop smoking, for even if we do find ways of selecting individuals who are at risk from airflow obstruction through cigarette smoking there are no grounds for believing that this same group will include those at risk from lung cancer, ischaemic heart disease or peripheral vascular disease.

Physical training in chronic bronchitis

The role that physical rehabilitation may play in the management of chronic bronchitis and emphysema has been extensively studied (Pierce et al., 1964; Paez et al., 1967; De Coster et al., 1972; Holten, 1972; Brunden, 1974) but little attention has been paid to the subject in clinical practice and teaching in Britain. The exercise programmes previously described have used intensive hospital training sessions, but recently a study from Edinburgh has shown that a simple unsupervised exercise programme used at home by patients with chronic bronchitis may enable them to carry out their usual activities with less distress and increase the range of their physical activities (McGavin et al., 1977).

This was a controlled study of 24 patients assessed with tests of ventilatory function, exercise performance on a bicycle ergometer and measurement of their 12-minute walking distance (McGavin et al., 1976). The training programme was graded stair-climbing activity: each of the 12 patients in the active group was asked to climb up and down a given number of steps for a given number of minutes at least once a day for five or more days each week. The most disabled group, unable to walk more than 800 metres in 12 minutes, started with 2 steps up and down for 2 minutes. The less disabled, who on average walked 1200 metres in 12 minutes at the outset, started with 5 steps for 5 minutes. The aim was to reach a daily target of 10 steps for 10 minutes, some of the more disabled patients only reached 10 steps for 5 minutes. All the patients were seen in the outpatient clinic at monthly intervals but the control group were not given exercise instruction. Many of the exercise group spontaneously claimed improvements in general well-being, breathlessness, cough and sputum volume and half of them reported an increase in the range of their general daily activities. There was no significant change in FEV_1 or FVC in either group, but there were significant improvements in work capacity on the bicycle ergometer and 12-minute walking distance in the exercise group compared with the controls. Their improvements were not accompanied by any changes in heart rate at rest or on exercise, nor by any changes in ventilation. The exercise group had significantly lengthened their stride with training. This has previously been reported with exercise programmes and is believed to be due to improved neuromuscular co-ordination (Paez et al., 1967).

McGavin et al. considered that the improvements achieved by their patients were valuable in helping them to achieve more within the limits of their disability, perhaps in part by giving them an increased tolerance for the sensation of dyspnoea. They have set out their exercises in a brief pamphlet which can be obtained from the Chest, Heart and Stroke Association. The ideal patient is one in whom breathlessness has begun to impinge on his daily activities and cause him to seek help. It seems unimportant whether the improvement in exercise performance is due to psychological or physiological effects. Any improvement which can be offered to disabled patients is valuable and this study demonstrates what can be achieved without complex apparatus or admission to hospital. Clearly motivation of the patient and an enthusiastic doctor are necessary, but the method seems ideally suited to use in general practice.

REFERENCES

Brundin A. (1974) Physical training in severe chronic obstructive lung disease. I, Clinical cause, physical work capacity and ventilation. II, Observations on gas exchange. *Scand. J. Respir. Dis.* **55**, 25.

CIBA Guest Sumposium (1959) Terminology, definitions and classification of chronic pulmonary emphysema and related conditions. *Thorax* **14**, 286.

De Coster A., Sergysels R. and Degre S. (1972) La readaptation à l'effort du handicape pulmonaire. *Acta Tuberc. Pneumol. Belg.* **63**, 68.

Doll R. and Hill A. B. (1964) Mortality in relation to smoking: ten years' observations of British doctors. *Br. Med. J.* **1**, 1399.

Doll R. and Peto R. (1976) Mortality in relation to smoking: 20 years' observations on male British doctors. *Br. Med. J.* **2**, 1525.

Fletcher C. M., Elmes P. C., Fairbairn A. S. et al. (1959) The significance of respiratory symptoms and the diagnosis of chronic bronchitis in a working population. *Br. Med. J.* **2**, 257.

Fletcher C. M., Peto R., Tinker C. et al. (1976) The natural history of chronic bronchitis and emphysema. London, Oxford University Press.

Holland W. W. and Reid D. D. (1965) The urban factor in chronic bronchitis. *Lancet* **1**, 445.

Holten K. (1972) Training effect in patients with severe ventilatory failure. *Scand. J. Respir. Dis.* **53,** 65.
McGavin C. R., Gupta S. P., Lloyd E. L. et al. (1977) Physical rehabilitation for the chronic bronchitic: results of a controlled trial of exercises in the home. *Thorax* **32,** 307.
McGavin C. R., McHardy G. J. R. and Lloyd E. L. (1977) *Exercise can help your breathlessness.* London, Chest, Heart and Stroke Association, Leaflet A177.
McGavin C. R., Gupta S. P. and McHardy G. J. R. (1976) Twelve-minute walking test for assessing disability in chronic bronchitis. *Br. Med. J.* **1,** 822.
Macklem P. T. (1972) Obstruction in small airways: a challenge to medicine. *Am. J. Med.* **52,** 721.
Macklem P. T. and Staff Division of United States Heart – Lung Institute (1974) Workshop on screening programme for early diagnosis of airway obstruction. *Am. Rev. Respir. Dis.* **109,** 567.
Medical Research Council (1965) Definition and classification of chronic bronchitis for clinical and epidemiological purposes: a report to the M.R.C. by their committee on the aetiology of chronic bronchitis. *Lancet* **1,** 775.
Medical Research Council (1966) Value of chemoprophylaxis and chemotherapy in chronic bronchitis. A report to the Medical Research Council by their working party on trials of chemotherapy in early chronic bronchitis. *Br. Med. J.* **1,** 1317.
Orie N. G. M., Sluiter H. T., De Vries K. et al. (1961) In: Orie N. G. M. and Sluiter H. J. (ed.), *Proceedings of the International Symposium on Bronchitis, Groningen,* p. 43.
Paez P. N., Phillipson E. A., Masangkay M. et al. (1967) The physiological basis of training patients with emphysema. *Am. Rev. Respir. Dis.* **95,** 944.
Pierce A. K., Taylor H. R., Archer R. K. et al. (1964) Responses to exercise training in patients with emphysema. *Arch. Intern. Med.* **113,** 28.
Reid L. (1954) Pathology of chronic bronchitis. *Lancet* **1,** 275.
Thurlbeck W. M. (1976) *Chronic Airflow Obstruction in Lung Disease.* Major Problems in Pathology Series, Vol. 5. Philadelphia, Saunders.
Van der Lende R. (1969) *Epidemiology of Chronic Non-specific Lung Disease (Chronic Bronchitis).* A critical analysis of three field surveys of CNSLD carried out in the Netherlands. Royal Vangorcum, Assen.

ADULT RESPIRATORY DISTRESS SYNDROME

During the war in Vietnam, medical personnel began to recognize a life-threatening form of progressive hypoxaemia in casualties suffering non-thoracic trauma (Collins et al., 1968). It soon became apparent that this condition could also develop following road traffic accidents and other civilian injuries (Olcott et al., 1971). More recently the list of causes has been extended to include fat and amniotic fluid embolism, septicaemia, acute viral pneumonia, inhaled irritants, blast injuries and cardiopulmonary bypass.

This type of progressive respiratory failure has been variously called 'shock-lung', 'wet lung' or 'congestive atelectasis' but present fashion favours 'adult respiratory distress syndrome' (ARDS). The main clinical features of the syndrome include tachypnoea, low arterial oxygen tension in the face of high inspired oxygen concentrations and diffuse patchy shadows on chest X-ray. Some authors have included all non-cardiogenic causes of pulmonary oedema as examples of ARDS (Solliday et al., 1976) but this may be unacceptable (Murray, 1975)

Characteristically there is a latent period between the injury and the onset of symptoms, although in patients with septicaemic shock the symptoms usually develop rapidly with the onset of circulatory failure. At first there may be few signs but with worsening hypoxaemia tachypnoea, tachycardia and signs of cerebral anoxia develop. Usually there are few abnormal signs in the lungs except in those cases associated with the inhalation of irritants or where local infection develops. The initial chest X-ray may appear normal with fat or amniotic fluid embolism, show diffuse 'fluffy' shadows following trauma or extensive shadowing in cases with viral pneumonia. In all but mild cases the progress of the condition is marked by extensive 'white-out' of the lung fields on serial X-rays.

Much of the details of pathology of ARDS have been gained through lung biopsies (Blaisdell, 1974; Teplitz, 1969) and experimental studies in animals (Hill et al., 1976; Lamy et al., 1976). In addition to interstitial and intra-alveolar oedema perivascular haemorrhage is usual and is sometimes accompanied by bleeding into alveoli. Thrombo-emboli in pulmonary vessels are a common feature and fibrin or fibrinogen hyaline membranes line the affected alveoli. Where the patient survives beyond the first few days fibroblast proliferation and widespread fibrosis usually develop.

Electron microscopy has revealed extensive changes of both type I and II alveolar pneumocytes and disruption of the surfactant layer. Details of pathogenesis of the condition gained from dog experiments may be of questionable relevance to man since in experimental studies in baboons similar lesions did not develop (Buckberg et al., 1971). It is thought that the two major mechanisms involved are spasm of small pulmonary veins and increased permeability of pulmonary capillaries. Both neurogenic and humoral mechanisms may contribute to the changes in the pulmonary veins.

Although pulmonary oedema may occur following cerebral injury (Theodore and Robin, 1975), experimental studies of the effects of cerebral hypoxia in dogs have given conflicting results (Moss et al., 1975; Kusajima, 1974). However, peripheral neural pathways may well be of importance in man for protection from pulmonary oedema by denervation of the lung has been reported (Flick et al., 1975). The humoral factors which may contribute to the development of the syndrome include serotonin released from platelet aggregates or ischaemic tissue, histamine, endotoxins, prostaglandins, lysosomal enzymes and various kinins and vasoactive peptides. It is suggested that such substances may be liberated in excess or inactivated abnormally by the lung following initial injury (Gillis, 1973; Junod, 1976). Whether substances such as serotonin exert their principal effects upon the pulmonary veins or upon the pulmonary arteries is not certain. Other mechanisms suggested for the initiation of lung injury in ARDS include direct damage to pulmonary epithelium by viral pneumonia, inhaled irritants or blast injuries (Freihofer et al., 1974; McCormick, 1975; McCaughey et al., 1973), drowning (Golden and Rivers, 1975) and inflammation caused by fatty acids released from hydrolysis of fat emboli (Parker et al., 1974).

Physiological disturbance

The physiological features of ARDS include reduction of lung compliance and increase of the dead space – tidal volume ratio resulting initially in hyper-ventilation with hypocapnia. There is gross widening of the alveolar-arterial oxygen tension gradient due to 'shunts' within the lungs from a number of causes including non-ventilated alveoli, poorly ventilated but perfused alveoli and in severe cases diffusion defects. The presence of a 'hyperoxic shunt' in which the magnitude of the effective 'shunt' increases as the inspired oxygen concentration is increased has been recognized (Markello et al., 1972); the degree of reversibility of the 'shunt' may be a useful prognostic feature (Lamy et al., 1976).

Treatment

Measures designed to prevent the development of ARDS in cases due to trauma include avoidance of over-transfusion and careful filtration when large volumes of stored blood are used. The role of continuous positive airway pressure (CPAP) in prophylaxis is uncertain. All patients require oxygen enrichment of inspired gases, aiming to give the lowest inspired oxygen concentration that will maintain adequate arterial oxygen tensions. Mechanical ventilation is necessary in most cases and careful attention to ventilator technique is necessary, it has been claimed that the use of maintained positive end-expiratory pressure is particularly helpful (Ashbaugh and Petty, 1973). Where mechanical ventilation fails to maintain adequate respiration extracorporeal membrane oxygenation has been used (Bartlett et al., 1974).

High doses of corticosteroids (e.g. intermittent injections of methyl-prednisolone 30 mg/kg) are generally advocated for treatment in the first 24 – 48 hours (Wilson, 1972), but opinion is divided as to their efficacy and the need for prolonged treatment (Sladen, 1976; Solliday et al., 1976).

Prognosis

Because of the diversity of causes of ARDS and uncertainty about the pathogenic mechanisms involved prognostic criteria are still under evaluation. The ease with which an improvement in arterial oxygen tension is achieved with the various measures available may be helpful in judging the likely outcome (Lamy et al., 1976). Recovery with normal lung function is possible but survivors commonly show a persistent restrictive ventilatory defect (Klein et al., 1976).

REFERENCES

Ashbaugh D. G. and Petty T. L. (1973) Positive end-expiratory pressure: physiology, indications and contraindications. *J. Thorac. Cardiovasc. Surg.* **65,** 165.
Bartlett R. H., Gazzaniga A. B., Fong S. W. et al. (1974) Prolonged extracorporeal cardiopulmonary support in man. *J. Thorac. Cardiovasc. Surg.* **68,** 918.
Buckberg G. D., Lipman C. A., Hahn J. A. et al. (1971) Pulmonary changes following haemorrhagic shock and resuscitation in baboons. *J. Thorac. Cardiovasc. Surg.* **59,** 450.
Collins J. A., Gordon W. C., Hudson T. L. et al. (1968) Inapparent hypoxaemia in casualties with wounded limbs: pulmonary fat embolism? *Ann. Surg.* **167,** 511.
Flick M. R., Kantzler G. B. and Block A. J. (1975) Unilateral pulmonary oedema with contralateral thoracic sympathectomy in the adult respiratory distress syndrome. *Chest* **68,** 736.
Freihofer A. F., Brooks S. M., Loudon R. G. et al. (1974) Functional effects of influenzal pneumonia. *Chest* **66,** Suppl. 36S.
Gillis C. N. (1973) Metabolism of vasoactive hormones by lung. *Anesthesiology* **39,** 626.
Goldon F. St C. and Rivers J. F. (1975) Thoughts on immediate care: the immersion incident. *Anaesthesia* **30,** 364.
Hill J. D., Ratcliff J. L., Parrott J. C. W. et al. (1976) Pulmonary pathology in acute respiratory insufficiency: lung biopsy as a diagnostic tool. *J. Thorac. Cardiovasc. Surg.* **71,** 64.
Junod A. F. (1976) The metabolic activities of pulmonary endothelial cells. *Pneumonologie* **153,** 169.
Klein J. J., Van Haeringen J. R., Sluiter H. J. et al. (1976) Pulmonary function after recovery from the adult respiratory distress syndrome. *Chest* **69,** 350.
Kusajima K., Ozdemir I. A., Webb W. R. et al. (1974) Role of serotonin and serotonin antagonist on pulmonary haemodynamics and microcirculation in haemorrhagic shock. *J. Thorac. Cardiovasc. Surg.* **67,** 908.

Lamy M., Fallat R. J., Koeniger E. et al. (1976) The pathologic features and mechanisms of hypoxaemia in adult respiratory distress syndrome. *Am. Rev. Respir. Dis.* **114**, 2.

McCaughey W., Coppel D. L. and Dundee J. W. (1973) Blast injuries to the lungs: A report of 2 cases. *Anaesthesia* **28**, 2.

McCormick P. W. (1975) Thoughts on immediate care: Immediate care after aspiration of vomit. *Anaesthesia* **30**, 658.

Markello R., Winter P. and Olszowka A. (1972) Assessment of ventilation – perfusion inequalities by arterial-alveolar nitrogen differences in intensive care patients. *Anesthesiology* **37**, 4.

Moss G. S., Newson B. and Das Gupta T. K. (1975) The normal electron histochemistry and the effect of haemorrhagic shock on the pulmonary sinfactant system. *Surg. Gynecol. Obstet.* **140**, 53.

Murray J. F. (1975) The adult respiratory distress syndrome (confessions of a 'lumper'). *Am. Rev. Respir. Dis.* **111**, 713.

Olcott C., Barber R. E. and Blaisdell F. W. (1971) Diagnosis and treatment of respiratory failure after civilian trauma. *Am. J. Surg.* **122**, 260.

Parker F. B., Racz G. B., Wax S. D. et al. (1974) The haemodynamics of experimental fat embolism and associated therapy. *Chest* **65**, Suppl. 545.

Sladen A. (1976) Methylprednisolone: pharmacological doses in shock lung syndrome. *J. Thorac. Cardiovasc. Surg.* **71**, 800.

Solliday N. H., Shapiro B. A. and Gracey D. R. (1976) Adult respiratory distress syndrome: clinical conference in pulmonary disease from North Western University —McGaw Medical Center, Chicago. *Chest* **69**, 207.

Teplitz C. (1969) The ultrastructural basis for pulmonary pathophysiology following trauma: Pathogenesis of pulmonary oedema. *J. Trauma* **8**, 700.

Theodore J. and Robin E. D. (1975) Pathogenesis of neurogenic pulmonary oedema. *Lancet* **2**, 749.

Wilson J. W. (1972) Treatment or prevention of pulmonary cellular damage with pharmacologic doses of corticosteroid. *Surg. Gynecol. Obstet.* **134**, 675.

RHEUMATOID DISEASE AND THE LUNGS

The changes in the lungs and pleura previously recognized in patients with rheumatoid disease including fibrosing alveolitis, necrobiotic nodules, pleural effusions and fibrosis (Ellman and Ball, 1948; Scadding, 1969). Published estimates of pulmonary involvement in rheumatoid disease have varied widely according to the methods of investigation used. With chest X-rays alone the prevalence was reported as 1·6 per cent (Walker and Wright, 1969) but when lung function tests were combined with X-rays almost 47 per cent of patients in one series showed evidence of pulmonary involvement (Franks et al., 1973). Until recently there have been few studies of pulmonary function in patients with rheumatoid disease but the typical findings have comprised a restrictive ventilatory defect with reduced carbon monoxide transfer, without airways obstruction (Franks et al., 1973; Davidson et al., 1974). Significant impairment of carbon monoxide diffusing capacity without airways obstruction has been reported in patients with rheumatoid arthritis with normal chest X-rays (Whorwell et al., 1975).

In one large survey patients with rheumatoid disease showed a higher incidence of bronchitis, bronchiectasis and pneumonia compared to controls with degenerative joint disease (Walker, 1967) and recently rapid development of severe airways obstruction was reported in a non-smoker with rheumatoid arthritis (Murray et al., 1967). A link between antitrypsin deficiency, airways obstruction and rheumatoid arthritis has been suggested (Collins et al., 1976). An excess of patients with the MS phenotype for alpha-1 antitrypsin deficiency was found in 26 of 43 (60·5 per cent) patients showing reduced maximum mid-expiratory flow rates (MMEF) but interpretation of these findings in relationship to rheumatoid disease is complicated because the majority of the patients in the affected group were cigarette smokers. Now a more convincing link between rheumatoid arthritis and progressive airways obliteration has been reported (Geddes et al., 1977). In this study 5 patients with rheumatoid arthritis and a sixth with circulating antinuclear factor without joint disease all developed progressive airway obliteration without symptoms of mucus hypersecretion and only two had been smokers. The presenting complaint in all patients was breathlessness without obvious cause, except in 1 patient in whom symptoms began after an apparent virus infection. Treatment with antibiotics, bronchodilators and corticosteroids was unhelpful and 5 patients died with respiratory failure, 5 – 18 months after the onset of symptoms. On examination all patients had widespread rales and a high pitched inspiratory squeak, best heard during quiet breathing. Lung function tests showed airflow obstruction in all patients, most marked in low lung volumes, with air trapping and poor gas mixing. Where measured, pulmonary compliance and carbon monoxide transfer coefficient (i.e. carbon monoxide transfer corrected for lung volume) were normal. Chest X-rays were 'surprisingly normal'.

At post mortem in 4 patients the major abnormality was fibrous narrowing or obliteration of bronchioles and small bronchi but alveolar ducts and alveoli were unaffected.

There were no granulomatous intraluminal polyps, usually associated with bronchiolitis obliterans. No certain cause for this uncommon form of widespread obliteration of airways was apparent except for the possible virus infection in 1 patient. Auto-immune inflammation was thought to be excluded as none of the patients had antibodies to any airway constituents and direct immunofluorescence of the lungs was negative. Drugs also seemed to be discounted as a cause, and although 3 of the patients had been treated with penicillamine before developing symptoms of lung disease the changes were identical in the other patients who had not received this drug. The authors suggested that the airways of patients with rheumatoid disease may react abnormally to inflammation after viral or unrecognized chemical bronchiolitis and cited abnormalities of T-cell function which have been identified in patients with rheumatoid arthritis as a possible contributory defect where virus infections are involved (Maini et al., 1975).

REFERENCES

Collins R. L., Turner R. A., Johnson A. M. et al. (1976). Obstructive pulmonary disease in rheumatoid arthritis. *Arthritis Rheum.* **19**, 623.
Davidson C., Brooks A. F. G. and Bacon P. A. (1974) Lung function in rheumatoid arthritis: A clinic survey. *Ann. Rheum. Dis.* **33**, 293.
Ellman P. and Ball R. E. (1948) Rheumatoid disease with joint and pulmonary manifestations. *Br. Med. J.* **2**, 816.
Frank S. T., Weg J. G., Harkleroad L. E. et al. (1973). Pulmonary dysfunction in rheumatoid disease. *Chest* **63**, 27.
Geddes D. M., Corrin B., Brewerton D. A. et al. (1977) Progressive airway obliteration in adults and its association with rheumatoid disease. *Q. J. Med.* **46**, 427.
Maini R. N., Scott J. T., Roffe L. et al. (1975) *Infection and Immunity.* Oxford, Blackwells, p. 579.
Scadding J. G. (1969) The lungs in rheumatoid arthritis. *Proc. R. Soc. Med.* **62**, 227.
Walker W. C. (1967) Pulmonary infections and rheumatoid arthritis. *Q. J. Med.* **36**, 239.

Walker W. C. and Wright V. (1969) Diffuse interstitial pulmonary fibrosis and rheumatoid arthritis. *Ann. Rheum. Dis.* **28,** 252.
Whorwell P. J., Wojtulewski J. A. and Lacey B. W. (1975) Respiratory function in rheumatoid arthritis. *Br. Med. J.* **2,** 175.

Surgical
RICHARD E. LEA FRCS

BULLOUS EMPHYSEMA

The value of surgical treatment in bullous emphysema is equivocal (Billig, 1968). The usual problem is that a patient undergoing investigation of dyspnoea is found to have emphysematous bullae. In these patients other lung disease is usually present and the difficulty is deciding whether the bullae are a major contributory factor in the shortness of breath.

In an attempt to resolve the problem a variety of tests has been advocated, from simple spirometry to angiography, bronchography, radioactive perfusion and ventilation scans and bronchospirometry. In spite of the variety of tests, many surgeons have found that subjective improvement did not correlate at all well with objective changes in pulmonary function. This discrepancy as Wesley (1972) explains is probably due to two factors. Firstly, any patient with chronic obstructive airways disease is likely to benefit subjectively from any intense medical treatment. Secondly, in many cases the period of follow-up has been too short so that the long term effect of operation on the disease process cannot be studied. In spite of the difficulties it has been shown that improvement can occur in all patients with moderate to severe symptoms provided the bullae occupy more than 30 per cent of a hemithorax (Forman et al., 1968; Boushy et al., 1969; Pride et al., 1970).

In selecting patients the greater the dyspnoea the greater the risks of operation. Nevertheless, it is in the most severely disabled patient (as Sung (1973) states) that the most dramatic improvement can be obtained. This is also seen in a case report by Harris (1976) in which a patient had both hypoxaemia and hypercapnia at rest.

The most important factor in all these patients is the state of the remaining lung. If there is a significant amount of compressed parenchyma available for re-expansion after the cyst is removed the patient is very likely to benefit by surgical treatment. It is important to differentiate between a bullous cyst causing lung compression and vanishing lung where the lung is destroyed (Richards, 1956). Although chest radiography including tomography can help in deciding whether lung compression is present it is not wholly satisfactory. Some authors have used lung perfusion scanning (Wesley, 1972; Parker, 1974), whereas others have preferred pulmonary angiography (Fitzgerald et al., 1974; Harris, 1976). If by either of these two methods crowding of the pulmonary vessels is demonstrated ablation of the cyst is likely to result in improvement of pulmonary function.

It is suggested by Wesley (1972) that the following criteria should be used in selecting the patients most likely to benefit from bullectomy.

1. The patient should have symptomatic and progressive dyspnoea.
2. The disease should be severe but localized, the bullae occupying 25 per cent or more of one hemithorax.

3. There should be radiological evidence of compressed lung tissue that can be re-expanded by removal of the bulla.
4. There should be evidence of regional imbalance with poor perfusion on the side of the lesion and relatively good perfusion in the contralateral side.
5. There should be a minimal inflammatory component of the disease process. Patients without marked cough and sputum production have the best postoperative response.

If these critera are followed and each patient has a full assessment of his pulmonary function both preoperatively and postoperatively then the confusion surrounding the value of surgery in bullous emphysema should disappear. It is essential that the postoperative assessment should continue over a number of years so that the natural progression of the disease can be observed.

REFERENCES

Billig D. M., Boushy S. F. and Kohen R. (1968) Surgical treatment of bullous emphysema. *Arch. Surg.* **97**, 744.
Boushy S. F., Billig D. M. and Kohen R. (1969) Changes in pulmonary function after bullectomy. *Am. J. Med.* **47**, 916.
Fitzgerald M. X., Keelan P. J., Cugwell D. W. et al. (1974) Long term results of surgery for bullous emphysema. *J. Thorac. Cardiovasc. Surg.* **68**, 757.
Foreman S., Weil H., Duke R. et al. (1968) Bullous disease of the lung: physiologic improvement after surgery. *Ann. Intern. Med.* **69**, 757.
Harris J. (1976) Severe bullous emphysema. *Chest* **70**, 658.
Parker F. P. (1974) Surgery in chronic lung disease. *Surg. Clin. North Am.* **54**, 1193.
Pride N. B., Hugh-Jones P., O'Brien E. N. et al. (1970) Changes in lung function following the surgical treatment of bullous emphysema. *Q. J. Med.* **39**, 49.
Richards D. W. (1956) The aging lung. *Bull. N.Y. Acad. Med.* **32**, 407.
Sung D. T., Payne S. and Black L. F. (1973) Surgical management of giant bullae associated with obstructive airways disease. *Surg. Clin. North Am.* **53**, 913.
Wesley J. R., Macleod W. M. and Mullard K. S. (1972) Evaluation and surgery of bullous emphysema. *J. Thorac. Cardiovasc. Surg.* **63**, 945.

MULTI-ORGAN SCANNING IN CARCINOMA OF THE BRONCHUS

The clinicians armamentarium is continually being expanded by modern technology, providing new methods of investigation. Many of these new methods require expensive apparatus and complex laboratory facilities, plus human expertise. All too often these tests become accepted as normal methods of investigation before their value has been assessed. This ready acceptance of unproved methods frequently leads to unjustified expense. At this time of financial restraint it is more than ever important that expensive and complex tests be carefully evaluated in terms of cost and effectiveness before being used routinely. One such example is isotope scanning of organs to identify unsuspected metastases. It is obviously sensible to exclude surgical treatment in any patient who has metastases from a carcinoma. Isotope scanning of organs, especially liver, brain, bone and lung, has been used as a method of screening in many centres. The value of the technique depends not only upon its accuracy in identifying distant metastases, but also in not producing false positives. A false positive would mean a patient being excluded from a chance of curative treatment.

The use of multi-organ scanning in lung cancer has recently been examined by Ramsdell et al. (1977) in 100 consecutive patients thought to have potentially resectable carcinoma of the bronchus. The study was to compare the accuracy of clinical assessment, including standard blood tests, against multi-organ scanning. The organs studied were liver, brain and bone. Of the 100 patients 47 were rejected as in these there was no histological proof of the diagnosis.

Liver scans

All patients with metastatic carcinoma of the liver and positive liver scans had clinical abnormalities. There were at least two false negatives, that is the scan failed to identify metastases. Three scans were falsely positive, that is the scanning suggested metastases but these were never subsequently confirmed.

Brain scans

In only 1 patient was there disagreement between a scan and clinical examination. In this patient a normal scan was associated with abnormal clinical signs. During the following month the neurological signs resolved. In no case was an unsuspected brain deposit diagnosed by brain scanning.

Bone scans

Assessment was rather more difficult in this investigation. Bone scanning and clinical evaluation agreed in 75 per cent. Of the negative scans all were truly negative. There were 23 patients with a positive scan, 13 of these being false positives. Only in 1 patient who had no clinical signs was unsuspected metastases identified.

In the 153 scans agreement between clinical signs and scanning was present in 128. Thus there were 25 scans that did not agree with the clinical findings. Of these there were two false negative scans and 16 false positives. In only 1 patient was an unsuspected secondary deposit found. In the 14 who had abnormal clinical signs a scan confirmed the presence of metastases.

It is apparent from this paper that multi-organ scanning is extremely useful in confirming clinical evidence of lung metastases to either the liver, brain or bone. When there is no clinical evidence the yield of unsuspected metastases is very low (0·7 per cent) and complicated by the high rate of false positives. It may well be that the latter could be reduced by better experience in the methods used. Nevertheless, the poor return in truly positive scans suggests that the routine use of multi-organ scanning in the absence of clinical signs is not justified. This does not mean a total abandonment but further research into increasing sensitivity and finding new methods of scanning for tumour metastases.

REFERENCE
Ramsdell J. W., Peters R. M., Taylor A. T. et al. (1977) Multi-organ scans for staging lung cancer: Correlation with clinical evidence. *J. Thorac. Cardiovasc. Surg.* **73**, 653.

THE MANAGEMENT OF PULMONARY METASTASES

The postoperative development of pulmonary metastases is often regarded as evidence of widespread dissemination of a malignant lesion. Although it is true that many patients subsequently show a rapid decline this is not always the case. Less well recognized is that the patient may die as a result of pulmonary metastases but not have other foci of disease Farrell (1935). There is undoubtedly a place for considering surgical resection if it can be shown that metastases are confined to the lungs. The type of case that might benefit is well described in an article by Holmes et al. (1977). In his article he examines the criteria for evaluation of patients with pulmonary metastatic disease. The first step in any patient who has pulmonary metastases after previous successful surgery is to exclude metastases elsewhere. There is no point in considering operation if the metastases are not confined to the lungs. In the past it has been suggested that operation should be considered only if there is a solitary pulmonary lesion. This, according to Holmes, is not necessary and patients with multiple or bilateral lung involvement should be considered.

The histology of the primary tumour is helpful in deciding whether the metastases are confined to the lungs. Certain tumours have a propensity to metastasize to lungs: they include osteogenic sarcoma, fibrosarcoma and the mesenchymal sarcomas. In contrast carcinomas such as breast, colon and stomach frequently metastasize to other organs before becoming widely disseminated and involving the lungs. Occasionally even in these patients the lung is the first site of metastasis and each case should be decided on its own merits.

The most important concept in deciding on surgical removal is the tumour doubling time (TDT): this is the time interval in days which it takes the tumour to double in size. A method was described by Collins et al. (1971) of measuring the TDT. The first 30 doublings in the life of a tumour produce a lesion 1 cm in diameter containing 109 cells with a mass of 1g.

A further 10 doublings increase the cells to 1012 with a mass of 1 kg and bring the patient to the termination of this disease. Assuming a constant growth rate some idea can be given on the course of the disease in that patient.

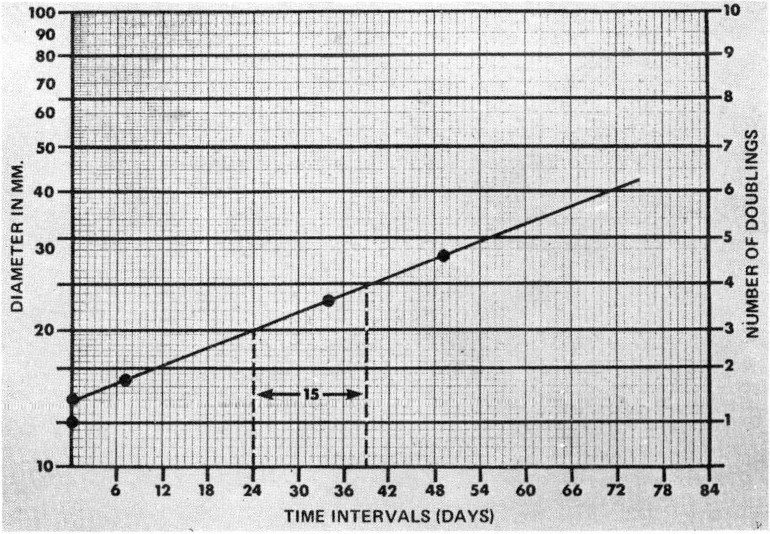

Fig. 1. Method of plotting TDT based on the direct measurement of the changing diameters of metastatic pulmonary nodules. (Reproduced from the *Journal of Thoracic and Cardiovascular Surgery.)*

The method of measuring the doubling time involves taking three chest X-rays at 2-weekly intervals, measuring the diameter and plotting the result on semi-logarithmic paper. The slope of the graph between two points represents the rate of tumour growth (*Fig.* 1).

The prognosis in relation to TDT was examined by Joseph et al. (1971). They found that there was good correlation between TDT and survival. The patients were divided into three groups: tumour with TDT less than 20 days, 20 – 40 days and TDT greater than 40 days, those patients with the larger TDT having the best prognosis. In those with a TDT greater than 40 days the 5-year survival was 63 per cent. In contrast, those with a TDT less than 20 days did not benefit by surgery. In a number of long term survivors bilateral thoracotomy as a stage procedure had been done. Conclusions to be drawn are that patients with pulmonary metastases should be considered for surgical treatment provided that: (1) The primary disease is controlled; (2) There is no evidence of metastases to other organs; (3) The TDT is greater than 40 days.

In patients with a TDT of less than 40 days surgical removal of metastases is not likely to benefit the prognosis. Holmes and his colleagues have combined removal with cytotoxic chemotherapy, but rightly state that it is highly experimental treatment and should be confined to centres with facilities for close supervision.

REFERENCES

Collins V. P., Morton D. L. and Adkins P. C. (1971) Variation in tumour doubling time in patients with pulmonary metastatic disease. *J. Surg. Oncol.* **3**, 143.

Farrell J. T. (1935) Pulmonary metastases: a pathologic, clinical roentgenologic study based on 78 cases seen at necropsy. *Radiology* **24**, 144.

Holmes E. C., Ramming K. P., Eilber F. R. et al. (1977) The surgical management of pulmonary metastases. *Semin. Oncol.* **4**, 65.

Joseph W. L., Morton D. L. and Adkins P. C. (1971) Prognostic significance of tumour doubling time in evaluating operability in pulmonary metastatic disease. *J. Thorac. Cardiovasc. Surg.* **61**, 23.

CHRONIC RHEUMATIC DISEASES

J. D. JESSOP MD, FRCPI, MRCP
and G. NUKI MRCP

OSTEOARTHROSIS

Degenerative joint disease remains the commonest form of arthritis amongst patients consulting their family doctor, attending rheumatology clinics or losing time from work in industry. Epidemiological studies over many years by Lawrence, and recent figures published by the Arthritis and Rheumatism Council in World Rheumatism Year (1977) indicate that about twenty million people in the U.K. have radiological evidence of osteoarthrosis (OA), of whom approximately 25 per cent may be expected to have symptoms. An appreciation of the magnitude of the problem coupled with advances in relevant basic sciences, such as connective tissue biochemistry and bio-engineering, has recently helped to focus the attention of research workers in many disciplines on underlying mechanisms which may be responsible for the development of OA in man and animals. A great deal of new knowledge has been amassed and concepts of the disease process are changing constantly, but the initial course or courses of this variety of joint failure remain uncertain. The aetiopathogenesis of OA was the subject of a small multidisciplinary International Symposium at the Welsh National School of Medicine in Cardiff in May 1977, and this review briefly summarizes the work presented.

Because the incidence of OA increases with age it has been common clinical practice to dismiss it as merely being related to the inevitable effects of 'wear and tear' on joints. Yet although hyaline articular cartilage does undergo changes with age, it is only in a relatively small percentage of cases that these changes progress to symptomatic idiopathic OA. Sokoloff (Stony Brook) underlined the difficulties of defining the precise starting point of OA by analysis of histopathological material, because of variations from the norm which appear early in multiple cartilage sites. He suggested that the dividing line between 'non-progressive age changes' and clinically significant OA was related to breaches of the osteoarticular junction. These led to subchondral cyst formation and microfractures in the articular cortex. Meachim (Liverpool) confirmed the wide variety of histological changes that may be found in operative specimens of articular cartilage. Deep splitting and fibrillation, abrasive wear and shearing damage as well as remodelling of subchondral bone can all precede the full-thickness cartilage loss and eburnation of exposed bone seen in late stage OA. Gardner (Manchester) emphasized the lack of information available on the variations of normal articular cartilage with such factors as age, sex and weight. A systematic study of postmortem femoral head cartilage revealed significant increases in articular cartilage thickness between the ages of 20 – 45 years in areas of the femoral head not typically the site of OA. The increase in thickness appeared to be an age response to normal mechanical stresses and strains and was accompanied by increases in compliance without predisposing to degenerative change and fibrillation.

Ehrlich (Boston) reviewed the biochemical changes observed in articular cartilage in OA. Early changes which are generally agreed include increases in water content and depletion of the proteoglycan matrix. The Boston work suggests that these changes are accompanied by increases in proteoglycan synthesis with reversion to a more primitive kind of cartilage matrix containing more chondroitin and less keratan sulphate. The increase in synthesis is proportional to the severity of the disease but a point of failure is ultimately reached when degradation by lysosomal enzymes and neutral proteoglycanases outstrips the process of cartilage repair. Although overall collagen content remains unchanged, their data suggest similar increases in collagen synthesis to a point of failure when collagenase digestion overcomes the repair potential of the chondrocytes. Other workers, however, challenged the biochemical data suggesting increased macromolecular synthesis. Maroudas (London) found no significant increase in sulphate uptake or glycosaminoglycan turnover in osteoarthrotic articular cartilage from the human femoral head, and Lust (Cornell) found that neither glycosaminoglycan nor collagen turnover were increased in degenerative articular cartilage from dogs prone to OA of the hips. His data suggested dramatic increases in the procollagen precursor content of degenerating cartilage.

Maroudas' work related the increased hydration of articular cartilage to the severity of histological damage, and was consistent with the concept of damage to the collagen network resulting in its failure to restrain the 'swelling pressure' of the proteoglycans. This fits well with the hypothesis of Freeman (London), who suggests that OA results from mechanical fragmentation of cartilage as a consequence of high contact pressures in joints and fatigue failure of the cartilage fibre network. Radin (Boston), on the other hand, believes that osteoarthrosis should be regarded as resulting from a proliferative rather than a degenerative response to biomechanical injury. Excessive stress from repetitive impulse loading leads to microfractures and stiffening of the subchondral bone, which he believes precede degeneration of the articular cartilage.

In order to examine the initial biochemical events in mechanically induced OA McDevitt and Muir (London) have studied an experimental model in the dog which closely simulates naturally occurring canine OA. Progressive histological changes indistinguishable from spontaneous OA follow cutting the anterior cruciate ligament of the knee which results in instability of the joint. Biochemical changes can be detected in articular cartilage long before histological lesions develop. The earliest changes include increases in water content and the extractability of proteoglycans and imply that profound alterations in cartilage metabolism precede the development of frank osteo-arthrosis. Clearly there are potential therapeutic implications if further research can show that these changes are reversible.

The importance of studying the human 'models' of osteoarthrosis provided by rare inborn errors of metabolism such as the mucopolysaccharidoses and alkaptonuria which may lead to degenerative joint disease was stressed by Harper (Cardiff) who reviewed the role of genetic factors. Studies of skeletal dysplasias emphasize dramatically how abnormal congruence of joints as well as trauma and joint instability can predispose to OA with very obvious orthopaedic implications for possible prevention. Moreover, it was of considerable interest to note that hip dysplasia and OA in dogs could be prevented by restricting food intake and weight gain during development (Lust, Cornell).

The term 'osteoarthrosis' implies that the primary pathological change in articular cartilage is degenerative, while osteoarthritis suggests inflammation. Dieppe (London) stressed how many clinical features of OA suggested an inflammatory component. An acute polyarticular onset with early morning stiffness and 'hot' Heberden's nodes are all reminiscent of inflammatory joint disease, as is the response to non-steroidal anti-inflammatory agents. The frequency of these inflammatory features was shown in a study of 100 consecutive cases. Of the 74 with knee involvement 54 (73 per cent) had effusions. In addition to the typical radiological features of OA, chondro-calcinosis was found in 4 patients, and other areas of abnormal calcification in and around joints were common. Samples of synovial fluid were examined from 34 patients. Calcium pyrophosphate dihydrate crystals were detected in 6 cases and hydroxyapatite nodules, frequently intracellular, in 9. Dieppe feels that crystal-induced inflammation from a variety of types of calcium phosphate mineral may be important in the pathogenesis of OA and suggests that crystals of apatite in particular, too small to be detected by polarizing light microscopy, but identifiable by scanning electron microscopy and energy dispersive elemental microanalysis, may be implicated. Some support for this hypothesis came from the work of Ali (London) who has found electron microscopic evidence of apatite-forming matrix vesicles in the mid zone of osteoarthrotic articular cartilage. These he feels may be both a source of the joint fluid crystals and the focus for the remodelling changes seen in calcified cartilage near the subchondral bone. Abnormalities of mineral metabolism were also suggested by Howell (Miami) who has shown pyrophosphate extrusion from osteoarthrotic articular cartilage *in vitro* as well as high concentrations of inorganic pyrophosphate in OA synovial fluids *in vivo*.

An immunological basis for cartilage damage in primary generalized OA was suggested by Cooke (Kingston, Canada), who found evidence for immune complexes containing immunoglobulins and complement components in immunofluorescence studies of articular cartilage biopsies. Complexes were detected in 51 per cent of 85 patients with idiopathic OA compared with 16 per cent of 32 patients with secondary OA and 92 per cent of 97 patients with rheumatoid arthritis. Histological examination of synovial tissue in the OA patients revealed lymphocytes and plasma cells consistent with local immune reactivity. A possible role for synovial membrane in the pathogenesis of OA was suggested by experiments of Jubb and Fell (Cambridge), who showed that synovial tissue can induce biochemical and histological changes in articular cartilage, in organ culture, which resemble some of the early changes in OA. Lest physicians might think that the answer to OA lies simply in the administration of anti-inflammatory drugs, it is salutary to note that Kalbhen (Bonn) was apparently able to induce severe degenerative changes in the articular cartilage of chickens following single intra-articular injections of near therapeutic concentrations of a number of non-steroidal anti-inflammatory agents.

Recent work on the aetiopathogenesis of OA suggests that degenerative joint disease can result from an interaction of a wide variety of genetic, biomechanical, biochemical and inflammatory factors. The realization that OA is not simply an inevitable consequence of ageing and 'wear and tear' of joints holds out hope for the possibility of preventive measures in the future.

REFERENCES

Nuki G. (ed.), *Aetiopathogenesis of Osteoarthrosis*. London, Pitman. In the press.

Ali S. Y. Mineral-containing matrix vesicles in human osteoarthrotic cartilage.
Cooke T. D. V., Bennett E. L. and Ohno O. Identification of immunoglobulins and complement components in articular collagenous tissues of patients with idiopathic OA.
Dieppe P. A., Huskisson E. C. and Willoughby D. A. The inflammatory component of OA.
Ehrlich M. G. and Mankin H. J. Biochemical changes in OA.
Freeman M. A. R. The pathogenesis of idiopthic ('primary') OA. An hypothesis.
Gardner D. L., Elliott R. J., Armstrong C. G. and Longmore R. B. The relationship between age, thickness, surface structure, compliance and composition of human femoral head articular cartilage.
Harper P. and Nuki G. Genetic factors in OA.
Howell D. S. Osteoarthritis: speculations on some biochemical factors of possible aetiological nature including cartilage mineralisation.
Jubb R. W. and Fell H. B. Changes resembling OA induced by the used culture medium of synovium in organ culture.
Kalbhen D. A. Drug-induced biochemical changes in cartilage metabolism: a new aspect of the aetiopathogenesis of osteoarthrosis.
Lust G. and Miller D. R. Biochemical changes in canine osteoarthrosis.
McDevitt C., Muir H. and Eyre D. Macromolecular biochemistry of cartilage in the initial stages of experimental canine osteoarthrosis.
Maroudas A. and Venn M. F. Biochemical and physico-chemical studies on osteoarthrotic cartilage from the human femoral head.
Meachim G. Ways of cartilage breakdown in human and experimental osteoarthrosis.
Radin E. L., Paul I. L. and Rose R. M. Osteoarthrosis as a final common pathway.
Sokoloff L. Ageing.

Lawrence J. S. (1977) *Rheumatism in Populations*. London, Heinemann.

SEXUALLY TRANSMITTED DISEASES

R. N. T. THIN MD, FRCP(Edin)

In his report for 1975, the Chief Medical Officer to the Department of Health and Social Security (1976) noted that more clinics for the treatment of Sexually Transmitted Diseases (STDs) had been re-named 'Departments of Genito-Urinary Medicine'. This had proved acceptable and may have been one reason for the improved recruitment of doctors to the specialty.

The report contained the numbers of cases seen in the clinics in England during the first six months of 1975 and compared them with the first six months of 1974. Figures for the second half of 1975 will appear in the next report. There was a slight fall in the numbers of fresh cases of syphilis and gonorrhoea but this was insufficient to warrant any relaxation of control measures. In contrast, the incidence of the other STDs had risen.

One important feature of the past year was several reports of penicillinase-producing isolates of gonococci. These will be described in the section on gonorrhoea.

An Editorial (1976) discussed the increased incidence of pelvic infection among women fitted with an intra-uterine contraceptive device (IUCD); pelvic infection seems to be four to five times more likely in these women than in other women. According to Westrom et al. (1976), at Lund, in Sweden, women who had never been pregnant and had an IUCD had seven times the risk of pelvic infection than other women. Pelvic infection appears more common among the socially disadvantaged and there is a case for taking a culture for gonococci from such women before inserting a device. Westrom et al. (1976) also suggested that there is a lower incidence of pelvic infection among women taking oral contraceptives.

Harnisch et al. (1977) studied 24 patients in Seattle, U.S.A., with acute epididymitis. They concluded that, in young men, the sexually transmitted organisms that cause urethritis, *Neisseria gonorrhoeae*, *Chlamydia trachomatis* and possibly *Ureaplasma urealyticum,* may also lead to acute epididymitis, but in older men Coliform and *Pseudomonas* organisms predominate.

REFERENCES

D.H.S.S. (1976) *On the State of the Public Health. The Annual Report of the Chief Medical Officer of the Department of Health and Social Security for the Year 1975.* London H.M.S.O., p. 47.
Editorial (1976) Risk of pelvic infection associated with intra-uterine devices. *Br. Med. J.* **3,** 717.
Harnisch J. P., Berger R. E., Alexander E. R. et al. (1977) Aetiology of acute epididymitis. *Lancet* **1,** 819.
Westrom L., Bengtsson L. P. and Märdh P. A. (1976) The risk of pelvic inflammatory disease in women using inter-uterine contraceptive devices as compared to non-users. *Lancet* **2,** 221.

SYPHILIS

An Editorial (1977) discussed the Jarisch-Herxheimer Reaction which may occur a few hours after starting therapy for syphilis. This reaction is more common in early than in late syphilis. There is fever and worsening of lesions due to cellular infiltration. The four phases of the reaction, prodrome, chill, flush, and defervescence, are typical of endotoxin-induced fever and recent studies suggest the presence of endotoxin which may depress complement. The Editorial (1977) noted the possibility of death occurring during the reaction in patients with localized late lesions of larynx, brain and the root of the aorta, and that the value of steroids in suppressing the reaction is not proved.

Grabau and his colleagues (1976) published an appraisal of their surgical treatment of syphilitic aortic regurgitation in London. They interpreted the high mortality as indicating a need for earlier surgical referral.

REFERENCES

Editorial (1977) The Jarisch-Herxheimer reaction. *Lancet* **1**, 340.
Grabau W., Emmanuel R., Ross D. et al. (1976) Syphilitic aortic regurgitation: an appraisal of surgical treatment. *Br. J. Vener. Dis.* **52**, 366.

GONORRHOEA

As already mentioned, a most important feature of the past year was the appearance of penicillinase-producing isolates of *Neisseria gonorrhoeae*. Previously, isolates only partly resistant to penicillin have been reported and this is due to chromosomal changes (McCormick, 1977). Three separate mutations are involved and at least one of these appears to change the cell wall so that it is less permeable to many antimicrobial agents in addition to penicillin; this explains why isolates partly resistant to penicillin may be partly resistant to other antibiotics. Penicillinase production, in contrast, is mediated by extra chromosomal DNA, called plasmid or R factor, and appears to be unrelated to resistance to other antibiotics.

The first penicillinase-producing gonococcus was reported from London by Phillips (1976). Similar strains were isolated elsewhere in London (Wilkinson et al., 1976), and in Liverpool, where 45 isolates were found in 1976 (Percival et al., 1976). By April 1977, 123 isolates had been reported in 19 states in the U.S.A. (McCormick, 1977). Such isolates have also been identified in Australia, Canada, the Ivory Coast, Japan, Netherlands, New Zealand, Norway, Phillipines, Republic of Korea, Singapore and South Africa, while epidemiological information suggests that infected patients have been present in Belgium, Ghana, Hong Kong, Oman and Thailand (World Health Organisation, 1976; Hallet et al., 1977; Piot, 1977).

The number of isolates showing this characteristic remains small in relation to the increasing numbers of fresh infections which continue to occur throughout the world. Penicillin remains the drug of first choice in the treatment of gonorrhoea in Britain and other countries where the prevalence of penicillinase-producing strains is low. However, follow-up examination after treatment is now more important than before, and if relapse occurs then it would be wise to change to another drug. The strains isolated in London are completely resistant to streptomycin but are sensitive to co-trimoxazole, kanamycin, spectinomycin and tetracycline (Editorial, 1976). Strains partly resistant to penicillin and other drugs are usually sensitive to spectinomycin, so when relapse occurs after penicillin, spectinomycin in a single dose of 2 or 4g intramuscularly is a useful, although expensive, alternative. Antibiotic sensitivity should be determined when relapse occurs and it is desirable to send isolates suspected of producing penicillinase to the appropriate reference laboratory. Vigorous contact tracing must also be carried out to minimize the spread of penicillinase-producing organisms.

Further important studies have been conducted on strains of gonococci causing disseminated gonococcal infection (DGI). Schoolnik et al. (1977), at Seattle, U.S.A., have shown that most gonococcal isolates from patients with DGI are resistant to the complement-dependent bactericidal action of human serum.

REFERENCES

Editorial (1976) Penicillinase-producing gonococci. *Lancet* **2**, 725.

Hallet A. F., Appelbaum P. C., Cooper R., Mokgokong S. and Monale D. (1977) Penicillinase-producing *Neisseria gonorrhoeae* from South Africa. *Lancet* **1**, 1205.

McCormick W. M. (1977) Treatment of gonorrhoea—is penicillin passé. *N. Engl. J. Med.* **296**, 934.

Percival A., Rowlands J., Corkill J. E. et al. (1976) Penicillinase-producing gonococci in Liverpool. *Lancet* **2**, 1379.

Phillips I. (1976) β-Lactamase producing penicillin resistant gonococcus. *Lancet* **2**, 656.

Piot P. (1977) Resistant gonococcus from the Ivory Coast. *Lancet* **1**, 857.

Schoolnik G. K., Buchanan T. M. and Holmes K. K. (1976) Gonococci causing disseminated gonococcal infections are resistant to the bactericidal action of normal human sera. *J. Clin. Invest.* **58**, 1163.

Wilkinson A. E., Seth A. D. and Rodin P. (1976) Infection with penicillinase-producing gonococcus. *Lancet* **2**, 1233.

World Health Organisation Weekly Epidemiological Record (1976) *Neisseria gonorrhoeae* producing β-Lactamase (penicillinase), vol. 51, 385.

NON-SPECIFIC GENITAL INFECTION

Study of *Chlamydia trachomatis* continued during the past year. Alani et al. (1977) reported *C.trachomatis* in 30 per cent of 385 men with non-gonococcal urethritis attending an STD clinic in London. The highest isolation rate of 68 per cent was in a selected group of men with a frank urethral discharge. This is a higher yield than previously reported and is similar to *C.trachomatis* isolation rates among patients with severe trachoma in hyper-endemic areas. The organism was isolated from only 3 per cent of 61 men without urethritis. 108 female contacts of the men were studied and significantly more pairs of sexual partners had the same chlamydial culture result than had different results. Isolation was more frequent among men admitting a casual sexual contact than in men claiming only regular partnerships.

Woolfitt and Watt (1977) isolated *C.trachomatis* from 26 per cent of 200 female patients attending an STD clinic in Manchester but from only 1 per cent of 200 female members of hospital staff. Märdh et al. (1977), at Lund in Sweden, described a study indicating that *C.trachomatis* is a common cause of acute pelvic infection.

Vaughan-Jackson et al. (1977) studied 49 men in London who developed non-gonococcal urethritis (post-gonococcal urethritis or PGU) after treatment for gonorrhoea. *C.trachomatis* was isolated from significantly more of them (53 per cent) than from those who did not develop PGU. This was interpreted as showing that *C.trachomatis* is a pathogen in the urethra. Results of cultures for *Ureaplasma urealyticum* (formerly called *T.mycoplasma,* see *Medical Annual* 1976, page 359) and *Mycoplasma hominis* indicated that these organisms are not pathogenic in the urethra. Piot (1976), in Antwerp, Belgium, also reported insignificant differences in the isolation of ureaplasmas from cases of gonorrhoea, non-gonococcal urethritis and controls; the distribution of serotypes was similar in the three groups. In contrast, Bowie et al. (1976), at Seattle, U.S.A., reported that ureaplasmas had a causative role in some cases of NGU, and this is supported by a human inoculation experiment described by Taylor-Robinson et al. (1977). Thus evidence for *C.trachomatis* as a cause of non-gonococcal urethritis is accumulating, but the role of ureaplasmas requires further evaluation.

Recent evidence indicates that *C.trachomatis* may cause respiratory infection in young infants and in one case the organism may have been acquired from the mother (Editorial, 1977).

REFERENCES
Alani M. D., Darougar S., Burns D. C. M. et al. (1977) Isolation of *Chlamydia trachomatis* from the male urethra. *Br. J. Vener. Dis.* **53**, 88.
Bowie W. R., Alexander E. R., Floyd J. F. et al. (1976) Differential response of chlamydial and ureaplasma-associated urethritis to sulphafurazole (sulfisoxazole) and amino-cyclitols. *Lancet* **2**, 1276.
Editorial (1977) *Chlamydia trachomatis* and the respiratory tract. *Lancet* **1**, 787.
Märdh P. A., Ripa T., Svensson L. et al. (1977) *Chlamydia trachomatis* infection in patients with acute salpingitis. *N. Engl. J. Med.* **296**, 1377.
Piot P. (1976) Distribution of eight serotypes of *Ureaplasma urealyticum* in cases of non-gonococcal urethritis, gonorrhoea and in healthy persons. *Br. J. Vener. Dis.* **52**, 266.
Taylor-Robinson D., Csonka G. W. and Prentice M. J. (1977) Human intraurethral inoculation of ureaplasmas. *Q. J. Med.* **66**, 309.
Vaughan-Jackson J. D., Dunlop E. M. C., Darougar S. et al. (1977) Urethritis due to *Chlamydia trachomatis*. *Br. J. Vener. Dis.* **53**, 180.
Woolfitt J. M. G. and Watt L. (1977) Chlamydial infection of the urogenital tract in promiscuous and non-promiscuous women. *Br. J. Vener. Dis.* **53**, 93.

VULVOVAGINAL CANDIDOSIS

Interest in vaginal candidosis continues. Hurley (1977), at a symposium in London, indicated that *Candida albicans* is not part of the normal vaginal flora and that its presence indicates morbidity. However, it is not clear how often genital *C.albicans* is sexually transmitted, and using a computer-based bank of data from an STD clinic in London, Thin et al. (1977) suggested that this was so in 39 per cent of women and 29 per cent of men. STDs frequently occur together and the discovery of genital yeasts should prompt a search for other STDs.

REFERENCES
Hurley R. (1977) Candidal vaginitis. *Proc. R. Soc. Med.* **70**, Suppl. No. 4, p. 1.
Thin R. N., Leighton M. and Dixon M. J. (1977) How often is genital yeast infection sexually transmitted? *Br. Med. J.* **3**, 93.

SEXUAL TRANSMISSION OF ENTERIC ORGANISMS

There have been several reports of the sexual transmission of organisms normally only affecting the bowel; these reports have mainly concerned homosexuals. Drusin et al. (1976) described epidemiological evidence for sexual transmission of shigellosis in New York, U.S.A.; Meyers et al. (1977) described a cluster of cases of sexually transmitted giardiasis in Seattle, U.S.A.; Dritz and Braff (1977) and Dritz et al. (1977) drew attention to the sexual transmission of shigellosis, amoebiasis, hepatitis A and B, and enteric fever, in San Francisco, U.S.A.

REFERENCES

Dritz S. K., Ainsworth T. E., Garrard W. F. et al. (1977) Patterns of sexually transmitted disease in a city. *Lancet* **2,** 3.
Dritz S. K. and Braff E. H. (1977) Sexually transmitted typhoid fever. *N. Engl. J. Med.* **296,** 1359.
Drusin L. M., Genwert G., Topf-Olstein B. et al. (1976) Shigellosis—another sexually transmitted disease. *Br. J. Vener. Dis.* **52,** 348.
Meyers J. D., Kuharic H. A. and Holmes K. K. (1977) *Giardia lamblia* infection in homosexual men. *Br. J. Vener. Dis.* **53,** 54.

SKIN DISEASES

TREVOR ROBINSON MA, MB, FRCP
and J. R. S. RENDALL MB BS, MRCP

ACNE: A DISEASE OF ZINC DEFICIENCY?

The pathophysiology of acne is very little understood. In recent years intensive research has concentrated on hormonal control of the pilosebaceous apparatus, bacterial flora of the skin and qualitative and quantitative sebum excretion studies. A new departure is the possible role of zinc in acne. This has been explored in two recent publications by Michaelsson et al. (1977), from Uppsala, Sweden. They noticed that the acne of a patient with the severe zinc deficiency syndrome acrodermatitis enteropathica cleared almost completely when treated with oral zinc sulphate. It has recently been shown (Smith et al., 1974) that zinc is required to maintain adequate levels of retinal binding protein (RBP) in the plasma of rats, possibly by influencing synthesis in the liver or its release from that site. It is suggested that RBP then controls the amount of vitamin A available for tissue uptake. Using this possible rationale as a starting point, the Swedish group have attempted to explore the role of zinc in man in two clinical studies.

The first study (Michaelsson, Juhlin et al., 1977) involved 38 male and 26 female patients aged between 13 and 25. Two-thirds were aged between 14 and 18. All but 3 had had acne for two years or more. Patients with only comedone acne were excluded, as were those who had had tetracyclines in the preceeding few months. The patients were randomly selected into four groups. Group 1 received 0·2 g of zinc sulphate daily (equivalent to 45 mg elemental zinc), Group 2 a placebo, Group 3 vitamin A 300 000 – 400 000 units daily and Group 4 zinc and vitamin A. If there was no improvement or deterioration after four weeks of treatment vitamin A was added to the zinc group (Group 1), zinc was added to the placebo group (Group 2) and the vitamin A group (Group 3). Group 4 continued with zinc and vitamin A throughout the study. An acne score was obtained by counting open and closed comedones, papules, pustules and cystic lesions in defined areas of the face and neck, the numbers being multiplied on an arbitrary scale of 0·5 for comedones to 4 for cysts. Separate synchronous assessment was undertaken by means of standardized photographs assessed blind by two layman who compared before and after treatment photographs, grading them on a 5-point scale. The study was concluded after 12 weeks.

Co-variance analysis of the four groups was carried out for comedones alone and for inflammatory lesions. No significant effect was seen with either zinc or vitamin A on comedones alone. Nor did vitamin A significantly affect the inflammatory lesions. The effect of zinc on inflammatory lesions was significant when analysed alone and became highly significant when both the zinc groups (1 + 4) were compared with both non-zinc groups (2 + 3). Using a separate statistical analysis the number of patients in each group who showed more than a 50 per cent improvement in inflammatory lesions was determined. Again there was a significant improvement in the zinc treated group, but none for the vitamin A group. Analysis of the photographic assessment became significant for the zinc group after eight weeks.

In a second study (Michaelsson, Vahlquist et al., 1977) serum zinc, RBP and vitamin A levels were determined in 173 acne patients (97 male and 76 female).

All patients were older than 15 years, as levels of RBP and probably zinc are often low in childhood and early puberty (Vahlquist et al., 1975). Patients who had had tetracyclines, vitamin A or other drugs were excluded. The patients were graded using a four-point clinical scale (Pillsbury et al., 1961), the last two of the four grades being termed 'moderately severe' and 'severe' respectively. A group of 74 age-matched controls were used from a similar social class and background. The patients were divided into two age groups, 15 – 19 and 20 years or over, in case late puberty influenced zinc levels of the former group. However, this did not prove to be the case.

In the less severe acne (Grades 1 and 2) there was no significant difference in either zinc or RBP levels compared with controls. Male and female patients in the severe Grades (3 and 4) had significantly lower levels of RBP than the control and these levels were lower than those found in Grades 1 and 2 patients. Male patients with Grade 3 and 4 acne had significantly lower zinc levels than the controls, but females did not. Patients with the most severe acne had lower levels of RBP than those with moderately severe disease. Serum zinc and RBP were positively correlated in females with Grade 1 and 2 acne. In males with the same degree of disease the correlation was not quite significant and no correlation was found in the most severe degrees.

If zinc has something to do with acne what might be the mechanism? There are at least three possibilities. Firstly, as suggested in these papers, zinc may be essential to maintain RBP and vitamin A levels. Secondly, zinc stabilizes macromolecules and biological membranes and may influence migration and phagocytosis of macrophages. As such it might interfere with the inflammatory process in acne. Finally, zinc is required for full activity of numerous enzyme systems, for example 17-β hydroxysteroid dehydrogenase. By such an action it might influence the androgen production of the pilo-sebaceous apparatus.

A major drawback to the first study was a failure to utilize the inflammatory and non-inflammatory types of acne to try to differentiate between the first and second possible modes of action of zinc; patients with comedones were specifically excluded from the trial, whereas if they had been retained, and had improved with zinc, support would have been gained for a vitamin A mediated mode of action as other evidence suggests that vitamin A is most effective in the comedone type of acne.

However, it seems from the data as presented that the reverse is true. Comedone lesions were little helped by zinc, but more severe inflammatory acne did improve, suggesting a possible role for zinc acting directly on inflammation.

The results of the second study were most difficult to interpret. The absence of any correlation between relatively non-inflammatory acne (Grade 1 and 2) and RBP/zinc levels compared with controls could again suggest that zinc's influence, if any, is on the inflammatory process rather than via an RBP – vitamin A effect. However, the RBP level was found to be progressively reduced the worse the acne, although the same was true for zinc only in males. Probably zinc is by no means the only influence on RBP level. The authors point out that zinc and RBP levels may be depressed by the inflammation of acne as both levels are known to fluctuate in systemic infection. Finally serum zinc and RBP levels may not be the best parameters of zinc and vitamin A status. Michaelsson and his group are convinced of the therapeutic efficacy of zinc and further longer term trials, involving more patients, are warranted. At the very least zinc provides a refreshing departure from the minute qualitative and quantative measurement of skin surface lipids!

REFERENCES

Michaelsson G., Juhlin L. and Vahlquist A. (1977) Effects of oral zinc and vitamin A in acne. *Arch. Dermatol.* **113**, 31.

Michaelsson G., Vahlquist A. and Juhlin L. (1977) Serum zinc and retinal-binding protein in acne. *Br. J. Dermatol.* **96**, 283.

Pillsbury D. M., Shelley W. B. and Kligman A. M. (1961) *A Manual of Cutaneous Medicine.* Philadelphia, Saunders, p. 273.

Smith J. E., Brown E. C. and Smith J. K. (1974) The effect of zinc deficiency on the metabolism of retinal-binding protein in the rat. *J. Lab. Clin. Med.* **84**, 692.

Vahlquist A., Rask P., Peterson P. A. and Berg T. (1975) The concentration of retinal-binding protein, prealbumin and transferrin in the sera of newly delivered mothers and children. *Scand. J. Clin. Lab. Invest.* **35**, 369.

PHLEBOTOMY AND CHLOROQUINE IN THE TREATMENT OF PORPHYRIA CUTANEA TARDA (PCT)

Swanbeck and Wennersten (1977), of the Karolinska Sjukhuset in Stockholm, have combined phlebotomy and chloroquine in the management of this uncommon but interesting disorder.

The liver is the main source of porphyrin products in PCT and great quantities of uroporphyrin and coproporphyrin are excreted. Sometimes the serum iron is raised and the iron-binding capacity is increased. Some as yet unknown genetic factor probably predisposes individuals to the disease, but alcohol ingestion, oestrogen hormones, hepatotoxic drugs and chemicals are common precipitating factors. Various treatments have been tried, including chelating agents, alkalinization of the urine, phlebotomy and chloroquine. Chloroquine can precipitate or aggravate PCT but it can also produce remission of symptoms and the correction of the biochemical abnormalities. Unfortunately this treatment can cause unpleasant side effects, such as nausea, vomiting, generalized abdominal pain, myalgia and fever. Treatment of PCT with chloroquine causes large amounts of porphyrins to be excreted in the urine, and may be regarded as a method of lowering the porphyrin load of the plasma and liver. The drawback of phlebotomy is the necessity for the patient to attend the hospital regularly, but in the combined treatment that these Swedish colleagues describe one to four venesections are performed before the administration of chloroquine. Equally high urinary porphyrin excretion is achieved with a marked reduction in side effects. These workers studied 11 patients (7 men and 4 women) with PCT. Their ages ranged from 25 to 70 years and all of them experienced photosensitivity and showed characteristic cutaneous stigmata. The duration of their disease ranged from 6 months to 10 years. Serum hepatic enzyme levels, serum iron and urinary uroporphyrin and coproporphyrin excretion were measured before treatment, estimated for 7 days during treatment and at about 1−2 and 3−4 months afterwards. The faecal porphyrin excretion and the serum erythroprotoporphyrin level were also recorded.

Chloroquine phosphate, 250 mg daily for 7 days orally, was given to each patient, but before starting this 1−4 venesections of 300 ml each were performed at 3−7-day intervals. One patient was given chloroquine without phlebotomy, and another had two courses of chloroquine, the first without preceding phlebotomy, at an interval of 2 years. These 2 patients developed fever, nausea, vomiting and myalgia. The second patient, who had a second course of chloroquine following phlebotomy, again developed fever, slight nausea and headache, but she stated that the treatment was much more tolerable on the second occasion. The other 9 patients who were venesected before chloroquine treatment had no serious side effects although 5 noticed slight nausea.

The serum iron levels, which were usually in the upper normal range, showed no change after phlebotomy during chloroquine therapy or soon thereafter. The porphyrin excretion values and serum hepatic enzyme levels did not alter significantly following venesection. In all the patients the urinary porphyrin excretion rose rapidly and the enzyme hepatic levels were at their highest by the end of the week of chloroquine therapy. The porphyrin excretion and serum hepatic levels fell rapidly during the first month following treatment, and then fell progressively over the next few months to well below the pretreatment levels. There was no obvious correlation between the number of venesections performed before treatment and the porphyrin excretion of hepatic enzyme levels.

It is not known how chloroquine produces its side effects in PCT, but iron 'intoxication' due to sudden release of iron from iron stores is an unlikely explanation as the serum iron levels in all patients were unaltered by treatment. Most of the patients had complained of malaise before treatment and almost all of them felt much better following therapy, and this effect lasted for some for at least a few months.

The authors rightly conclude that their combined treatment offers advantages over either venesection alone, which is tedious for both patient and doctor, and chloroquine alone with its rather unpleasant side effects.

REFERENCE
Swanbeck G. and Wennersten G. (1977) Treatment of porphyria cutanea tarda with chloroquine and phlebotomy. *Br. J. Dermatol.* **97**, 77.

PUVA: APPLICATIONS IN THE MANAGEMENT OF VITILIGO AND MYCOSIS FUNGOIDES

PUVA therapy (Psoralen and Ultra Violet A Light) for psoriasis was discussed in the last *Medical Annual* (1977, p. 300). Two reports concerning its application in vitiligo and mycosis fungoides have recently been published.

PUVA for vitiligo

Treatment for vitiligo remains tedious and unsatisfactory. However, the range of options open to patients has gradually increased. Vitiliginous areas may be stained by the use of dyes and protected by sunscreening agents. Topical halogenated steroid applied to limited areas may be useful in promoting repigmentation, although systemic absorption, local steroid atrophy and also cost limit usefulness on large areas. Psoralen (isomer of furocoumarins, derivatives of coumarin – benzopyrone) was introduced in 1947 (El Mofty, 1948) following observations on the effectiveness of local herbal remedies in Egypt which proved to contain these agents. Topical applications of either a psoralen mixture (Meladinine paint) trimethylpsoralen (trioxsalen, TMP) or

8-methoxypsoralen (methoxsalen, 8-MOP), combined with exposure to natural sunlight or black light, has been shown to be effective (Kelly and Pinkus, 1955; Fulton et al., 1969; Africk and Fulton, 1971), but limitations due to severe phototoxic blistering are often found.

A comparison of trioxsalen and methoxsalen systemically administered and combined with black light has recently been reported (Parrish et al., 1976). Twenty-six patients were exposed to UVA 2 hours after ingestion of one of the drugs at a dosage of 40 mg. Half the patients were treated with each drug. Irradiation was delivered using fluorescent bulbs producing 320–390 nm wavelengths. A plastic filter was incorporated to remove wavelengths below 320 nm. Initial exposure was 2 Joules/sq cm increasing by 1 J increments every third treatment to a maximum of 12 J/sq cm. Patients were treated 2–3 times per week. When the phototoxic reaction was too severe (erythema, marked itching or desquamation, 48–72 hours after exposure) incremental increase was postponed until the reaction subsided. Because such reactions were more common with methoxsalen, patients reached maximum exposure more quickly with trioxsalen.

Patients received similar quantitites of both drugs and UVA exposure. The resulting repigmentation was extremely similar and equivalent to a group treated previously with trioxsalen and natural sunlight. Four of the trioxsalen group and 2 of the methoxsalen group obtained more than 75 per cent repigmentation of affected areas. For 50 – 75 per cent improvement the figures were 5 and 4 respectively. Non-responders were 3 for the trioxsalen group and 4 for the methoxsalen group. The other patients achieved less than 50 per cent repigmentation or only follicular improvement. All the patients in the methoxsalen group experienced intermittent erythema throughout the treatment period of 12–14 months. Transient pruritus, desquamation and nausea occurred much more commonly than with the patients taking trioxsalen.

The mechanism of action of psoralens in vitiligo is unknown, and the stimulation of melanogenesis may not necessarily be related to the phototoxic effect. Although the numbers of patients were small this study suggests that trioxsalen may be as capable of stimulating repigmentation with less risk of serious phototoxicity than methoxsalen, an important consideration when treatment may be prolonged and high levels of supervision unavailable. The trial demonstrates once again the often unsatisfactory effect of even prolonged therapy for vitiligo.

PUVA for mycosis fungoides

The treatment of mycosis fungoides (MF) was reviewed in the last *Medical Annual* (1977, p. 303). Another application for photochemotherapy has been found in this condition. A number of therapeutic manoeuvres are effective in early MF but treatment is least helpful in the systemic form of the disease. Early premycotic eruptions may require observation alone but are sometimes responsive to topical halogenated steroids and also to ultraviolet light. True infiltrative MF may still be responsive to steroids and ultraviolet light, but usually either topical nitrogen mustard therapy or electron beam (B ray scatter) techniques are required. It is dealing with this plaque type MF that photochemotherapy seems to be most effective.

A study describing the effect of photochemotherapy on 12 patients with MF has recently been published (Roenigk, 1977). Diagnosis was established in 8 women and 4 men aged 27−82 years by multiple skin biopsies. Patients with systemic involvement (as shown by bone-marrow biopsy, gastrointestinal X-rays, liver and brain scans and lymph node biopsies) were excluded from the trial. Laparotomy was carried out in only 1 patient. Methoxsalen was given in standard dosage 2 hours before exposure to ultraviolet A light (dosages: up to 50 kg body-weight 20 mg, 51−65 kg 30mg, 66−80 kg 40 mg, over 80 kg 50 mg). UVA was delivered from a number of different machines, but all emitting continuous UVA between 320 and 400 nm. Initial exposures of 1·5−3 J/sq cm were given according to ability to tan. Minimum dosage increments of 0·5 J/sq cm were made at each treatment. Treatment was given three times weekly and the final clearing dose used as maintenance at a frequency between twice-weekly and every alternate week. Assessment was made by means of photographs and repeat biopsies from closely related sites. Seven patients with plaque MF cleared after a mean dose of 1·8 J and have been maintained clear for greater than a year. Four patients required radiotherapy for isolated tumour lesions while their plaque lesions cleared with PUVA. One patient's treatment was complicated by erythroderma but was ultimately controlled.

This study and that of Gilchrist et al. (1976) demonstrate the effectiveness of PUVA in plaque type MF and such therapy may ultimately prove to be the treatment of choice for this form of the disease. Comparative trials between extensive topical nitrogen mustard, electron beam and PUVA therapy are likely to be hindered by the relative rarity of the disease and PUVA is clearly not applicable to late stage systemic disease where chemotherapy is often ineffective. The mechanism of action of PUVA in MF is not clear, but tumour inhibition due to this treatment has been demonstrated in several different experimental systems. Probably phototoxic products react with the pyrimidine bases of DNA inhibiting cell division.

This mode of action, which seems to be separate from that in vitiligo, is probably the relevant one in psoriasis and might conceivably be of use in other chronic inflammatory skin conditions, for example chronic lichenified eczema and lichen planus. Empirical trial in such conditions may be undertaken in the future as the availability of PUVA spreads.

REFERENCES

Africk J. and Fulton J. (1971) Treatment of vitiligo with trimethylpsoralen and sunlight. *Br. J. Dermatol.* **84**, 151.
El Mofty A. M. (1948) Preliminary clinical report on the treatment of leucoderma with Ammi Majus Linn. *J. Egypt. Med. Ass.* **31**, 651.
Fulton J. E., Leyden J. and Papa C. (1969) Treatment of vitiligo with topical methoxsalen and blacklite. *Arch. Derm.* **100**, 224.
Gilchrist B. A., Parrish J. A. and Tannenbaum L. (1976) Oral methoxsalen photochemotherapy of Mycosis fungoides. *Cancer* **38**, 683.
Kelly E. W. and Pinkus H. (1955) Local application of 8-methoxypsoralen in vitiligo. *J. Invest. Dermatol.* **25**, 453.
Parrish J. A., Fitzpatrick T. B., Shea C. et al. (1976) Photochemotherapy of vitiligo. *Arch. Dermatol.* **112**, 1531.
Roenigk H. H. (1977) Photochemotherapy for mycosis fungoides. *Arch. Dermatol.* **113**, 1047.

STEROID AEROSOL TREATMENT OF ORAL LICHEN PLANUS

The treatment of oral lichen planus with local steroid preparations is now established practice. The efficacy of hydrocortisone hemisuccinate and betamethasone valerate pellets and triamcinolone acetonide in orabase has been investigated in controlled and uncontrolled trials and, on the whole, it has been found that improvement is limited to erosive areas. Betamethasone valerate is the most topically active steroid of those mentioned above, but it is not generally available in a form suitable for oral use. There is, however, an aerosol preparation (Bextasol) available for the treatment of asthma which delivers a metered dose of 100 μg of betamethasone valerate. When fitted with an adapter, as used in the treatment of rhinitis (Archer et al., 1975), this aerosol is suitable for oral use, and Tyldesley and Harding (1977) have assessed this novel form of treatment in oral lichen planus.

Twenty-three patients attending an oral medicine clinic in Liverpool with symptoms of pain or discomfort due to oral lichen planus were entered into the trial. Diagnosis rested principally on the clinical picture, but biopsies were performed if there was any doubt. Five were classed as having the non-erosive form of the disease, 17 the minor erosive form and 1 the major erosive form. The duration of symptoms was, on average, 2 years (maximum 20 years), but some patients with symptoms of recent onset were included. Sixteen patients were female and 7 male: the average age was 49 years (range 36 – 72 years).

Patients were randomly allocated to active or placebo treatment in a double-blind manner. Two puffs of aerosol 4 times a day were administered to the affected area. The active aerosol delivered a daily dose of 800 μg of betamethasone valerate and the placebo aerosol contained only the propellants, Arcton-11 and 12. Following initial assessment and entry into the trial, patients were reassessed at 2, 4 and 8 weeks, and the extent of the lesion, discomfort or pain, and response to therapy were noted. The main criterion for assessment for those with erosions was crater size, but a more subjective overall assessment was used for non-erosive cases. All patients were swabbed at each visit for the detection of fungal growth. Twelve patients took the active drug and 11 the placebo. Twenty patients completed the study. Overall, 8 improved on the active drug with 3 showing no change, and 2 improved on placebo with 7 showing no change ($P<0\cdot05$, by χ^2 analysis). Eight patients in the actively treated group and 7 in the placebo group were found to have *Candida albicans* in their mouths without any sign of clinical infection. One patient developed acute pseudomembranous candidiasis on aerosol treatment which responded to treatment withdrawal and amphotericin lozenges, and subsequent re-introduction of treatment did not result in relapse.

Of the 7 patients showing no change on placebo treatment, 5 were given active aerosol on an open basis at the end of the trial. Three of these patients showed a marked improvement at 8 weeks, 1 showed moderate improvement and 1 no change.

The results of this trial suggest that an aerosol of micronized betamethasone valerate was successful in treating the majority of patients with non-erosive or minor erosive oral lichen planus. The most impressive response was obtained with minor erosive disease, in which lesions started to regress within 2 weeks of starting treatment. The full trial dose, set at 800 μg, was not, in fact, taken by most patients for more than a few days, as it was often found that with the healing of the erosions it was frequently possible to discontinue the use of aerosol temporarily.

On the whole, the treatment of oral lichen planus is unsatisfactory at present, and the availability of this effective aerosol must represent a considerable advance.

REFERENCES

Archer G. J., Thomas A. K. and Harding S. M. (1975) Intranasal betamethasone valerate in the treatment of season rhinitis. *Clin. Allergy* **5**, 285.

Tyldesley W. R. and Harding S. M. (1977) Betamethasone valerate aerosol in the treatment of oral lichen planus. *Br. J. Dermatol.* **96**, 659.

THE TREATMENT OF PERSISTENT PALMOPLANTAR PUSTULOSIS WITH CLOMOCYCLINE

The management of persistent palmoplantar pustulosis (PPP) is well known to be very difficult, and any addition to the therapeutic armoury has to be welcome. The problem is complicated by the fact that it is probable that diseases of different aetiological complexion are contained within this rather general, but for the present convenient, group term. This may well explain why a particular line of therapy is very effective in a small number of cases, and apparently quite ineffective in the remainder. However, at present these suggestions are conjectural and only further detailed study will provide the answers that we need.

Ward and her co-workers (1976) describe the results of clomocycline (Megaclor) treatment of 60 patients with PPP in a double-blind cross-over trial, each patient receiving 3 months each of clomocycline and placebo in random order. Forty patients completed the trial. Twenty-two failed to respond to either treatment, 15 improved on clomocycline, 2 improved on placebo and 1 improved on both treatments. These significant results ($P = 0\cdot003$) suggest that clomocycline may suppress pustulation in some patients. The 22 non-responder's were compared with eighteen 'responders' for sex, age, length of history and associated psoriasis, but no significant differences were found. Further follow-up of both groups suggested that comocycline used over a long period favourably influenced the course of the disease in the 'responder' group.

The trial was carried out on patients with an established clinical diagnosis of PPP who were attending the skin outpatients department of three hospitals (St John's Hospital for Diseases of the Skin, Charing Cross Hospital and Central Middlesex Hospital). Diagnosis was based on the presence of chronic, recurring, sterile pustulation on the palms and/or soles with characteristic cyclical changes in the pustules from yellow to brown, followed by shedding of the dry scale. Patients were admitted to the trial, if the disease had been seen to be active by one of the physicians, for at least 2 months, providing that pustules and macules were bigger than 2 mm and the patients had not had tetracyclines during the preceding 3 months.

Sixty patients were entered, of whom 48 were women, mean age $52\cdot4$ years $\pm12\cdot3$, and 12 men, mean age $45\cdot6$ years $\pm13\cdot8$. The patients were told that treatment was being evaluated that might help some cases and their co-operation for at least 6 months was sought. Further detail of the methods used can be obtained from the original paper, but assessment of PPP by the method the authors describe was found to be practical and reproducible. In the 30 patients who were separately judged by two observers there was complete agreement in 58 of 60 assessments made.

Of 60 patients entering the trial 20 failed to complete treatment. Of the remaining 40 patients, 22 failed to respond to either treatment, i.e. showed no preference ($=$non-responders); 15 improved on clomocycline and failed to respond to placebo, i.e. showed preference for clomocycline; 2 improved on placebo and failed to respond to clomocycline, i.e. showed preference for placebo; 1 improved on both treatments, i.e. showed no preference. Thus 17 patients expressed a preference for one of the treatments, and of these 15 showed a preference for clomocycline and 2 for placebo. All the 15 patients who responded to clomocycline either failed to respond to placebo if this was given first or relapsed on placebo when it was given second. The probability of getting by chance 15 preferences for clomocycline from a total of 17 is very small ($P = 0 \cdot 003$), and so there is a highly significant difference between the effectiveness of clomocycline and placebo in a proportion of patients who suffer from PPP. Comparison of 18 'responders' with 22 'non-responders' failed to show any obvious clinical reason for the different effect of treatment in the two groups.

Of the 20 patients who failed to complete the trial, 6 failed to attend at some stage, 14 discontinued with side effects. One of these was a placebo and complained of heartburn. The 13 on clomocycline complained of nausea and vomiting (6), vaginal thrush (1), constipation (1), heartburn (1), miscellaneous symptoms (4).

The condition of the 'responders' was compared to the 'non-responders' after follow-up lasting from 6 months to 2½ years. A significant portion of those who initially responded had maintained their improvement: 9 of 18 as compared to 3 of 22 'non-responders'. After 1−2 years 28 patients were still pustulating, 19 from the 'non-responders' and 9 from the 'responders'. Six of the latter had relapsed without treatment following the trial, and 3 of those remained better on further clomocycline therapy, relapsing when it was stopped. Ten of the 19 'non-responders' had further treatment with tetracyclines, to no avail.

The authors rightly stress the difficulties of assessing the effect of treatment in PPP. The importance of pustulosis as the main index of activity is corroborated by the natural history of this disease or group of diseases. As spontaneous remission occurs so, gradually, fewer pustules are produced, itching and soreness diminish, and there then may follow a longish period of redness and scaling before the skin returns to normal. The clinical picture varies considerably from patient to patient, but in any one individual it is usually strikingly consistent with respect to the area involved, the morphology of the pustules and the amount of erythema and dyskeratosis. This, together with the need to treat as many patients as possible, suggested the use of patients as their own controls in a cross-over trial design.

Twenty-two of 40 patients completing the trial were apparently not improved, suggesting that at least 50 per cent of patients are likely to be unresponsive to tetracyclines. Although 18 patients improved during treatment (15 on clomocycline, 3 on placebo, including 1 who improved on both), the numbers are small. Nevertheless, statistical analysis is consistent with the view that pustulosis was suppressed by clomocycline in these 15 patients. As an alternative, consideration as to whether these 15 patients might have improved spontaneously was given by the authors. Most previous work suggests that spontaneous remission is relatively low in PPP. Hellgren and Mobacken (1971) stated that 75 per cent of patients were still pustulating after 5 years. Enfors and Molin (1971) found 75 per cent of 248 patients to have symptoms more than 10 years after onset. Of 82 patients observed for 4−6 months, only 7 per cent had cleared. During the 6 months of this present trial the 3 placebo reactors may represent spontaneous remissions as may also the 1 non-responder who subsequently cleared, giving a comparative figure of 10 per cent. If, on the other hand, all the patients who responded in the 6-month period are considered to have improved spontaneously an incidence of 45 per cent recovery obtains, and this is highly unlikely. In addition, only 12·5 per cent of the 40 patients who completed the trial gave a past history of spontaneous healing of the lesions of one or more limbs lasting for 3 months or more.

No significant difference could be found in the clinical features of 'responders' and 'non-responders', but the authors rightly note that PPP may not be a homogeneous disease entity. Some patients show a more eczematous response with severe itching, vesicle formation and often lichenification in addition to pustulation: 9 patients showed these features. A further group of patients with PPP may represent pustular bacterid, which is a rare, usually self-limiting variant, and only 1 patient in this trial fell into this category. These groups may well have a different pathogenesis from the main bulk of PPP.

A disappointingly large proportion of patients failed to complete the trial. Rather unexpectedly, 12 patients complained of nausea, vomiting and heartburn, and 7 of the 8 of those who had to be withdrawn from the trial were taking clomocycline.

It is well known that patients may vary widely in their response to drugs. This may be due to the disease being treated, the responsiveness of the disease to the drug or its plasma concentration (Rawlins, 1974). Nothing is known about tissue responsiveness to tetracyclines in PPP. A variation in serum level between the groups the authors feel is unlikely and the results of their further studies on this are awaited with interest.

The authors conclude that although the numbers in this trial are too small to be entirely conclusive, there was good evidence that some cases of PPP benefit from oral tetracycline.

REFERENCES

Enfors W. and Molin L. (1971 Pustulosis palmaris et plantaris. *Acta Derm. Venereol.* **51**, 289.

Hellgren L. and Mobacken H. (1971) Pustulosis palmaris et plantaris. *Acta Derm. Venereol.* **51**, 284.

Rawlins M. D. (1974) Variability in response to drugs. *Br. Med. J.* **4**, 91.

Ward J. M., Corbett M. F. and Hanna M. J. (1976) A double-blind trial of clomocycline in the treatment of persistent palmoplantar pustulosis. *Br. J. Dermatol.* **95**, 317.

GENERAL SURGERY

O. J. A. GILMORE MS, FRCS,
FRCS(Edin)

ABDOMINAL WOUND DEHISCENCE

Any surgical incision through the layers of the abdominal wall is associated with a small but definite risk of dehiscence. In the early postoperative period the integrity of a wound is maintained entirely by the sutures used in its closure. These sutures have to withstand all mechanical stresses applied to the wound until healing starts. The wound begins to gain strength after a lag phase of four to five days. It then rapidly gains strength over the next ten days or so, during the incremental phase. The rate of gain in strength then diminishes as it enters the plateau phase of healing.

There are three types of abdominal dehiscence: superficial, deep and complete. Superficial dehiscence occurs when the skin and subcutaneous tissues part, this usually occurs when the skin sutures are removed and occurs in approximately one-third to a half of all infected wounds. Deep dehiscence is when the deep, that is the muscle layers or the linea alba, separate resulting in an incisional hernia. The usual causes of deep dehiscence are suture failure or infection. The incidence varies from approximately 1 per cent in uncontaminated wounds to nearly 10 per cent in deeply infected wounds. Although there are very few reports in the literature on the incidence of incisional hernia, a recent study showed the overall incidence to be 5 per cent, just over half the cases being due to suture failure and half due to infection (Leaper et al., 1977).

In complete dehiscence all layers of the abdomen part, with the result that the abdominal viscera protrude and approximately a quarter of the patients die. Complete dehiscence is commonest in the 50 – 80-year-old age group, with a peak in the 60s. It is commoner in males than in females, and in vertical (paramedian and midline) incisions than in transverse or oblique incisions. It is also commoner in the upper rather than the lower abdomen. The majority of complete dehiscences occur during the second postoperative week. The three main factors which interfere with healing, and which thus result in dehiscence, are infection, ischaemia and increased intra-abdominal pressure. Increased intra-abdominal pressure usually results from postoperative coughing, vomiting or abdominal distension.

In the past a 5 – 7 per cent rate of disruption was considered inevitable by many surgeons and it was thought that this rate was unaffected by the suture material or technique used. Some surgeons, however, have achieved long series of laparotomies with few disruptions, often less than 1 per cent (Abel and Hunt, 1948; Spencer et al., 1963). The use of heavy non-absorbable sutures, inserted with large bites, is a common feature in the closures employed by such workers.

Jenkins (1976) recently claimed that burst abdomen is nearly always mechanical in origin. He pointed out that during the first few days of convalescence abdominal distension may lengthen a vertical wound by 30 per cent. He has shown that the smaller the initial bite and the greater the interval between bites, the shorter will be the total length of suture relative to the length of the wound. A large bite of heavy material therefore obviously distributes stresses on a larger suture/tissue interface than does a small, fine, neat stitch. Jenkins' results suggest that for a continuous stitch the straight length of material should be at least four times that of the wound and the bites should be at least 1 cm deep and sewn closely together.

The type of suture material used has also been reviewed following the discovery that catgut can be unreliable due to its inability to retain its tensile strength for sufficient time for the tissues to heal. Just over a decade ago its disintegration was the cause of 15 out of 18 burst abdomens examined (Standevan, 1955), while another survey ten years later reported 11 bursts with 5 deaths out of 107 paramedian incisions closed in layers with No. 1. chromic catgut (Goligher et al., 1975). If catgut is to be used for closure of the abdomen it should be supported by interrupted nylon retention sutures, which may be removed after two weeks.

Wire, although difficult to use, results in virtual abolition of wound disruption (Spencer et al., 1963) but today monofilament polypropylene, having the same general properties and advantages as wire, is preferable because it is better tolerated by the patients, especially in the late postoperative period. Recently, monofilament polyethylene has also become popular. It is strong and handles well, slides easily through delicate tissues, knots securely, is inert and rarely causes sinus formation (Hermann, 1974).

The main discussion today, however, centres on whether abdominal wounds should be sutured in layers or by mass one-layer closure. Paramedian incisions are best closed in layers and it is recommended that large bites of tissue are taken (Jenkins, 1976) and that a continuous everting mattress suture is used because it is stronger than an over-and-over suture (Haxton, 1965). One-layer suturing is especially suited to the closure of midline incisions (Tagart, 1967; Nayman, 1976). If it is used in paramedian incisions then a rectus split approach is required which damages the rectus muscle. A recent study concluded that there was no difference in the results of layered closure with retention sutures compared with a single layer mass closure, and that infection was the main cause of dehiscence (Irvin et al., 1977). It seems clear, therefore, that for surgeons to further reduce their rates of dehiscence, no matter what their method of closure, they must think mechanically while they sew and employ an effective method of wound infection prophylaxis.

REFERENCES

Abel A. L. and Hunt A. H. (1948) Stainless steel wire for closing abdominal incisions and for repair of herniae. *Br. Med. J.* **2**, 379 – 382.
Goligher J. C., Irvin T. T., Johnston D. et al. (1975) A controlled clinical trial of three methods of closure of laparotomy wounds. *Br. J. Surg.* **62**, 823 – 829.
Haxton H. A. (1965) The influence of suture materials and methods on the healing of abdominal wounds. *Br. J. Surg.* **52**, 372 – 375.
Hermann R. E. (1974) Abdominal wound closure using a new polypropylene mono-filament suture. *Surg. Gynec. Obstet.* **138**, 84 – 86.
Irvin T. T., Stoddard C. J., Greaney M. G. et al. (1977) Abdominal wound healing—a prospective clinical study. *Br. Med. J.* **2**, 351 – 352.
Jenkins T. P. N. (1976) The burst abdominal wound: a mechanical approach. *Br. J. Surg.* **63**, 873 – 877.
Leaper D. J., Pollock A. V. and Evans M. (1977) Abdominal wound closure: a trial of nylon, polyglycolic acid and steel sutures. *Br. J. Surg.* **64**, 603 – 606.
Nayman J. (1976) Mass single layer closure of abdominal wounds. *Med. J. Aust.* **1**, 183 – 186.
Spencer F. C., Sharp E. H. and Jude J. R. (1963) Experiences with wire closure of abdominal incision in 293 selected patients. *Surg. Gynec. Obstet.* **117**, 235 – 238.
Standevan A. (1955) Small-bowel obstruction following partial gastrectomy. *Br. J. Surg.* **43**, 104.

Tagart R. E. (1967) The suturing of abdominal incisions. A comparison of monofilament nylon and catgut. *Br. J. Surg.* **54**, 952 – 957.

DIAGNOSTIC ERROR IN ACUTE APPENDICITIS

The diagnosis of acute appendicitis is considered by many to be simple, but alas this is not always the case. Acute appendicitis is the commonest diagnosis made in the United Kingdom in patients with acute abdomen. Hospitals serving a population of 250 000 can expect to admit 250 patients with the diagnosis of acute appendicitis each year. At operation, however, some of these patients will be found to have a normal appendix; their symptoms being due to other causes.

Although many people have written on the diagnosis and misdiagnosis of appendicitis, documentation of the incidence of conditions mimicking appendicitis is sparse. A study in the Reading Hospital, England, in which an emergency appendicectomy was carried out through a gridiron incision in 444 consecutive patients, sought to determine the incidence of genuine appendicitis, diagnostic error and the conditions which mimic appendicitis (Gilmore et al., 1975). After each operation the surgeon recorded the operative findings, in particular the state of the appendix and other organs.

Of the 444 patients in the study, 346 had an acutely inflamed gangrenous or perforated appendix. The surgeon's diagnosis of acute appendicitis was therefore correct in 78 per cent of patients. The surgeon was likely to be wrong twice as often in female as in male patients, only 70 per cent of the females having genuine appendicitis compared with 85 per cent of the males. The incidence of gangrenous appendix was the same in both sexes, but perforation was twice as common in males as in females.

The incidence of diagnostic error, although always greater in females, varied with the patient's age (*Fig.* 1). Thirty two per cent of girls under 21 were

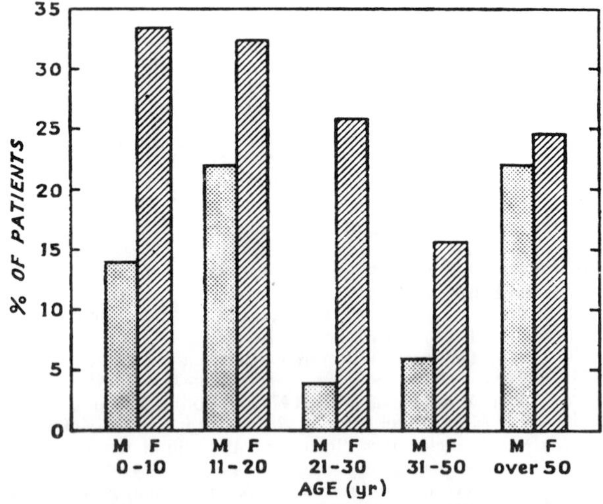

Fig. 1. Frequency of diagnostic error, in patients diagnosed as having appendicitis, related to age and sex of patient. (By kind permission of the *Lancet.*)

found to have a normal appendix compared with 19 per cent of boys in the same age-group. Of the 82 men aged 21 – 50, only 4 did not have acute appendicitis. Errors in diagnosis were particularly common during the first two decades and in the over 50s, in whom acute sigmoid diverticulitis was quite often the cause of the patients' symptoms.

The mimicking condition most frequently presenting itself in children under 11 was non-specific mesenteric adenitis. Constipation, tubo-ovarian or related disorders, such as ruptured, twisted or bleeding ovarian cysts and salpingitis, were often misdiagnosed as appendicitis in females between the ages of 11 and 20. Gynaecological conditions, however, also frequently mimicked appendicitis in women over the age of 30. Other conditions misdiagnosed as acute appendicitis included small-bowel obstruction, Crohn's disease, tuberculous ileitis, acute cholecystitis, acute Meckel's diverticulitis and urinary tract infection. Conditions known to present as acute appendicitis, including pneumonia, perforated peptic ulcer, ectopic pregnancy, acute pyelonephritis, ureteric colic, carcinoma of the caecum, gastroenteritis and idiopathic torsion of the omentum were either not seen or were correctly diagnosed. In 24 patients (5·5 per cent) no diagnosis at all was made. The other interesting finding was how the diagnostic accuracy of the surgeons involved (range 54 – 95 per cent) varied according to their experience.

Postoperative complications, both early and late, may follow the removal of a normal appendix. Chest infection, aspiration pneumonia, urinary retention, early intestinal obstruction, stress ulceration, paralytic ileus, generalized peritonitis, pelvic abscess, deep-vein thrombosis and late intestinal obstruction, have all been recorded. During pregnancy spontaneous abortion is a common complication. Every effort must therefore be made to reduce the number of unnecessary appendicectomies. Great care must be taken over the details of the history. A thorough clinical examination, including a rectal and, where necessary, a vaginal examination, is vital. Even today, too few surgeons do a vaginal examination on patients with acute abdomen. In cases of doubt, reappraisal at intervals is essential, for a classic presentation is unusual. The conditions which mimic appendicitis, and the types of patients in whom these occur, must be carefully considered. Finally, the gridiron incision is the incision of choice, since it is less liable to complications, including sepsis, than the paramedian (Gilmore and Sanderson, 1975) and when centred over the point of maximum tenderness it is adequate for dealing with the majority of conditions which mimic appendicitis.

REFERENCES

Gilmore O. J. A. and Sanderson P. J. (1975) Prophylactic interparietal povidone-iodine in abdominal surgery. *Br. J. Surg.* **62**, 792.

Gilmore O. J. A., Brodribb A. J. M., Browett J. P. et al. (1975) Appendicitis and mimicking conditions. *Lancet* **2**, 421.

TROPICAL DISEASES

MAJOR-GENERAL W. O'BRIEN
OBE, MD, FRCP

VIRUS DISEASE IN THE TROPICS

In perhaps no other field of tropical medicine has the perspective changed so much as that in regard to viral infections. Vaccination has been successful to a varying extent in controlling such lethal diseases as smallpox, yellow fever and poliomyelitis. However, to balance these successes other new serious viral infections have come to light, whilst dengue fever, long known as a nuisance to expatriates, has now taken on the guise of a killing disease in native children.

Many tropical virus diseases share the epidemiological characteristics of other tropical infections in that there is a primary animal host and the disease is transmitted by an insect vector. The response to these virus infections appears to be dominated by the immunological reaction of the host. Thus in many of the animal hosts there is complete immunological tolerance to a chronic viraemia, whilst in man viraemia induces immunological disaster. Progress in the fields of immunology and virology have done much to advance our understanding of these conditions. It is perhaps also of interest that two of these infections came to light in small mission hospitals in Africa.

DENGUE

Dengue fever is endemic in many parts of Southern Asia, the Pacific and the Caribbean. Until recently it had been a nuisance rather than a serious medical problem and indeed it has been suggested that the immunity of Southern Asia from yellow fever may have been due to dengue acting as an immunological barrier (Theiler and Anderson, 1975). Multiple infections in childhood, when dengue produced only a mild illness, resulted in immunity in indigenous adults and overt illness was largely confined to foreigners. However, since the 1950s extensive outbreaks of urban dengue in native children have been characterized by a severe haemorrhagic state and medical shock, which have often proved fatal (Halstead, 1966).

The dengue virus is a mosquito-borne arbovirus of the B Group, or in more modern terms is a togavirus of the flavivirus genus. It is a very small virus containing a single molecule of RNA enclosed in a tightly fitting envelope. There are at least four serological types. Isolation of the virus is difficult. It grows in cell cultures of monkey and hamster kidney but cytopathogenic changes do not develop readily and because of this dengue challenge techniques have been introduced. Mice inoculated with a suspect serum are challenged 21 – 28 days later with a known lethal dose of mouse-adapted dengue virus. If the mice survive, it is presumptive evidence of dengue virus infection in the original serum. A modification of this principle is based on the fact that a very small amount of dengue virus will protect stable grevet kidney cells from the cytopathogenic effects of viruses such as poliomyelitis virus and ECHO 9 (Halstead et al., 1964; Sukhavachana et al., 1966). Following infection, neutralizing antibody and haemagglutination-inhibition antibody appear after 7 days and complement-fixing antibody after 14 – 21 days. In practice serological diagnosis is often complicated by previous dengue or other

Group B virus infections causing an anamnestic reaction. Primary dengue infection is identified by an absent or a low titre of antibodies in acute sera and the sequential development of IgM antibody followed by IgG antibody in convalescence. Secondary dengue infection is characterized by complement-fixing antibody broadly reactive to Group B viruses in acute and early convalescent sera. The position is further complicated by the fact that Chikungunya virus carried by the same mosquito not infrequently infects simultaneously. As the former virus is more easily identified, virological misdiagnosis is liable to occur.

The vector of urban dengue is the *Aedes aegypti* mosquito which was introduced into Asia from Africa about the beginning of the century. This mosquito is highly anthrophilic and breeds in artificial water containers in and around houses. The common practice of storing water in large jars provides abundant breeding sites. As a result dengue is now widespread in the coastal areas of India and southeast Asia and has spread to inland cities and towns along lines of communication. The female mosquito feeds indoors during daylight hours and at dusk. There appears to be no natural animal reservoir of infection beyond man. Viraemia precedes the onset of the illness in man by 6 − 18 hours and then lasts for a further 3 days. *Aedes aegypti* become infective 11 − 14 days after an infected blood feed and then remain infective for life.

The mosquito introduces its proboscis directly into a capillary beneath the skin and injects infected saliva. During the incubation period of 4 − 6 days viral multiplication ensues in the vascular endothelium and in reticulo-endothelial cells. Virus liberated from these cells gives rise to a viraemia which precipitates the systemic phase of the illness. In classic dengue there is a sudden onset of chills, fever, severe frontal and retro-orbital headache, accompanied by generalized aches and pains particularly felt in the lumbar-sacral region. Fever remains high for 3 − 4 days, and falls suddenly only to rise again within 24 hours for a further 2 − 3 days, the so-called 'saddle-back fever'. Upper abdominal pain and vomiting are common as are upper respiratory symptoms accompanied by signs of bronchitis. An alteration in taste is a common symptom. There is increasing suffusion of the face and congestions of the conjunctivae accompanied by photophobia. A macular or maculopapular rash appears on the second day involving the trunk, arms and thighs and a macular rash may also accompany the secondary rise in fever. At this time also petechiae may be seen on the extremities and buccal mucosa, epistaxis is not uncommon and the tourniquet test may be positive. There is leucopenia and the pulse rate falls steadily. There is, however, considerable variation in the severity of attacks and indeed in the clinical features themselves and the classic syndrome is often seen only in a minority of patients in any outbreak. Thus in many patients there is a 7-day fever without any break, with or without a rash, whilst in others, especially children, there is only a very short non-specific febrile illness or even no clinical manifestations in the presence of proved viraemia. Convalescence may be prolonged and be accompanied by depression.

A quite different clinical response to dengue infection was first noticed in Manila in 1953 (Quintos and Lim, 1954). The patients were all native children under the age of 15 years and were usually aged 3 − 6 years. The illness was accompanied by severe haemorrhage and often fatal medical shock. Another epidemic followed in Manila in 1956 with 1207 cases and a 6 per cent mortality. Outbreaks confined to the rainy season have been reported from Bangkok since 1958, occurring annually with peaks every 2 years. In the period 1958 – 63 there were 10 367 cases reported from that city, with 694 deaths. Retrospective study of case histories has suggested that the condition had been prevalent in Bangkok since 1950. Other large outbreaks occurred in Hanoi in 1958, South Vietnam in 1963 and 1973, Burma in 1970, 1971 and 1972, and in Singapore in 1973. These figures refer to hospital admissions and in the outbreak a very much larger number of individuals were found with minor illness. The incidence was not affected by race, sex or socio-economic status except so far as it was not seen in severely malnourished children. All four types of dengue virus have been incriminated but the majority of infections were with Dengue Type 2.

The onset in these children was with a minor febrile illness with upper respiratory symptoms, headache, anorexia, vomiting and abdominal pain. Nevertheless, they often remained ambulatory until the third or fourth day (Halstead, 1966). Then most recovered, but in a proportion there was rapid deterioration which resulted in their admission to hospital. There was a sudden appearance of weakness and collapse with restlessness, sweating, a flushed face, warm trunk and cold clammy extremities. The skin might appear purple from peripheral vascular stasis. Petechiae were found on the forehead, hands and feet and in some cases there was a macular or maculopapular rash. There was tachycardia, a weak thready pulse, the heart sounds were faint, the arterial bood pressure was low or unrecordable and the pulse pressure was less than 20 mm Hg. The liver was enlarged but not tender. Severe melaena or haematemesis were the usual haemorrhagic manifestations. Deaths usually occurred on the 4th or 5th day and were preceded by unresponsive shock and coma. If the child survived this period there was a steady and fairly rapid recovery.

Laboratory investigation revealed a prolonged bleeding time with thrombocytopenia, maturation arrest of megakaryocytes in the bone-mrrow, an increased haemocrit reading and a mild leucocytosis due to haemoconcentration. There was hypoproteinaemia and liver function tests were abnormal in parallel with the severity of the condition. Autopsy revealed evidence of capillary dysfunction with tissue oedema, clear or blood-tinged fluid in serosal cavities, focal and subserosal haemorrhage, gastrointestinal haemorrhage, focal hepatic necrosis and infiltration of the portal tracts with lymphocytes and plasma cells. It was seldom possible to isolate the virus, and serological testing indicated secondary dengue infection in the great majority of cases. Serum complement concentration was markedly reduced.

Treatment was with intravenous electrolyte solutions, plasma, blood and platelet transfusion, oxygen, hydrocortisone and phentolamine was used with apparent effect. It was important to withhold fluids during the recovery phase when extracellular fluid was returning to the circulation.

It was difficult to understand why dengue viruses, usually benign, are now causing a severe and often fatal illness. Dengue with haemorrhage and shock had previously been reported during large epidemics in non-endemic areas, but such cases were rare in predominantly classic attacks. During the 1956 epidemic of haemorrhagic dengue fever in Manila 2 dengue viruses were isolated with antigenic components which differed from Types 1 and 2 previously identified. These at first were considered to be variants with a greatly increased virulence and were designated Types 3 and 4. However, it soon became apparent that all 4 types of dengue virus could be associated with dengue haemorrhagic fever.

Halstead (1966) and Halstead et al. (1967) suggested that haemorrhagic dengue with shock was the result of a hyperimmune response in individuals sensitized by a previous dengue infection. The condition was only seen in areas where multiple dengue-type infections were endemic, it was never seen in short-term residents and it was accompanied in the great majority of cases by an accelerated secondary antibody response leading to rapid disappearance of dengue virus from the blood. Dengue haemorrhagic fever and dengue shock syndrome in Asian children was due to sequential infections with heterologous types of dengue virus: the first dose sensitized the patient, the second dose caused immunological catastrophe. The Report of an International Collaborative Study (1973) supported this hypothesis. The rapid onset of a short-lasting, rapidly reversible state as well as the lack of histopathological vascular lesions suggested a pharmacologically active mediator. The association with a previous attack of dengue due to a heterologous-type virus was supported by the anamnestic antibody response seen in most patients, leading to a high concentration of antidengue IgG antibody in the blood early in the course of the disease. It was likely that this in turn gave rise to circulating antigen-antibody complexes. Viraemia was rarely found and then only in the presence of low titres of haemagglutination-inhibition antibody. Fifty-three out of 55 patients investigated had secondary dengue infection with a rapid geometric increase in antibody concentration. Two patients had primary infections, both were infants of mothers who had circulating dengue antibody and the infants had presumably acquired maternal IgG antibody transplacentally. All but 1 of 36 patients who developed the dengue shock syndrome had circulating dengue antibody at the time of shock. A marked depression of serum levels of complement components was found and the fall correlated with the severity of the disease. C3, C3 proactivator, C4 and C5 were involved. Activation of C3 and C5 was known to be accompanied by dissociation of low molecular weight peptides which had the capacity to release histamine and were very potent permeability-increasing factors. The low platelet counts, reduced fibrinogen levels and the presence of circulating split products, as well as preliminary evidence of reduced Hageman Factor, provided strong evidence for disseminated intravascular coagulation as the cause of the haemorrhage. The following mechanisms were likely to be involved: dengue infection in a patient with pre-existing antibody, an immune pathological process involving immune complexes, massive complement activation, liberation of vasoactive peptides and initiation of intravascular blood coagulation.

This, however, may not be the whole story. Severe and fatal haemorrhagic dengue has been described in primary dengue infections. Barnes and Rosen (1974) recorded an epidemic with these features in young patients on a Pacific island which had not been exposed to dengue for 25 years. Scott et al. (1976) also described fatal haemorrhagic dengue with shock in primary dengue infection but these patients also showed complement depletion, suggesting an immunological mechanism.

REFERENCES

Barnes W. J. S. and Rosen L. (1976) Fatal haemorrhagic dengue and shock associated with primary dengue infection in a Pacific island. *Am. J. Trop. Med. Hyg.* **25**, 866.

Halstead S. B. (1976) Mosquito-borne haemorrhagic fevers of South and Southeast Asia. *Bull. WHO* **35**, 3.
Halstead S. B., Sukhavachana P. and Nisalak A. (1964) Assay of mouse adapted dengue viruses in mammalian cell cultures by an interference method. *Proc. Soc. Exp. Biol. Med.* **115**, 1062.
Halstead S. B., Nimmannitya S. and Yamarat C. et al. (1967) Haemorrhagic fever in Thailand; recent knowledge regarding etiology. *Jap. J. Med. Sci. Biol.* **20**, 96.
Quintos F. N. and Lim L. E. (1954) *St Thomas's J. Med.* **9**, 319.
Report of an International Collaborative Study (1973) Pathogenetic mechanisms in dengue haemorrhagic fever. *Bull. Wld Hlth Org.* **48**, 117.
Scott R. M., Nimmannitya S., Bancroft W. H. et al. (1976) Shock syndrome in primary dengue infections. *Am. J. Trop. Med. Hyg.* **25**, 866.
Sukhavachna P., Nisalak A. and Halstead S. B. (1966) Tissue culture techniques for the study of dengue viruses. *Bull. Wld Hlth Org.* **35**, 65.
Theiler M. and Anderson C. R. (1975) The relative resistance of dengue-immune monkeys to yellow fever virus. *Am. J. Trop. Med. Hyg.* **24**, 115.

JAPANESE ENCEPHALITIS

Japanese encephalitis is another disease caused by a Group B arbovirus which is a cause of death in Asian children. In countries located between 23 and 43 N latitude which have generally temperate climates (Japan, Korea, Taiwan) transmission occurs mainly in the late summer and human encephalitis epidemics are a regular and serious occurrence (Grossman et al., 1973). In areas with generally tropical climates (Sarawak, Malaysia, Southeast Asia, India) transmission is endemically maintained throughout the year and only sporadic cases occur.

The epidemiology of endemic Japanese encephalitis has been studied in a land Dyak village in Sarawak (Bendell, 1970; Heathcote, 1970; Hill, 1970; Simpson et al., 1970; Bowen et al., 1975; and Simpson et al., 1976). The village consisted of 80 dwellings with 500 inhabitants. In close proximity to the village were well established rice fields with piggeries and the whole was surrounded by forest forming a discrete ecosystem. It was estimated that 6 per cent of the human population became infected each year and that 80 per cent had become infected by the age of 20 years.

Pigs were infected throughout the year at a rate 20 times as great as in man. Infection between pigs was transmitted mainly by *Culex gelidus* mosquitoes which fed only on pigs and to a lesser extent by *Culex tritaeniorhynchus* which fed on both pigs and man. At the time of flooding of the rice fields in September and October prior to planting, conditions became optimal for breeding of *C.tritaeniorhynchus* and an explosive increase in the number of these mosquitoes occccurred. This in turn resulted in a sharp increase in pig infections, an enormous increase in infected *C.tritaeniorhynchus* and a much greater liability of human infection by this night-biting mosquito. The pig acted as a maintenance host in a cycle involving *C.gelidus* mosquitoes and also acted as an important amplifier host towards the end of the year in a cycle involving *C.tritaeniorhynchus*.

Another study of the epidemiology of this infection was undertaken in 1970 in the Chinagmai Valley of Thailand, an area considered to be intermediate between temperate (epidemic) and tropical (endemic) Japanese encephalitis infection. Again the annual rate of infection in man was estimated at 6 per cent and nearly the whole population had been infected by the age of 30 years. The annual rate of infection represented approximately 29 000 infections in a population of 484 000. Of these 100 were clinical infections necessitating admission to hospital and of these 23 died. Two-thirds of these patients were male and the peak age of incidence was 5 – 9 years, only 6 per cent of the patients being over 30 years of age.

In 1969 there had been a double epidemic of Japanese encephalitis and dengue. Confirmation of the diagnosis in 1970 was by positive serology. Seventy-five per cent of the patients showed a primary response with a significant rise in haemagglutination-inhibition antibodies between acute and convalescent sera, but in 25 per cent there was a secondary type response to Group B arbovirus antigens, which was interpreted as a new Japanese encephalitis infection in patients previously infected with dengue. In spite of this cross response, previous infection with dengue appeared to give no protection against Japanese encephalitis infection (Grossman et al., 1973 a, b and c).

Like dengue Japanese encephalitis affects adult expatriates visiting or serving in endemic areas. It was an important cause of death amongst British military personnel in southeast Asia and an outbreak occurred amongst U.S. marines in Nham Phong, Thailand, during July – August 1972 (Benenson et al., 1975). Thirteen marines became sick with meningo-encephalitis. On investigation 9 showed a fourfold or greater rise in haemagglutination-inhibition antibodies to Japanese encephalitis virus, whilst 3 had high antibody titres in acute sera. Serological investigation of a large sample of apparently fit marines showed that more than a quarter had recently been infected. There was an apparent to inapparent infection ratio of 1:63. The highest incidence of infection was in men of security units who had been more exposed to night-biting mosquitoes.

REFERENCES

Bendell P. J. E. (1970) Japanese encephalitis in Sarawak; studies on mosquito behavior in a Land Dyak village. *Trans. R. Soc. Trop. Med. Hyg.* **64**, 497.

Benenson M. W., Top F. H., Gresso W. et al. (1975) The virulence to man of Japanese encephalitis virus in Thailand. *Am. J. Trop. Med. Hyg.* **24**, 974.

Bowen E. T. W., Simpson D. I. H., Platt G. S. et al. (1975) Arbovirus infection in Sarawak, October, 1968 – February, 1970; human serological studies in a Land Dyak village. *Trans. R. Soc. Trop. Med. Hyg.* **69**, 182.

Grossman R. A., Edelman R., Chiewanich P. et al. (1973) Study of Japanese encephalitis virus in Chiangmai Valley, Thailand; II Human clinical infections. *Am. J. Epidemiol.* **98**, 121.

Grossman R. A., Edelman R., Willhight M. et al. (1973) Study of Japanese encephalitis virus in Chiangmai Valley, Thailand. III Human seroepidemiology and inapparent infections. *Am. J. Epidemiol.* **98**, 133.

Grossman R. A., Gould D. J. Smith T. J. et al. (1973) Study of Japanese encephalitis virus in Chiangmai Valley, Thailand; I Introduction and study design. *Am. J. Epidemiol.* **98**, 111.

Heathcote D. H. U. (1970) Japanese encephalitis in Sarawak; studies in juvenile mosquito populations. *Trans. R. Soc. Trop. Med. Hyg.* **64**, 483.

Hill M. N. (1970) Japanese encephalitis in Sarawak; studies on adult mosquito populations. *Trans. R. Soc. Trop. Med. Hyg.* **64**, 483.

Simpson D. I. H., Bowen E. T. W., Platt G. S. et al. (1970) Japanese encephalitis in Sarawak; virus isolation and serology in a land Dyak village. *Trans. R. Soc. Trop. Med. Hyg.* **64**, 503.

Simpson D. I. H., Smith C. E. G., Marshal T. F. de C. et al. (1976) Arbovirus infections in Sarawak; the role of the domestic pig. *Trans. R. Soc. Trop. Med. Hyg.* **70**, 66.

CHIKUNGUNYA VIRUS

Another virus, a member of Group A of the arboviruses, has been responsible for outbreaks of a short-term fever superficially resembling dengue in southeast Asia. The condition was first recognized in Tanganyika (Robinson, 1955). A characteristic feature was joint pains of frightening severity which completely immobilized some patients. A local name, 'chikungunya', was applied meaning 'that which bends up'. The outbreak was explosive, involving 60 – 80 per cent of the population of some villages within 2 – 3 weeks, and *Aedes aegypti* was thought likely to be the vector. Other features were an irritating maculopapular rash, bradycardia and leucopenia. Joint pains might recur for up to 4 months. McIntosh et al. (1963) described a small outbreak in a party of white Rhodesians who had spent a night in a hut. The illness was confined to those who had not used mosquito nets and African servants who slept outside were not affected. An incubation period of 3 days was followed by a sudden dramatic onset of fever with severe joint pains which when involving the feet were crippling. An irritating measles-like rash appeared on the 4th day just as the fever was abating.

During 1964 several cities in India were struck by epidemics of dengue-like fever. In several outbreaks dengue viruses were proved to be responsible, but in Vellore and Madras City the epidemics were found to be due primarily to chikungunya virus. The Vellore epidemic (Carey et al., 1969) began in August, reached a peak in October and ended in December, a period which corresponded closely to the season for dengue outbreaks. No subsequent cases were reported for at least 4 years and there was serological evidence that the last outbreak had been 30 years previously: 274 patients were found to have been infected with chikungunya virus alone, 14 with both chikungunya and dengue virus either simultaneously or sequentially and 6 with dengue virus alone. There was a sudden onset of fever, headache and severe pain in the joints, this last being the dominant complaint. These pains mainly affected the small joints of the hands, wrists and feet but frequently occurred in the knees as well. Early on there was a diffuse erythematous flush over the face and upper chest and toward the end of the febrile phase (3rd to 5th day) most patients developed a diffuse maculopapular, irritating rash which lasted for 48 hours. At the same time many patients developed enlarged and tender inguinal nodes and also many reported a tingling or burning sensation in the pinnae, which were red, swollen and infiltrated. Only a small proportion of chikungunya patients exhibited haemorrhagic phenomena, which ranged from epistaxis and bleeding gums to melaena, but in no case was the bleeding severe. Tourniquet tests were generally negative.

All the adult patients recovered uneventfully although a number experienced persistent, intermittently incapacitating joint pains for several months. However, nearly a third of the 39 proved chikungunya infections in infants and children were associated with convulsions and in several these were more persistent than was usual with simple febrile convulsions. One child died following a number of seizures and 2 children had persistent neurological defects. Laboratory diagnosis was relatively simple since the virus could always be recovered from the blood during the first 48 hours. Haemagglutination-inhibition antibody appeared between the 4th and 6th days and reached a peak during the 2nd week; complement-fixing antibody appeared later and reached a peak in the 3rd month. Chikungunya fever at Vellore was not just another 'dengue-like' fever. Arthralgia was its most prominent feature in contrast to myalgia in dengue. Furthermore, the post-chikungunya patient, although burdened with persistent arthralgia, was usually ready to return to work within a week in contrast to the prolonged period of asthenia so common after dengue. The strikingly enlarged and tender inguinal lymph nodes and the red, swollen ears were other distinguishing features.

The effects of dengue and chikungunya infections in children in Bangkok were contrasted by Nimmannitya and Mansuwan (1966) and Nimmannitya et al. (1969). The onset of chikungunya was more acute so that 70 per cent of admissions to hospital were on the first day of the illness and the febrile course was shorter. Convulsions and an erythematous maculopapular eruption were much more common in chikungunya. Petechial haemorrhage, epistaxis and a positive tourniquest test were common in both but a confluent petechial rash, gastrointestinal bleeding and shock were only seen in dengue patients.

REFERENCES

Carey D. E., Myers R. M., DeRanitz C. M. et al. (1969) The 1964 chikungunya epidemic at Vellore, South India, including observations on concurrent dengue. *Trans. R. Soc. Trop. Med. Hyg.* **63**, 434.

McIntosh B. M., Harwin R. M., Paterson H. E. et al. (1963) An epidemic of chikungunya in South-Eastern Rhodesia. *Centr. Afr. J. Med.* **9**, 351.

Nimmannitya S., Halstead S. B., Cohen S. N. et al. (1969) Dengue and chikungunya virus infection in man in Thailand 1962 – 1964. 1, Observations on hospitalized patients with haemorrhagic fever. *Am. J. Trop. Med. Hyg.* **18**, 954.

Nimmannitya S. and Mansuwan P. (1966) Comparative clinical and laboratory findings in confirmed dengue and chikungunya infections. *Bull. WHO* **35**, 42.

Robinson M. C. (1955) An epidemic of virus disease in Southern Province, Tanganyika Territory, in 1952 – 53: 1, Clinical features. *Trans. R. Soc. Trop. Med Hyg.* **49**, 28.

THE ARENOVIRUSES

Murphy et al. (1969) and Rowe et al. (1970) designated a family of viruses having common morphological and antigenic characteristics as arenoviruses. These were small RNA viruses approximately 100 nm in diameter which when viewed under the electron microscope contained a variable number of electron dense particles indistinguishable in size and shape and density from ribosomes. These granules resembled grains of sand (*arenaceous* = sandy). The viruses were stable and grew readily in Vero (African green monkey) cell cultures in which a cytopathogenic effect was seen in 4 – 5 days after inoculation. This group of viruses had probably existed for thousands of years infecting rodents in which they cause viraemia without overt disease, immunological tolerance having given rise to a stable symbiotic situation.

The best known member of this group of viruses is the virus of lymphocytic choriomeningitis. In recent years other viruses of this group have been shown to cause serious infection in man. This infection is usually acquired through contamination of grain stores by rodent urine. The basic pathology caused by these viruses is through an active immunological reaction to the virus resulting in damage to capillary blood vessels with leakage of plasma and blood. This in turn results in hypovolaemia, haemoconcentration, arterial hypotension, oliguria and haemorrhage, a situation similar to that seen in haemorrhagic dengue.

Such a virus is the Junin virus which has caused regular autumn epidemics of haemorrhagic fever amongst maize harvesters in the Argentine since 1953. After an incubation period of 10 – 12 days there is a gradual onset of fever which lasts 7 – 15 days. Drowsiness, pallor, facial oedema, conjunctival injection and palpebral oedema are common findings and there may also be lymphadenopathy, tremor and constipation. Bleeding gums, epistaxis, haematemesis and melaena are the haemorrhagic manifestations. A slow pulse is characteristic and in severe cases there may be a precipitous drop in arterial blood pressure, with oliguria and anuria (Simpson, 1972). The Machupo virus, another member of this group, caused a single very severe epidemic in Bolivia. In a population of 2,500 there were 470 cases and 142 deaths, and again the clinical features included fever, leucopenia, a haemorrhagic rash and medical shock. In both these infections the common field mouse was considered to be the primary host and the virus was conveyed to man through contamination of grain by infected mouse urine.

The latest addition to the arenoviruses pathogenic for man is the Lassa fever virus (Buckley and Casals, 1970). This disease was reviewed in the *Medical Annual* of 1976 (p. 375) and it is clear that the clinical features are very similar to those of other known arenovirus infections. The condition is limited to West Africa and two special features are a pharyngeal eruption and a marked tendency to cause severe infections in hospital and laboratory workers. More recently an outbreak of Lassa fever has been described from the Eastern Province of Sierra Leone, which unlike those previously reported was not a hospital epidemic, most of the patients being infected in the community (Frazer et al., 1974; Monath et al., 1974). It differed also in that the outbreak was not short and explosive but lasted over a year and appeared to involve many generations of cases. The mortality rate in patients admitted to hospital was 12 per cent compared with previous reported mortalities of 30 – 50 per cent. This lower mortality was attributed to a high index of clinical suspicion, with the resulting admission of relatively mild cases. Serological testing of the population suggested many mild or even subclinical infections which would otherwise have gone unrecognized.

The multimammate rat *Mastomys nataliensis,* widely distributed south of the Sahara, a prolific breeder adapted to life in houses and in the open, has been confirmed as the primary host. In the rainy season it may leave the fields and seek shelter and food within houses and this may explain the peak incidence of infection in man in Sierra Leone. Low levels of sanitation, the customary storage of grain and other foodstuffs within houses, and the ample shelter for these rats in houses constructed of mud and thatch are thought to be important epidemiological factors.

REFERENCES

Buckley S. M. and Casals J. (1970) Lassa fever; a new virus disease of man from East Africa. 3, Isolation and characterisation of the virus. *Am. J. Trop. Med. Hyg.* **19,** 680.
Frazer D. W., Campbell C. C., Monath T. P. et al. (1974) Lassa fever in the Eastern Province of Sierra Leone 1970 – 1972. 1, Epidemiologic studies. *Am. J. Trop. Med. Hyg.* **23,** 1130.
Monath T. P., Maher M., Casals J. et al. (1974) Lassa fever in the Eastern Province of Sierra Leone, 1970 – 1972. 2, Clinical and virological studies in selected hospital cases. *Am. J. Trop. Med. Hyg.* **23,** 1140.
Murphy F. A., Webb P. A., Johnson K. M. et al. (1969) Morphological comparison of Machupo with lymphocytic choriomeningitis virus; basis for a new taxonomic group. *J. Virol.* **4,** 535.
Rowe W. P., Murphy F. A., Bergold G. H. et al. (1970) Arenoviruses; proposed name for a newly defined virus group. *J. Virol.* **5,** 651.
Simpson D. I. H. (1972) Arbovirus diseases. *Br. Med. Bull.* **28,** 10.

THE MARBURG VIRUS

In 1967 there was an outbreak of a new tropical virus infection in man involving workers in factories in Marburg, Frankfurt and Belgrade who were producing vaccines and sera. All the workers affected had had direct contact with blood, organs or cell cultures of African green monkeys recently imported from Uganda. In addition a doctor and a nurse who had been caring for the patients became ill, as did the wife of a patient. Nearly a quarter died.

After an incubation period of 5 – 7 days there was an abrupt onset of fever, malaise, prostration, myalgia and severe headache. Fever remained around 40 °C for 6 days and then gradually fell. There was nausea, vomiting and diarrhoea and a characteristic rash developed. The latter was a maculopapular eruption involving the trunk, face and upper arms and which later coalesced into a diffuse erythema. At the same time the palate showed a dark red colouring and half the patients had conjunctivitis. Patients were noted to be sullen, aggressive, confused or to show impairment of consciousness whilst death was preceded by coma. A feature in severe cases was a haemorrhagic state with bleeding from the gums, nose, puncture lesions and the gastro-intestinal tract. There were no mild or subclinical infections (Martini, 1969). Laboratory findings included thrombocytopenia, leucopenia with atypical plasmacytoid lymphocytes, hypoproteinaemia and high SGOT levels. Convalescence was often prolonged and liver puncture at this time revealed single cell necrosis and moderate fatty degeneration with a focal increase in Kuppfer cells.

African green monkeys were extremely susceptible to infection when inoculated by whatever route, all dying within 13 days of inoculation but often appearing fit until shortly before death. All the monkeys exhibited viraemia and the saliva and urine was infective (Simpson, 1969). An infective agent was isolated in Germany which produced characteristic cytoplasmic inclusions in tissue cultures, a cytopathogenic effect in certain cell lines, but was larger than any known virus.

The next reported outbreak of this condition was from Johannesburg (Gear et al., 1975). In February 1975 a young Australian man, who had been hitch-hiking through Rhodesia and who had been bitten or stung 6 days previously by an unknown agent, was admitted to a Johannesburg hospital with a severe febrile illness from which he died. Two days after his death his female travelling companion became sick. A nurse who had attended both patients and who had assisted in intratracheal intubation and bronchial suction of the first patient also became ill. Both women recovered.

The illness in these patients was in almost all respects similar to that seen in Marburg in 1967. There was a sudden onset of fever, malaise, headache and myalgia. Nausea, vomiting, abdominal pain and diarrhoea followed as did a maculopapular rash. The patients were lethargic and depressed. Severe bleeding occurred in the first patient and massive haematemesis and melaena led to his death. This bleeding was associated with thrombocytopenia, low plasma fibrinogen and high fibrinogen degradation product levels, strongly suggesting disseminated intravascular coagulation. The other 2 patients had minor haemorrhagic episodes which may have been controlled by early treatment with heparin. There was leucopenia, atypical plasmacytoid lymphocytes and the acquired Pelger – Huet anomaly of neutrophils strongly suggesting a virus infection. The plasma SGOT concentration was very high. Autopsy in the first patient revealed profuse bleeding from the gastrointestinal tract and lungs as well as patchy but extensive degeneration of hepatocytes. Following inoculation of material obtained from throat swabs, blood and organs obtained at autopsy, into Vero cell cultures, cytoplasmic inclusions and particles morphologically and antigenically indistinguishable from the Marburg agent were found. The 2 patients who recovered showed a rising titre of blood antibodies to the Marburg agent.

In 1976 sporadic cases of haemorrhagic fever were reported from the Southern Sudan followed by an outbreak of a similar condition in Northern Zaire. The epidemic in Zaire increased in intensity with a disturbingly high percentage of cases reported amongst hospital personnel, suggesting case-to-case infection. It seems that the clinical features were essentially similar to those reported from the 2 previous outbreaks. Material for virological study was despatched to the Center for Disease Control, Atlanta, to the Micro-biological Research Establishment, Porton, and to the Institute of Tropical Medicine, Antwerp. The infecting agent was isolated and was found to consist of large filamentous virus particles 100 nm in diameter and 300 – 1 500 nm in length. They were similar to the particles isolated in Germany following the 1967 outbreak and Vero cell cultures showed the characteristic inclusions. However, immunofluorescent antibody studies gave only a weak reaction to the previous Marburg agent isolates and because of this the virus was provisionally termed the 'Ebola virus'. Ebola is the name of a small river in Zaire (Bowen et al., 1977; Johnson et al., 1977; and Pattyn et al., 1977).

REFERENCES

Bowen E. T. W., Platt G. S., Lloyd G. et al. (1977) Viral haemorrhagic fever in Southern Sudan and Northern Zaire. *Lancet* **1**, 571.
Gear J. S. S., Cassal G. A., Gear A. J. et al. (1975) Outbreak of Marburg virus disease in Johannesburg. *Br. Med. J.* **4**, 489.
Johnson K. M., Webb P. A., Lange J. V. et al. (1977) Isolation and partial characterization of a new virus causing acute haemorrhagic fever in Zaire. *Lancet* **1**, 569.
Martini G. A. (1969) Marburg agent disease in man. *Trans. Soc. Trop. Med. Hyg.* **63**, 295.
Pattyn S., Jacob W., van der Groen G. et al. (1977) Isolation of Marburg-like virus from a case of haemorrhagic fever in Zaire. *Lancet* **1**, 573.
Simpson D. I. H. (1969) Marburg agent disease in monkeys. *Trans. R. Soc. Trop. Med. Hyg.* **63**, 303.

UROGENITAL TRACT

A. G. MORGAN BSc, MD, MRCP
J. CUNNINGHAM BM, MRCP
M. J. VANDENBURG BSc, MB, BS, MRCP
V. L. SHARMAN MA, MB, BChir, MRCP
J. P. MITCHELL TD, MS, FRCS, FRCSE
R. C. L. FENELEY MChir, FRCS
P. H. ABRAMS FRCS
M. O. SYMES MD

Medical

THE TREATMENT OF GLOMERULONEPHRITIS

A. G. MORGAN BSc, MD, MRCP

Despite many enthusiastic attempts to treat glomerulonephritis, success has been elusive and recent reviews of the subject make gloomy reading. The object of the present article is not to add to the glooom but to point cautiously to two new approaches to therapy which promise to brighten the future.

Although uncertainty about the natural history of glomerular disease has often made assessment of the effect of treatment difficult, most authorities accept that the likelihood of spontaneous recovery is slim when a patient with rapid deterioration of renal function has a biopsy in which more than 70 per cent of glomeruli contain extracapillary crescents. Rapidly progressive glomerulonephritis (RPGN) of this type may complicate a number of systemic disorders or may occur as an isolated syndrome. It is uncommon, yet many workers have published the results of their efforts to treat it—usually with anti-inflammatory, immunosuppressive, anti-platelet and anticoagulant drugs. Such combinations have been chosen empirically because immunological factors are obviously involved in the disease and because crescent formation is associated with fibrin deposition. An overall impression from publications ont he subject suggests that a common factor in cases showing improvement is the use of anticoagulants. Opinions vary, though. Kincaid-Smith (1975) stated, 'Our experience since we have been using heparin in such patients differs so strikingly from experience before we used heparin that we hesitate to do a controlled trial.' By contrast Suc et al. (1976) conclude, 'Our results suggest that the risks involved in the treatment of patients with RPGN with heparin far outweigh the potential benefits.' Robson et al. (1977) make a suggestion that may help to resolve this disagreement. Reasoning that the syndrome may be heterogeneous and that coagulation may play a more important role in some patients than in others, they selected patients for anti-coagulant treatment only when they found persistent evidence of intravascular coagulation. Out of 183 children who presented with acute glomerulo-nephritis, 6 with severe glomerular changes on biopsy also had evidence of increased fibrinogen breakdown shown by plasma fibrinogen chromatography. They were treated with anticoagulants, starting with intravenous heparin and changing to phenindione after three days: all received azathioprine and dipyridamole in addition. Azathioprine was continued for one year, anticoagulants for two, and all patients were followed up for a minimum of one year after that. In all 6 patients glomerular filtration rate improved convincingly (often to normal) and the improvement was maintained when treatment was stopped. The authors consider carefully the possibiity that all their patients had improved spontaneously and conclude that this is highly unlikely. They appear to have shown that progression to renal failure can be prevented in selected patients with RPGN. This conclusion needs to be tested by a controlled trial, but since the treatment was uniformly effective in cases whose prognosis would generally have been considered very poor, a statistically significant result might be obtained in a trial containing relatively few patients.

Anticoagulants can only be effective in glomerulonephritis by suppressing one of the tissue-damaging mechanisms whilst the underlying disease process runs its course. RPGN is probably a form of acute soluble immune complex disease and more fundamental treatment is still not possible. But if the disease is naturally self-limiting why not remove the immune complexes from the circulation as soon as they are formed and thus protect the kidneys until the danger is past? This daunting task has been attempted by Lockwood et al. (1977), following earlier work in which similar logic was applied to the therapy of Goodpasture's syndrome. Frequent (often daily) plasma exchange was carried out in 9 patients with RPGN. On each occasion 4 litres of plasma were removed and replaced by plasma-protein fraction (mostly albumin), a technologically advanced procedure requiring an indwelling arteriovenous shunt and access to a cell separator. This treatment was combined with steroids, cyclophosphamide and sometimes azathioprine. Renal function in 5 of the 9 patients improved soon after the start of this regime and in several a test for circulating immune complexes indicated a fall after plasma exchange. After a variable time—one to two weeks in most patients—plasma exchange was stopped and treatment continued with steroids and immunosuppressive drugs alone. The results are encouraging: at the time of the report 6 of the 9 patients were still alive up to 40 weeks after the start of treatment and renal function appeared to be stable. The treatment is still experimental of course, but a longer, controlled study is planned and its results will be awaited with interest.

REFERENCES

Kincaid-Smith P. (1975) *The Kidney. A Clinico-pathological Study.* Oxford, Blackwell, p. 272.

Lockwood C. M., Rees A. J., Pinching A. J. et al. (1977) Plasma exchange and immunosuppression in the treatment of fulminating immune-complex crescentic nephritis. *Lancet* 1, 63 – 67.

Robson A. M., Cole B. R., Kienstra R. A. et al. (1977) Severe glomerulonephrites complicated by coagulopathy: treatment with anticoagulant and immunosuppressive drugs. *J. Pediatr.* **90**, 881 – 892.

Suc J. M., Durand D., Conte J. et al. (1976) The use of heparin in the treatment of idiopathic rapidly progressive glomerulonephritis. *Clin. Nephrol.* **5**, 9 – 13.

SOME CLINICAL ASPECTS OF RENAL TRANSPLANTATION

J. CUNNINGHAM BM, MRCP

The development of renal transplantation as a treatment for end stage renal failure has posed a number of new and, in some cases, unique medical problems.

Pre-transplant phase

Pre-transplant assessment of the recipient is undertaken in the hope that risk factors thought to affect graft or patient well-being can be identified and, if possible, corrected before the transplant is performed.

Pre-transplant nephrectomy. Hitherto it has been the practice to subject patients with a history of urinary tract infection, chronic pyelonephritis with or without documented infection, polycystic disease, or vesico-ureteric reflux to bilateral nephro-ureterectomy prior to transplantation. This policy is now being questioned and a recent report from Glasgow (Calman et al., 1976) draws attention to the significant mortality (9 per cent) and morbidity resulting from this procedure, and re-examines some of the indications for it. Bilateral nephrectomy did not protect against urinary infection in either pyelonephritic or glomerulonephritic patients. However, vesico-ureteric reflux and bacteriuria remain absolute indications for pre-transplant bilateral nephro-ureterectomy.

Peptic ulceration. The association between steroid therapy and peptic ulceration is widely accepted, although a retrospective analysis of 42 studies has failed to confirm an association between steroid therapy and gastro-intestinal bleeding (Conn et al., 1976). A history of peptic ulceration or proved peptic ulcer would be expected to lead to a high risk of post-transplant gastrointestinal problems, of which bleeding and perforation are the most serious, both carrying a high mortality (Owens et al., 1976). However, a report of 54 patients in whom pre-transplant barium and acid secretion studies were undertaken suggested that these investigations have little predictive value (Chisholm et al., 1977). The use of H_2 receptor antagonist drugs in the early post-transplant period may prove beneficial. Although controlled studies are not yet available, there is some evidence that the incidence of postoperative bleeding can be reduced to near zero by using cimetidine prophylactically (Jones et al., 1977).

Blood transfusion. Transfusion of the potential recipient has hitherto been avoided as far as possible, on the assumption that exposure to foreign leucocytes would enhance graft rejection by the production of lymphocyto-toxic antibodies. However, several reports have shown that graft survival is in fact significantly better in patients who have previously received blood transfusions (Opelz et al., 1974; Festenstein et al., 1976; Perkins et al., 1977; Uldall et al., 1977). As a result of these observations, some units now routinely transfuse their potential recipients. This policy, while probably improving the outlook of those patients who are transplanted, may induce multi-specific antibodies in a few patients, rendering the acquisition of a suitable kidney extremely unlikely.

Donor preparation. Preoperative attention to the potential donor before death attempts to ensure that the kidneys remain in good condition until the last possible moment, by maintenance of blood pressure, preservation of urine flow and avoidance of sepsis. Further donor 'pre-treatment' in the form of massive doses of steroids and cytotoxic drugs given a few hours before death is now being assessed by several units. The rationale is that donor leucocytes are inevitably transplanted with the kidney and, being highly immunogenic, may lead to rejection. Early results are encouraging but inconlcusive (Zincke et al., 1977). Because such treatment involves the administration of a lethal dose of cytotoxic drug to the donor several hours before the kidneys are removed, new ethical and medicolegal problems are raised.

Early post-transplant phase

The immediate postoperative period is fraught with hazards to both graft and recipient. The possible interactions of recent surgery, rejection, uraemia, immunosuppression and infection are varied and dangerous. Peptic ulceration has been alluded to and will not be discussed further.

Major sepsis, often involving opportunistic organisms, is the commonest cause of death in most published series and local sepsis predisposes to the breakdown of the vascular and urinary anastomoses. The unusually low mortality from sepsis in one series of 100 transplants may be related to the low maintenance dose of steroid used during the first 60 days (McGeown et al., 1977).

Infection is also important: both bacterial and common viral infections may precipitate rejection episodes (Gabriel et al., 1976).

Late post-transplant phase

Glomerular disease in the graft. It is surprising that the transplanted kidney often appears to thrive in a recipient whose own kidneys have been damaged by circulating immune complexes, as in some types of nephritis, or by an unknown but presumably persistent factor as in diabetes mellitus. However, there is increasing evidence that parenchymal lesions, other than those of rejection, may be frequent and result in graft failure. The most commonly encountered lesion has the appearance of mesangio-capillary glomerulo-nephritis under light microscopy and is seen in most long-surviving grafts. It appears whether or not the recipient's original disease involved the glomeruli, suggesting that it is a manifestation of the host's response to the graft (Mathew et al., 1975; Petersen et al., 1975; Cameron et al., 1977). Immune globulins, usually IgM, complement and fibrin may be seen. The condition has been termed 'graft glomerulopathy' and its histological appearance renders the identification of true recurrent glomerulonephritis most difficult. The latter is most likely to occur following anti-glomerular basement membrane disease, mesangio-capillary glomerulonephritis, crescentic nephritis, and in particular 'dense deposit' disease (Turner et al., 1976). Severe graft dysfunction as a result of recurrent glomerulonephritis or 'graft glomerulo-pathy' is the exception rather than the rule. The probability of recurrent disease appears to be greater following transplantation between identical twins than following allografting (Glassock et al., 1968; Noel et al., 1975).

The diagnosis of recurrent glomerular disease is further complicated by the finding of a strong association between vesico-ureteric reflux into the transplanted kidney, histological evidence of glomerular change and late graft failure (Mathew et al., 1977). Although the refluxing patients did not show an increased incidence of urinary infection, it is unclear whether the combination of reflux with infection confers a worse prognosis than reflux alone. Functionally, these kidneys showed microscopic haematuria, proteinuria and progressive impairment of glomerular filtration. Histologically they showed mesangio-capillary changes in the glomeruli, but no evidence of chronic rejection. These findings suggest that the importance of creating a non-refluxing type of ureteric implant into the bladder may have been under-estimated.

Diabetes mellitus. Specific diabetic vascular lesions have been seen in kidneys transplanted into diabetics, but there is no evidence that these lesions contribute to the poorer than average results of transplantation in such patients (Mauer et al., 1976).

Bone disease. The almost invariable derangement of calcium, phosphate and vitamin D metabolism seen in uraemic and dialysis patients would be expected to resolve following successful renal transplantation. Such is not always the case and two recent reports (Chatterjee et al., 1976; Pletka et al., 1976) have documented the persistence of hyperparathyroidism in 66 per cent of 76 patients and of hypercalcaemia in 27 per cent of 60 patients, all with good graft function. There was no evidence that the hypercalcaemia was detrimental to the graft, but the incidence of aseptic necrosis of the femoral head was high in the hypercalcaemic patients (7 out of 16) compared with those who were normocalcaemic (3 out of 44). This complication is not seen in primary hyperparathyroidism, suggesting a potentiation of this particular side effect of steroid therapy by hyperparathyroidism or hypercalcaemia.

Potassium. Hyperkalaemia following transplantation is usually associated with acidosis, poor renal function or rejection episodes. Sometimes it is encountered in isolation and a prospective study of 4 such patients (De Fronzo et al., 1977) has demonstrated normal responsiveness of the renin – angiotensin – aldosterone system to sodium depletion and hydrochlorothiazide and abnormally small kaliuretic responses to exogenous mineralocorticoids, frusemide and acetazolamide. All these abnormal responses may be restored to normal by prior administration of hydrochlorothiazide, which also restored the serum potassium to normal levels.

Malignant disease. A worrying, but quantitatively small hazard to long term graft survivors is the increased incidence of malignant disease to which they are subject. An analysis of 6297 cases (Hoover et al., 1973) shows that this increase is largely due to lymphomas which were 35 times more common than would be expected, and in particular to reticulum cell sarcoma which was 350 times as common as expected. Involvement of the central nervous system, which is normally extremely uncommon, was a prominent feature in these patients. Other reports have documented an increased incidence of solid and reticulo-endothelial tumours (Sheil et al., 1977; Sloan et al., 1977). Possible explanations for this phenomenon include loss of immune surveillance, an oncogenic effect of immunosuppressive drugs and chronic immuno-stimulation from the graft.

REFERENCES

Calman K. C., Bell P. R. F., Brigge J. D. et al. (1976) Bilateral nephrectomy prior to renal transplantation. *Br. J. Surg.* **63**, 512 – 516.
Cameron J. S. and Turner D. R. (1977) Recurrent glomerulonephritis in allografted kidneys. *Clin. Nephrol.* **7**, 47 – 54.
Chatterjee S. N., Friedler R. M., Berne T. V. et al. (1976) Persistent hypercalcaemia after successful renal transplantation. *Nephron* **17**, 1 – 7.
Chisholm G. D., Mee A. D., Williams G. et al. (1977) Peptic ulceration, gastric secretion and renal transplantation. *Br. Med. J.* **1**, 1630.
Conn H. O. and Blitzer B. L. (1976) *N. Eng. J. Med.* **294**, 473 – 479.
De Fronzo R. A., Goldberg M., Cooke C. R. et al. (1977) Investigation into the mechanism of hyperkalaemia following renal transplantation. *Kidney Int.* **11**, 357 – 365.
Festenstein J., Sachs J. A., Paris A. M. I. et al. (1976) Influence of HLA matching and blood transfusion on outcome of 502 London Transplant Group renal-graft recipients. *Lancet* **1**, 157 – 161.
Gabriel R. et al. (1976) *Nephron* **16**, 282 – 286.
Hoover R. and Fraumeni J. F. (1973) Risks of cancer in renal transplant recipients. *Lancet* **2**, 55.

Jones R. H. et al. (1978) *Br. Med J.* **1**, 398 – 400.
McGeown M. G., Loughridge W. G. G., Alexander J. A. et al. (1977) One hundred kidney transplants in the Belfast City Hospital. *Lancet* **2**, 648 – 651.
Mathew T. H., Kincaid-Smith P. and Vikraman P. (1977) Risks of vesico-ureteric reflux in the transplanted kidney. *N. Engl. J. Med.* **297**, 414 – 418.
Mathew T. H. et al. (1975) *Am. J. Med.* **59**, 177 – 190.
Mauer S. M., Bar osa J., Vernier R. L. et al. (1976) Development of diabetic vascular lesions in normal kidneys transplanted into patients with diabetes mellitus. *N. Engl. J. Med.* **295**, 916 – 920.
Opelz G. and Terasaki P. I. (1974) *Lancet* **2**, 696.
Owens M. L., Wilson S. E., Saltzman R. et al. (1976) Gastrointestinal complications after renal transplantation. *Arch. Surg.* **111**, 467 – 471.
Perkins H. A. and Salvatierra O. (1977) Correlation of renal allograft survival with previous blood transfusion. *Transplant. Proc.* **9**, Suppl. 1, 209 – 210.
Petersen U. P., Olsen T. S., Kissmeyer-Nielsen F. et al. (1975) Late failure of human renal transplants. An analysis of transplant disease and graft failure among 125 recipients surviving for one to eight years. *Medicine (Baltimore)* **54**, 45.
Pletka P. G., Strom T. B., Hampers C. L. et al. (1976) Secondary hyperparathyroidism in human transplant recipients. *Nephron* **17**, 371 – 381.
Sheil A. G. R. (1977) Cancer in renal allograft recipients in Australia and New Zealand. *Transplant. Proc.* **9**, 1129 – 1132.
Turner D. R., Cameron J. S., Bewick M. et al. (1976) Transplantation in mesangio-capillary glomerulonephritis with intramembranous 'dense deposits'. Recurrence of disease. *Kidney Int.* **9**, 439.
Uldall P. R. et al. (1977) *Lancet* **2**, 316 – 319.
Zincke H. and Woods J. E. (1977) *Surg. Gynecol. Obstet.* **145**, 183 – 188.

CONVERTING ENZYME INHIBITOR

M. J. VANDENBURG BSc, MB, BS, MRCP

In 1965 Ferreira isolated an extract from the venom of *Bothrops Jararaca,* containing a number of peptides (Ferreira, 1965), which has been shown to inhibit the conversion of angiotensin 1 (A1) to angiotensin 2 (A2). The most potent and long-acting of the peptides was a nonapeptide which has been synthesized and its amino-acid sequence established by Ondetti at the Squibb Institute and by others. This nonapeptide, SQ20881, has been shown to be an inhibitor of A1 converting enzyme (CE), and blocks the effect of A1 in animals and in man. It also blocks the degradation of the vasodilator bradykinin by inhibiting the enzyme kininase 2, which has been shown to be identical with converting enzyme.

SQ20881 may be used to study the role of the renin-angiotensin system in blood pressure control. Other compounds have already been used to try to elucidate this role. Propranolol depresses the release of renin and has been shown to depress blood pressure in proportion to the initial level of plasma renin, although others have been unable to confirm this. Saralasin, an octapeptide competitive inhibitor of A2, has also been used extensively but suffers from the disadvantage of possessing A2 agonist activity which causes a pressor response in some subjects who have low plasma renin activity.

CE inhibitors have been shown to reduce the blood pressure in animal models where abnormalities of the renin-angiotensin system are thought to be important, but not in those where changes in circulating volume are postulated as being the major factor contributing to the maintenance of the high blood pressure (Miller et al., 1972). SQ20881 has been shown to be active when given intravenously, subcutaneously and intramuscularly; however, it is not active when given orally. An oral CE inhibitor is undergoing evaluation in trials and its effect when given to normal subjects has been reported (Ferguson et al., 1977).

CE inhibition has been used to try to determine the role of the renin-angiotensin system in normal subjects. In sodium-depleted volunteers it had no consistent effect on the blood pressure in either the upright or the supine position but did cause a rise in plasma renin without an associated rise in aldosterone. In sodium-depleted normal subjects it caused a marked fall in blood pressure on tilting with a rise in plasma renin and a fall in aldosterone (Sancho et al., 1976). The rise in renin may be reduced by propranolol (Willard, 1976).

When given to subjects with various forms of hypertension it often caused a sustained fall in blood pressure. The fall was shown to be most marked in subjects with high plasma renin, but, in contrast to saralasin, it did have an effect in the majority of patients with essential hypertension with normal plasma renin. Hypertensive patients with chronic renal failure in whom circulatory volume overload was thought to be present did not respond (Gavras et al., 1974). Subsequently it was demonstrated that in a similar group of 64 hypertensive patients, again of mixed aetiology, the fall in blood pressure obtained correlated well with the initial plasma renin, and the hyperreninaemia produced. All patients with a high initial plasma renin and most with a normal level of renin responded (Case et al., 1977). Both papers showed that sodium depletion, induced by dietary restriction, diuretic therapy or dialysis, caused an exaggerated hypotensive response to the converting enzyme inhibitor.

It has been argued that the fall in blood pressure is due to blockade of the renin-angiotensin system alone and that inhibition of bradykinin degradation plays no part. However, it has recently been shown that administration of a CE inhibitor induces a prolonged elevation of plasma bradykinin when given to hypertensive patients (Williams and Hollenberg, 1977) whereas in normal subjects the increase was absent (Sancho et al., 1976) or only transient (Mersey et al., 1977). This may indicate that hypertensive patients metabolize bradykinin differently from normal subjects, perhaps owing to decreased levels of alternate degrading enzymes , or to a relative difference in the affinity of the converting enzyme for SQ20881, A1 and bradykinin. Therefore, in hypertensive patients CE inhibition, with SQ20881, cannot be used alone to evaluate participation of the renin-angiotensin system in the elevation of blood pressure.

CE inhibition with SQ20881 has been used to treat severely hypertensive patients (Johnson et al., 1975). In 12 patients who were given intravenous CE inhibitor for a period of 2 – 7 days good blood pressure control was obtained in all those with high plasma renin and half those whose plasma renin was normal. Again diuresis and dialysis were shown to enhance the hypotensive effect. It has also been given to patients with pre-eclamptic toxaemia who remained hypertensive after delivery. It had no effect on the blood pressure unless they were salt-depleted, thereby demonstrating that A2 is not directly involved in the aetiology of pre-eclamptic toxaemia.

CE inhibition has also been shown to increase renal blood flow despite a reduction of blood pressure. This was associated with a rise in plasma bradykinin (Williams and Hollenberg, 1977).

Future uses of converting enzyme inhibition

The compound will continue to be used as an investigational tool to elucidate pathogenic mechanisms in hypertension, particularly the roles of the renin-angiotensin and the bradykinin-kallikrein systems.

There may also be a place for CE inhibition in the assessment of renin-dependent hypertensive patients as a screening procedure before more invasive investigations such as arteriography, as it is known that the fall in blood pressure it produces is proportional to the initial level of plasma resin.

There is no doubt that SQ20881 is a powerful antihypertensive drug, whether through its potentiation of vasodilator, or inhibition of vasoconstrictor mechanisms. Very few side effects have been reported. It has caused two local reactions, both transient, but there has been no evidence of damage to renal, hepatic, cardiac or bone marrow function. It has caused profound hypotension when combined with diuretic therapy and ganglionic blockade (Duhme et al., 1974), although this might have been anticipated since all the systems known to maintain blood pressure were interfered with.

The author has given SQ20881 successfully to a patient with severe refractory renal hypertension for 5 months, and it is likely that when an oral CE inhibitor is generally available it will be an effective hypotensive drug in resistant cases of high-renin hypertension.

REFERENCES

Case D. B., John W. M., Keim H. J. et al. (1977) Possible role of renin in hypertension as suggested by renin-sodium profiling and inhibition of converting enzyme. *N. Engl. J. Med.* **296**, 641 – 646.

Duhme D. W., Sancho J., Athanosoulis L. et al. (1974) Hypotension during administration of angiotensin converting enzyme inhibitor SQ20881. *Lancet* **1**, 408 – 409.

Ferguson R. K., Turini G. A., Brunner H. R. et al. (1977) A specific orally active inhibitor of angiotensin converting enzyme in man. *Lancet* **1**, 775 – 778.

Ferreira S. H. (1965) *Br. J. Pharmacol.* **24**, 163 – 169.

Gavras H. et al. (1974) *N. Engl. J. Med.* **219**, 817 – 821.

Johnson J. G., Black W. D., Vukovitch R. A. et al. (1975) Treatment of patients with severe hypertension by inhibition of A – C-Enzyme. *Clin. Sci. Mol. Med.* **48**, 533 – 563.

Mersey J. H., Williams G. H., Hollenberg N. K. et al. (1977) Relationship between aldosterone and bradykinin. *Circ. Res.* **40**, Suppl. 1, 84 – 88.

Miller E. D., Samuels A. I., Haber E. et al. (1972) Inhibition of angiotensin conversion in experimental renovascular hypertension. *Science* **177**, 1108 – 1109.

Sancho J., Re R., Burton J. et al. (1976) The role of the renin – angiotensin – aldosterone system in cardiovascular homeostasis in normal human subjects. *Circulation* **53**, 400 – 405.

Willard D. A. (1976) Effects of beta blockade and angiotensin infusion on SQ20881-induced hyperreninemia in sodium depleted subjects. *77th Annual Meeting of the American Society for Clinical Pharmacology and Therapeutics, March 19, 1976, Seattle, Washington, U.S.A.*

Williams G. H. and Hollenberg N. K. (1977) Accentuated vascular and endocrine response to SQ20881 in hypertension. *N. Engl. J. Med.* **297**, 184 – 188.

DIALYSIS ENCEPHALOPATHY

V. L. SHARMAN MA, MB, BChir, MRCP

Recently a new neurological syndrome has been recognized in patients receiving maintenance haemodialysis therapy. Since the original report of this condition from Denver (Alfrey et al., 1972) a similar syndrome has been observed in dialysis units in Europe, Japan and Australia, and in other centres in the U.S.A. The disease is a significant cause of death in patients in some haemodialysis centres.

Dialysis encephalopathy may occur at any time after starting haemodialysis treatment but is unusual in the first year. It usually presents with stuttering or slurring of speech occurring towards the end of each dialysis and this is followed later by dysarthria, dysphasia and dyspraxia which may progress over a few months, making speech unintelligible. Myoclonic jerks are common and all patients eventually develop a global dementia. Personality changes, paranoid thinking, psychosis, delirium and seizures may occur. The EEG is always markedly abnormal, showing paroxysmal high voltage theta and delta waves with frequent bursts of spike and slow waves. Brain histology is non-specific and often minimal. The syndrome is nearly always progressive and usually ends in death 3 – 15 months after its onset (Burks et al., 1976).

Haemodialysis patients are exposed to the double risk of depletion of essential factors or accumulation of toxic substances and the widespread prescription of aluminium hydroxide to control hyperphosphataemia in dialysis patients focused attention on aluminium as a cause of the syndrome. It was originally assumed that the aluminium was excreted as insoluble aluminium phosphate in the faeces with negligible absorption of metal. However, some years ago Berlyne et al. (1970) showed increased aluminium levels in the blood of some uraemic patients taking aluminium hydroxide and subsequently suggested that this could lead to toxic effects (Berlyne et al., 1972). Further studies have shown a positive balance of 100 – 568 mg per day of aluminium in uraemic patients given aluminium hydroxide (Clarkson et al., 1972) and a marked rise in serum aluminium when it is given to normal subjects (Kaehny et al., 1977). It has been known for several years that aluminium may be retained in the bones of dialysis patients, even when aluminium hydroxide has not been given (Parsons et al., 1971), but the role of aluminium in the aetiology of dialysis encephalopathy was only recently suggested by the finding of four times the concentration of aluminium in the grey matter of patients who had died of the syndrome compared with a control group of non-encephalopathic patients undergoing dialysis (Alfrey et al., 1976).

The source of aluminium in patients with dialysis encephalopathy was originally assumed to be oral aluminium hydroxide, but this did not explain the disorder in patients with the syndrome who had never taken this treatment, nor its absence in the large numbers of patients taking aluminium hydroxide without developing toxic effects, nor the fact that 70 per cent of cases of the syndrome reported in the United Kingdom were derived from only four dialysis units. This situation was clarified by Flendrig et al. (1976 a and b) who described the experience of two dialysis centres in Holland. These centres used the same dialysis equipment and procedures and the same source of tap water, yet in one unit 6 patients developed encephalopathy whereas those in the other unit were spared the condition. Measurement of the dialysate fluid aluminium concentration revealed a seventeenfold difference between the two centres and it was concluded that this explained the different incidence of the syndrome. The source of aluminium was two aluminium anodes forming part of a cathodic protection system against corrosion in the boiler supplying the water to one centre but not the other. Over a period of two years the anodes had completely eroded forming a precipitate of aluminium hydroxide at the bottom of the boiler.

Further supportive evidence for the importance of the composition of dialysate fluid has come from Sheffield (Platts et al., 1977). The water supplying the homes of patients with encephalopathy was found to contain significantly less calcium and fluorine and significantly more aluminium and manganese. The concentration of aluminium in the water supply of 8 of the 10 patients with encephalopathy was at least twice that found in the water supply to patients without encephalopathy. In addition, 5 pairs of patients in the Sheffield area had used the same houses for dialysis and of these patients 3 pairs had developed encephalopathy, strongly suggesting an environmental cause for their disease.

A close association between encephalopathy and bone disease has been recognized. Ward et al. (1976) described 14 patients with encephalopathy in Newcastle, 13 of whom had renal osteodystrophy with severe osteomalacia and a low serum alkaline phosphatase concentration. This form of osteomalacia is thought to be due to phosphate depletion. In 4 patients the progress of the dementia was halted by withdrawing aluminium treatment and adding phosphate to the dialysate, suggesting that phosphate depletion may be an important exacerbating factor.

It is difficult to dissociate aluminium overload from phosphate depletion since the latter is a direct consequence of the former, but it is of interest that all the Newcastle patients who developed encephalopathy were dialysing in an area where the water content of aluminium was high. Since the recent installation of deionizers, to remove aluminium from the water supply, in the homes of all patients receiving home dialysis treatment in the Newcastle area, no further cases of encephalopathy have been seen.

The case against aluminium is not yet totally proved as it is possible that aluminium needs another factor to cause disease or is a marker for an undetermined toxin in the water supply. However, the evidence is slowly becoming more convincing.

REFERENCES

Alfrey A. C., Mishell J. M., Burks J. et al. (1972) Syndrome of dyspraxia and multifocal seizures associated with chronic haemodialysis. *Trans. Am. Soc. Artif. Intern. Organs* **18**, 257 – 261.
Alfrey A. C., LeGendre G. R., Kaehny W. D. (1976) The dialysis encephalopathy syndrome: possible aluminium intoxication. *N. Engl. J. Med.* **294**, 184 – 188.
Berlyne G. M., Ben Ari J., Pest D. et al. (1970) Hyperaluminaemia from aluminium resins in renal failure. *Lancet* **2**, 494 – 496.
Berlyne G. M., Yagil R., Ben Ari J. et al. (1972) *Lancet* **1**, 564 – 567.
Burks J. S., Alfrey A. C., Huddlestone J. et al. (1976) *Lancet* **1**, 764 – 768.
Clarkson E. M. et al., (1972) *Clin. Sci.* **43**, 519 – 531.
Flendrig J. A., Kruis H., Das H. A. (1976a) *Lancet* **1**, 1235.
Flendrig J. A., Kruis H., Das H. A. (1976b) Aluminium intoxication: the cause of dialysis dementia? In: Robinson B. H. B., Vereerstraeten P. and Hawkins J. B. (ed.), *Proceedings of the European Dialysis and Transplantation Association,* Vol. 13. London, Pitman Medical, pp. 355 – 361.
Kaehny W. D. et al. (1977) *N. Engl. J. Med.* **296**, 1389 – 1390.
Parsons V. et al. (1971) *Br. Med. J.* **4**, 273 – 275.
Platts M. M., Goode G. C., Hislop J. S. (1977) Composition of the domestic water supply and the incidence of fractures and encephalopathy in patients on home dialysis. *Br. Med. J.* **2**, 657 – 660.
Ward M. K., Pierides A. M., Fawcett P. et al. (1976) Dialysis encephalopathy syndrome. In: Robinson B. H. B., Vereerstraeten P. and Hawkins J. B. (ed.), *Proceedings of the European Dialysis and Transplantation Association,* Vol. 13. London, Pitman Medical, pp. 348 – 354.

Surgical

THE INCIDENCE OF CALCULUS DISEASE

J. P. MITCHELL TD, MS, FRCS, FRCSE

In recent years the possible epidemiological factors in the aetiology of urinary calculi have attracted increasing attention. In the underdeveloped countries today, as in Europe 200 years ago, the incidence of vesical calculus was common and probably much greater than that of renal calculi (Batty Shaw, 1970). In areas of East Anglia the condition was 10 times as common as in London—50 per cent of the victims being children and by far the majority being young boys. Various causes have been suggested from Vitamin A deficiencies to recurrent dehydration from endemic gastroenteritis. Many children in endemic stone areas have hypercalciuria, hypophosphaturia (inorganic phosphate), and a low urinary pH. Gaches et al. (1975) have suggested that the hardness of water at a specific pH may offer one possible explanation of the curious distribution of endemic areas in which communities with otherwise identical living standards were shown to have a high incidence of stone in childhood when the water supply had a calcium level of 200 parts per million of Ca CO_3 with a pH of $8 \cdot 0$, whereas neighbouring communities with different water supplies showed a negligible incidence of stone. In Europe the relative disappearance of the vesical calculus has been attributed to dietary and nutritional factors as well as improvements in standards of hygiene (Thomas, 1949; Andersen, 1962). The animal protein content of the diet may be the principal contributing factor (Andersen, 1972).

In contrast the renal stone has shown a steady increase from the turn of the last century until the present day in countries of Western Europe, North America, Japan, and Australia. The earliest appreciation of this change was by Hedenberg (1951), who made a study of renal and ureteric stone in Sweden from 1911 to 1938. Various writers have commented on the effects of the World Wars on the incidence of stone in the upper urinary tract and have each shown in surveys of different Western Countries that the number of cases fell during each war and particularly in the initial post-war period (Boshamer, 1961; Schumann, 1963; Andersen, 1972), only to increase again at an even more rapid rate as soon as the period of dietary stringency was over. Despite the fact that urinary tract infection is more common in the female, stone in the upper urinary tract is twice as common in the male during middle life. Finally, renal calculi have a much higher recurrence rate than do vesical calculi, as shown by Williams (1963) and Blacklock (1969); in fact it would appear that the incidence of recurrence is directly proportional to the length and accuracy of the investigators' follow-up (Williams, 1977).

Improvements in diagnostic methods and surgical techniques presumably can account for some of the increase in recognition of stone in the upper tract, but it is worthy of note that diagnoses of stone in the kidney were made long before the discovery of X-rays. The account appears in the writings of John Aubrey, where he described the Mariner of Bristowe, who was operated on for stone in the kidney by Dominic de Marchetti at Padua in the year 1680 (Murphy, 1969).

Environmental factors of climate, brackish water supply, ultraviolet light (Parry and Lister, 1975), and occupation (such as the sedentary worker, or the labourer in a hot dry atmosphere) can all contribute as localizing effects in endemic stone areas. As well as the probable variation in ethnic predisposition and life-style, the principal feature in analysis of the epidemiology of stone seem to point to nutrition and diet being the common denominator. Historical trends, and geographic and familial associations all suggest the significance of nutrition and diet in the epidemiology of both upper and lower urinary tract stones (Blacklock, 1976). The disappearance of the vesical calculus on improved protein diet has been well illustrated by Pavone et al. (1965); in their series from Sicily they also showed transient reappearance of the vesical calculus during the Second World War, when protein intake again fell for a 6-year interval.

As regards the upper urinary tract, stone appears to be a disease which is on the increase in the more affluent countries, where there has been a steady increase of animal protein, animal fat, and refined sugar in the diet, which has, at the same time, shown a marked diminution of fibre. Much speculative evidence has been presented to support each and all of these four dietary factors. These are well surveyed by Blacklock (1976) who points out that Andersen (1972), in presenting his theory that the increase in renal stone may be due to increase in dietary animal protein, has in fact quoted from the areas which also have the greatest sugar intake.

Cleave (1974) has suggested that renal stone should be included in the 'saccharine diseases' syndrome, and, in support, has shown the parallel graphs of sugar intake and renal stone both diminishing in each of the World Wars. Blacklock and Macleod (1974) have shown increased calcium absorption in renal stone formers; carbohydrates can increase intestinal absorption of calcium (Vaughan and Filer, 1960); increasing and decreasing carbohydrate in the form of refined sugar can correspondingly vary the amount of calcium in the urine in healthy normal individuals. In addition, small variations in urinary oxalate can be shown to correlate with the carbohydrate in the diet, though the possible explanations are hypothetical.

Only time will show whether today's propaganda to promote a high fibre diet with emphasis on bran and fresh fruit while also reducing the refined sugar and animal fats will bring with it a corresponding reduction in the incidence of renal calculi. At the same time the increasing cost of tea may help to reduce the oxalate content of our diet.

It seems likely in the future that epidemiological studies will throw more light on the aetiology of stone than have the studies carried out in stone clinics in the Western World, where patients with recurrent calculus disease are invariably placed on multiple therapy (Rose, 1977) in the form of increased fluid intake, low calcium diet, and one or more drugs to vary the pH, treat infection, or adjust the urinary or blood chemistry.

REFERENCES

Andersen D. A. (1962) Nutritional significance of primary bladder stones. *Br. J. Urol.* **34,** 160.
Andersen D. A. (1972) Environmental factors in the aetiology of urolithiasis. In: *Urinary Calculi: International Symposium.* Basle, Karger, pp. 130–144.
Batty Shaw A. (1970) The Norwich school of lithotomy. *Med. Hist.* **14,** 221.
Blacklock N. J. (1969) The pattern of urolithiasis in the Royal Navy. In: *Renal Stone Research Symposium.* London, Churchill, p. 33.
Blacklock N. J. (1976) Epidemiology of urolithiasis In: Williams, D. I. and Chisholm, G. D. *Scientific Foundations of Urology,* vol. 1. London, Heinemann Medical, p. 235.

Blacklock N. J. and Macleod M. (1974) 47-Calcium absorption in urolithiasis. *Br. J. Urol.* **46,** 377.
Boshamer K. (1961) The calculus areas of the world. In: *Handbook of Urology,* vol. 10. Berlin, Springer Verlag, p. 34.
Cleave T. L. (1974) *The Saccharine Disease.* Bristol, Wright.
Gaches C. G. C., Gordon I. R. S., Shore D. F. and Roberts J. B. M. (1975) Urinary lithiasis in childhood in the Bristol Clinical Area. *Br. J. Urol.* **47,** 109.
Hendenberg I. (1951) Renal and ureteric calculi: a study of the occurrence in Sweden during 1911 to 1938. *Acta Chir. Scand.* **101,** 17.
Murphy L. J. T. (1969) Reported by Mitchell J. P. In: *The History of Urology.* Springfield, Ill., Thomas, p. 78.
Parry E. S. and Lister I. (1975) Sunlight and hypercalciuria. Lancet **1,** 1063.
Pavone M., Piazza B. and Medonia S. (1965) Modification of statistical indices of urolithiasis in Sicily. *Rass. Urol. Nephrol.* **3,** 17.
Rose G. A. (1977) Biochemical aspects of urinary stones. *Proc. R. Soc. Med.* **70,** 517.
Schumann H. J. (1963) Die Haufigkeit der Urolithiasis im Sektionsgut des Pathologischen Institutes St. George, Leipzig. *Zentrabbl. Allg. Pathol.* **105,** 88.
Thomas J. M. R. (1949) Vesical calculus in Norfolk. *Br. J. Urol.* **21,** 20.
Vaughan O. W. and Filer L. J. (1960) The enhancing effects of certain carbohydrates on the intestinal absorption of calcium in the rat. *J. Nutr.* **71,** 10.
Williams R. E. (1963) Long term survey of 538 patients with upper urinary tract stones. *Br. J. Urol.* **35,** 416.
Williams R. E. (1977) Renal calculus follow-up. Communication to joint meeting of British Association of Urological Surgeons and Association of Surgeons, Royal College of Surgeons, 1 April 1977.

URODYNAMIC STUDIES AS A SERVICE COMMITMENT

R. C. L. FENELEY MChir, FRCS
P. H. ABRAMS FRCS

During the past two decades, the need for clinical measurement has been recognized in many branches of medicine. In urology, the need for an accurate diagnosis in functional disorders, and voiding problems in particular, has resulted in the rapid development of equipment and methods enabling the measurements of pressure and flow in the urinary tract. Such pressure – flow measurements are known as urodynamic studies. They have now passed the stage of pure research interest and are coming to be regarded as an essential part of the investigation of many urological patients.

A high proportion of patients referred for a urological problem present with lower urinary tract symptoms. These symptoms include those of frequency, urgency, incontinence, and urine flow problems. In many cases the conventional investigations of bacteriology, radiology, and endoscopy fail to provide a satisfactory explanation for the patient's symptoms. Urodynamics, as the name implies, provides dynamic evidence as to the function of the patient's lower urinary tract. This has led to a revision of attitudes in treating several groups of patients, in particular the older male patient with prostatism and the parous middle-aged woman with incontinence. The need for more accurate diagnosis has been highlighted by the recent publications of papers quoting a proportion of disappointing results for prostatectomy and repair operations respectively (Abrams, 1977; Stanton, 1977). Urodynamics have shown in these two groups of patients how failure to recognize abnormalities of bladder activity have led to poor case selection for surgery.

Urodynamic concepts

The control of continence and micturition depends on the synergic balance between bladder or detrusor activity on the one hand and the outflow resistance provided by the bladder neck, the urethra, and the para-urethral structures on the other.

In dynamic terms, continence of urine may be expressed as follows:

$$\text{Intrinsic detrusor pressure} \quad < \quad \text{Maximum urethral pressure}$$
$$\text{(Approximately 10 cm } H_2O) \qquad \text{(Approximately 50 cm } H_2O)$$

During micturition, detrusor pressure rises above the urethral pressure, and urine flow measurements can be recorded. Urodynamic studies consist of an analysis of these parameters by measurement of detrusor pressures during filling and voiding, together with urethral pressures and urine flow.

Urodynamic studies

Urodynamic investigations have developed as a result of the enthusiasm of workers from several specialties, and provide an interesting example of the benefits that accrue from an interdisciplinary approach. The International Continence Society, now in its seventh year, has provided the forum for discussions which have led to the development of urodynamics as an essential study in urology. In this Society, clinicians, physiologists, physicists, and physiotherapists meet to present their work. Urodynamic studies are now service investigations in the fields of Urology, Gynaecology, Neurology, Geriatrics, Spinal Injury, and Paediatric Surgery.

THE TECHNIQUES

The equipment necessary for urodynamic studies is relatively expensive and requires specially trained medical and technical staff. Hitherto, most units have been confined to major urological centres.

Most pressure measurements involve the use of fluid-filled catheters in the bladder and rectum. These are connected to strain gauge pressure transducers and hence to recording equipment.

Urine flow rate may be measured using a variety of methods. Von Garrelts' weight transducer method is well tried and reliable, and provides a simultaneous display of flow and volume voided (Von Garrelts, 1957).

Although pressure – flow studies form the basis of urodynamic investigations, more sophisticated equipment providing synchronous video cystography and pelvic floor electromyography during the filling and voiding phases, may yield further information (Bates et al., 1970).

Bladder studies are undertaken by means of the filling and voiding cystometry with continuous recording of intravesical pressure, abdominal pressure, subtracted detrusor pressure, and urine flow rate (*Fig.* 1). These measurements are usually made via a fine urethral catheter but the suprapubic route is occasionally preferred. Intravesical pressure is the total pressure within the bladder but since this is influenced by changes in abdominal pressure, detrusor pressure is derived by subtraction of the abdominal pressure recorded via a rectal catheter. These three pressures are displayed simultaneously.

During the filling phase the volume at which the patient experiences an initial desire to micturate and the point when urgency of micurition occurs are recorded. The inflow is completed at this point.

The bladder should normally fill to a capacity of about $300-500$ ml at a destrusor pressure of less than 15 cm H_2O without evidence of leakage.

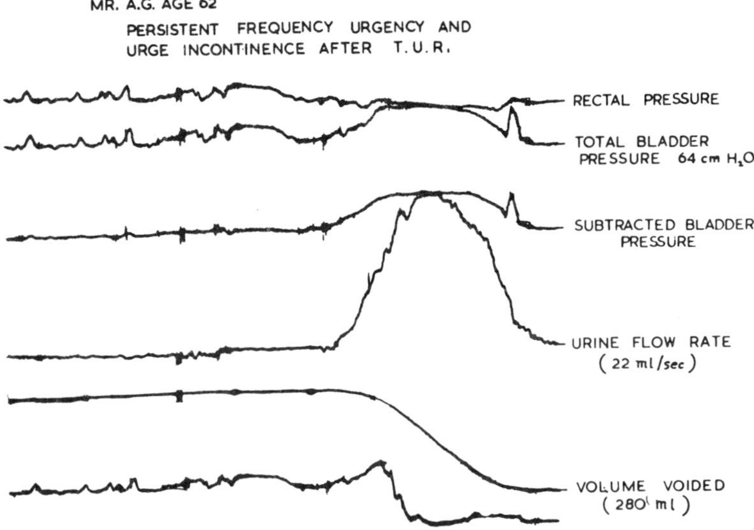

Fig. 1. To illustrate recording of abdominal pressure, total bladder pressure, urine flow rate and volume voided.

When the filling phase has been completed, the voiding phase commences. During micturition, continuous recording is made of the detrusor pressure, urine flow rate, and the volume voided. The detrusor pressure normally rises to about $40-60$ cm H_2O in men and $30-50$ cm in women. Maximum flow rates of $20-30$ ml per second are within the normal range. Women tend to produce flow rates at or above the upper limit of this range whereas the flow rates of men tend to be lower.

The urethral pressure profile is a method of assessing bladder outflow resistance. It is performed by withdrawing a fine catheter along the length of the urethra. This catheter is irrigated slowly and continuously with saline which escapes from two small openings on either side of its tip. The resistance of the saline flow varies according to the pressure exerted by the urethral wall at the catheter side holes. By recording the pressure change, a measure of urethral resistance is obtained. The outline of this tracing is termed the urethral pressure profile and the site of maximal urethral pressure is normally situated at the level of the external urethral sphincter, with levels of about $50-60$ cm H_2O. The patient may be asked to squeeze the urethra as if attempting to hold urine and by this manoeuvre may increase the urethral pressure to as much as 120 cm H_2O. Subsidiary rises of pressure may be recorded at the bladder neck or in the prostatic urethra. These increases in pressure are thought to represent the intrusion of the bladder neck or prostate into the urethral lumen (*Fig.* 2).

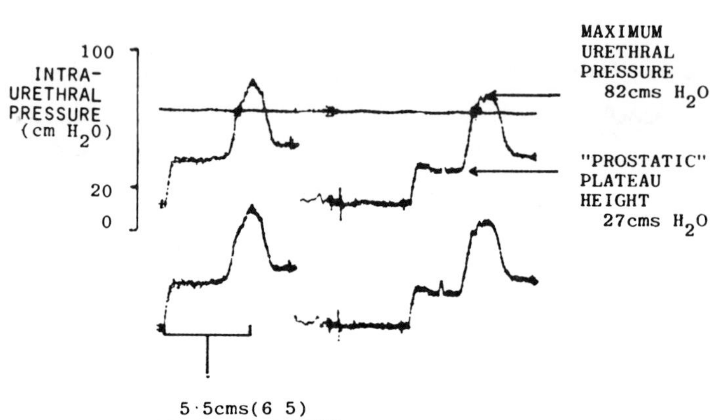

Fig. 2. Urethral pressure profile in a male patient with prostatic obstruction.

THE CLINICAL APPLICATION OF URODYNAMIC STUDIES

With the introduction of this method of assessing lower urinary tract problems, new criteria and classifications of common urological problems have been made possible. The measurement of urine flow avoids the embarrassment of observing the patient's urinary stream with the inevitable

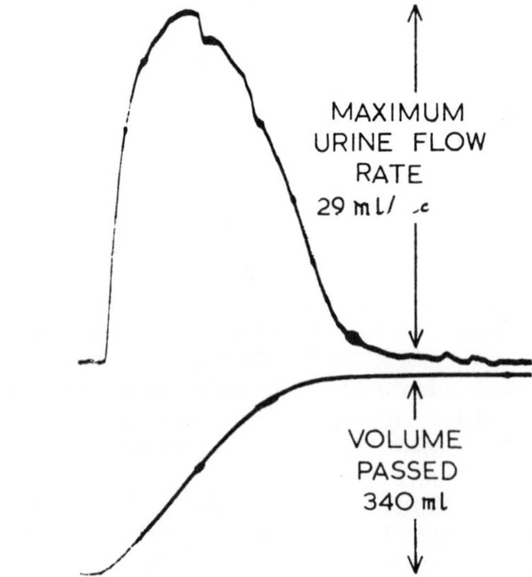

Fig. 3. A normal urine flow rate.

psychological inhibitory effect. The urine flow rate is a simple means of recording graphically the rate and volume of the urinary flow and provides a useful screening investigation in the Out-patient Clinic when voiding problems are suspected (*Fig.* 3).

DETRUSOR ABNORMALITIES

Detrusor abnormalities may be revealed during the filling phase of cystometry which measures the functional capacity of the bladder. This may be shown to be reduced or abnormally large. Particular attention has been focused on the finding of the unstable bladder. The condition is associated with bladder contractions during filling, with detrusor pressures above 15 cm H_2O which the patient is unable to inhibit (*Fig.* 4). They occur with or without the patient's awareness of urgency to micturate.

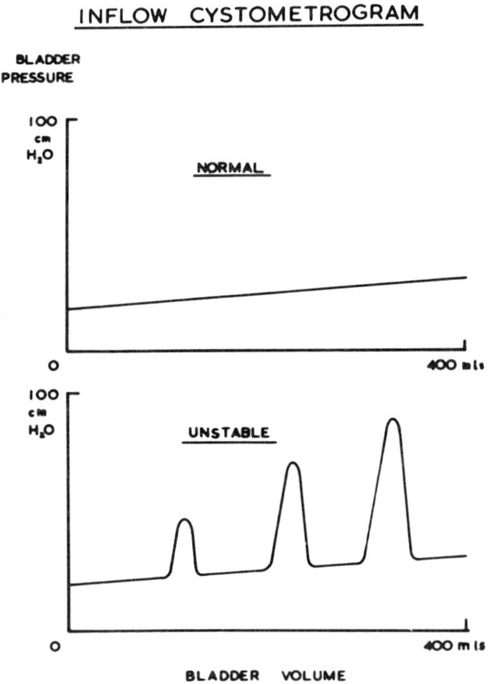

Fig. 4. Representing a normal cystometrogram and an unstable cystometrogram.

Bladder instability may be demonstrated when the patient is under investigation for frequency, urgency and urge incontinence of urine and thus it occurs in a wide group of clinical problems. It is commonly found in cases of enuresis, and also in a proportion of patients with prostatism and stress/urge incontinence. Furthermore, a high percentage of patients under investigation for unresolved symptoms following unsuccessful prostatic or gynaecological surgery have been shown to have this condition.

OUTFLOW PROBLEMS

Outflow abnormalities may be related to the detrusor or the outflow tract. Voiding cystometry, urine flow rates, and the urethral pressure profile give a clear analysis of the ability of the bladder to empty. The volume of residual urine is measured before and after cystometry. A high detrusor pressure with a low or intermittent urine flow suggests obstruction in the outflow tract, whereas a low detrusor pressure with poor urine flow indicates an abnormality of detrusor contraction.

By analysis of these urodynamic parameters, more accurate diagnosis of lower urinary tract problems is now possible. Many groups of common clinical conditions have been studied in detail, and it would be beyond the scope of this article to give more than brief examples of the importance of urodynamic application. For example, the assumption that the elderly man with frequency and urgency has outflow obstruction may be incorrect, as a reduced functional bladder capacity or an unstable bladder may be the cause of his symptoms. In many elderly patients with symptoms of frequency, urgency, and incontinence, bladder instability is a frequently recognized condition and may or may not be associated with outflow obstruction.

Amongst the group of women with stress and stress/urge incontinence, urodynamic investigations have allowed more accurate selection of patients for surgery. It has been shown that the operative results in those patients with unstable bladders are so poor that surgery should be avoided. The clinical differentiation between pure stress and stress/urge incontinence in women has always been a pitfall in clinical practice, and in this field urodynamics have made a valuable contribution. Geriatric incontinence and voiding problems in neurologically abnormal patients are further examples in which urodynamic studies help to define the detrusor or outflow abnormalities which may be present.

THE CLINICAL COMMITMENT TO URODYNAMIC STUDIES

The development of urodynamic investigations has clarified the basic physiological abnormalities in a wide group of micturition disorders which had previously defied accurate analysis. The demonstration of bladder instability as a factor involved with the large group of patients of all ages experiencing frequency, urgency, and incontinence problems should allow a more logical foundation for their therapeutic management.

Furthermore, these studies have contributed useful parameters which may be considered in certain grey areas of clinical judgement such as the prostatic group in men or the stress/urge incontinence group in women. By introducing accurate scientific definitions to diagnosis, selection for operative or non-operative treatment should be improved, and the results of clinical management may be more critically assessed.

The time necessary for the investigation of a patient is between 30 and 40 minutes. With experience it is possible to shorten the investigation by undertaking selective studies. For example, in the elderly male patient a urine flow measurement and a residual urine estimation may be all that is required. When there is doubt whether the patient is obstructed or not, it is necessary to perform both inflow cystometry and a pressure – flow analysis of micturition.

At present, urodynamic units are mainly confined to the larger medical centres. In order that all patients may benefit from these investigations it is important that urodynmic screening becomes available in District General

Hospitals. The minimum investigation is that of urine flow measurement. It is probably desirable that the facility for inflow cystometry is also available in order to demonstrate the presence of bladder contractions during filling.

REFERENCES

Abrams P. H. (1977) Prostatism and prostatectomy: the value of urine flow rate measurement in the preoperative assessment for operation. *J. Urol.* **117,** 10.
Abrams P. H., Farrar D. J., Turner Warwick R. T. et al. (1977) The objective results of elective prostatectomy. Communication to Meeting of British Association of Urological Surgeons, Aberdeen, 1977.
Bates C. P., Whiteside C. G. and Turner Warwick R. T. (1970) Synchronous cine/pressure/flow cystourethrography with special reference to stress and urge incontinence. *Br. J. Urol.* **42,** 714.
Stanton S. L., Williams J. E., Ritchie D. et al. (1977) The urodynamic analysis of failed incontinence surgery in the female. Communication to Meeting of British Association of Urological Surgeons, Aberdeen, 1977.
Von Garrelts B. (1957) Intravesical pressure and urine flow during micturition in normal subjects. *Acta Chir. Scand.* **114,** 49.

MAJOR ADVANCES IN THE MANAGEMENT OF UROTHELIAL TUMOURS DURING THE LAST DECADE

J. P. MITCHELL TD, MS, FRCS, FRCSE

The major advances in the field of urothelial tumours during the last 10 years can be summarized under three headings: first, a better understanding of the natural history of the disease, including an assessment of the true value of histology and cytology; secondly, the conviction of certain bladder carcinogens; and thirdly, the number of stimulating new concepts on treatment which, though still in an immature state, offer to us some real hope of improvement in therapy within the next few years.

In 1969 the Bristol Bladder Tumour Registry presented its report, which was a survey of urothelial tumours in the South West of England over a period of 15 years (Miller et al., 1969). One of the problems that bedevils any survey of bladder tumours is the difficulty of developing a true lingua franca, hence the attempts to obtain international agreement on the International Union against Cancer (U.I.C.C.) for the urothelium (Wallace et al., 1975). Even though the principles of the T.N.M. classification of bladder tumours is supported by nearly all urologists in this country, it must nevertheless be admitted that the dividing line between T2 and T3 and again between T3 and T4 is anything but clear-cut when any group of cases is analysed (*Fig.* 5).

Much of the scepticism on the histology of transitional cell tumours was due to the inadequacy of the biopsies, as taken by the minute cystoscopic biopsy forceps, which could only remove at the most the tips of a few fronds. These were then extracted in a very damaged state, from which no pathologist could be expected to interpret sufficient information to grade the tumour.

The histological grading of a tumour was thought to vary in different parts of the tumour. For example, the periphery of a papilloma could be very different from the pedicle in histological appearance. Secondly, the histology of the periphery of the tumour would give no indication of the probability of invasion and, thirdly, the histology of the bladder tumours was thought to be changing constantly from one grade to another. With these preconceived ideas on bladder tumour histology it was no wonder that histological grading was not at first accepted in the International T.N.M. Classification.

The size of biopsy sections was improved with the introduction of larger biopsy forceps, which could still be introduced via an endoscopic sheath of comparatively small size. Most of the bladder biopsies taken for the Bristol Bladder Tumour Registry were obtained by means of the resectoscope.

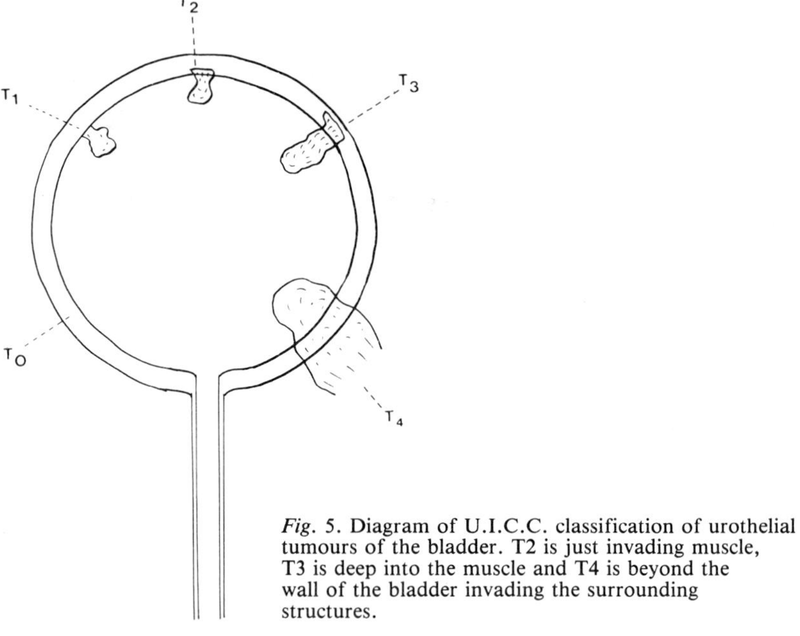

Fig. 5. Diagram of U.I.C.C. classification of urothelial tumours of the bladder. T2 is just invading muscle, T3 is deep into the muscle and T4 is beyond the wall of the bladder invading the surrounding structures.

Although the margins of such biopsies were slightly coagulated with the diathermy, the sections were still large enough to give the pathologist a satisfactory amount of undamaged tissue, and from this it was shown that a biopsy of the periphery of the tumour was, in fact, representative of the grading of the whole tumour throughout. It was also of interest to note that the endoscopic appearance of necrosis on the tips of the fronds was, in fact, a fairly consistent indication of the probability of invasion of the basement membrane, even through the mucosa into muscle. When tumours were resected in toto, cuts with the resectoscope dug well into the bladder wall would subsequently confirm or disprove the evidence of invasion. It is gratifying to note that now the International T.N.M. Classification has been extended to include histological grading.

Most pathologists and urologists are now agreed that truly benign tumours of the bladder wall are rare, probably somewhere in the region of 2–3 per cent at the most. A low-grade transitional cell carcinoma has obvious transitional epithelium more than five cells thick, with a regular basement cell showing palisade appearance. Some variation in size and shape of the cells and of the nuclei and occasional mitotic figures may be seen. An average grade tumour has transitional epithelium more than five cells thick, with an irregular basement cell, and nuclei tending to be circular and varying in size and density. More frequent mitoses could be seen. A high-grade tumour was one in which transitional epithelium was only just identifiable as such, there was a great variation in size and shape of the cells and the nuclei, and tumour giant cells could be seen with many very darkly staining nuclei and frequent mitoses. The distinction between low-grade and average grade is much more clear-cut than the distinction between average and high. This problem was not as serious as may appear at first becaue the ultimate prognosis between average and high was almost identical, except in the speed of progress. The ultimate outcome of low and average tumours showed a much more distinct difference.

The patient may occasionally develop a new tumour, totally different in endoscopic appearance and, unfortunately, always of a higher grade. It has been possible in very few cases to find two separate tumours of different grade co-existing within the bladder at the same time but by far the majority of recurrences show that for any one individual the characteristics of different generations of tumour are exactly the same, and often the area of bladder wall affected is the same for many years.

For over 25 years beta-naphthylamine has been incriminated as a bladder carcinogen. Its known source was at an intermediate stage in the production of aniline dyes, but, more recently, the rubber industry has also exposed its workers to this chemical. For 10 years it has been recognized officially as an industrial hazard, but other members of the benzine ring with the NH_2 appendage have been suspected. The evidence against smoking as a bladder carcinogen is rather more circumstantial (Cole et al., 1971). The finding of amino-phenols in the urine of regular smokers has suggested the possibility of some disorder in the metabolism of tryptophane. Rose and Wallace (1973) have quoted a higher level of chemiluminescent products in the urine of smokers than in non-smokers. Certain substances, when coming into contact with urothelium, develop this property of chemiluminescence. This production of visible or ultraviolet light is thought to cause intracellular changes which may go on to malignancy. Two aromatic amines, magenta and auramine, are under suspicion. Magenta is manufactured from orthotoludine, which may itself be a carcinogen. Johannsen et al. (1974) have produced evidence in Sweden that taking large quantities of phenacetin is associated with urothelial tumours. The effect of phenacetin on the kidney, producing a drug nephropathy, has been fully described in the past, but this is the first suggestion of the drug being carcinogenic. The related analgesic, Panadol, may very well come under suspicion. Lastly, the drinking of coffee has been claimed to have shown an association with cancer of the lower urinary tract (Cole et al., 1971).

Turning now to the treatment of bladder tumours, it has been shown that the most successful line of approach for the tumour under $2 \cdot 5$ cm diameter is a transurethral resection removing the whole tumour and a partial thickness of the bladder wall at the base of the tumour. If the histology of the tumour shows low grade, with or without superficial invasion of the bladder wall, then probably transurethral resection will be sufficient to destroy the tumour. If the histology is average or high grade the surgery is supplemented by radiotherapy.

We are left with three major problems in the management of bladder tumours: first the T3, T4 advanced tumour; secondly, the patient with multiple papillomatosis of low grade histology; and, thirdly, the somewhat indeterminate condition of carcinoma in situ, classified under U.I.C.C. as TIS.

To deal with these in the reverse order: carcinoma in situ, although agreed and accepted as an entity by all urologists and pathologists, has a slightly vague boundary from mucosal hyperplasia. Macroscopically, the bladder usually shows an unpleasant and suspicious patchy lesion. Failure to respond to radiotherapy in any form or intracavity treatment leaves only one course open, namely total cystectomy. This is nearly always an extremely hard decision to make in a patient who is showing no frank proliferative tumour of the bladder wall, but the prognosis of carcinoma in situ is universally agreed to justify such drastic surgery.

The real problem arises in the patient with symptoms, yet with a bladder mucosa which could pass as normal on endoscopy. Because of the symptoms a quadrant biopsy is taken. If this is returned as carcinoma in situ few surgeons would be prepared to embark on total cystectomy in the absence of any abnormality visible on endoscopy. Histology of specimens removed at total cystectomy show the distribution of carcinoma in situ throughout the bladder can be very irregular, and therefore a negative quadrant biopsy could miss these areas. Hence the possibility of carcinoma in situ being present, or the random biopsy specimen which proves positive despite no abnormality on endoscopy, demands repeated endoscopy at least at 6-monthly intervals for a period of 3 years, which is the accepted limit for carcinoma in situ to become manifest.

Multiple papillomatosis is the term used for several tumours of equal size co-existing on the bladder mucosa. The aetiology is very suggestive of either a generalized spontaneous change in the urothelium, or a simultaneous carcinogenic activity. The tumours are nearly always low grade, but only a few can be completely eradicated by transurethral resection. On the whole, the tumours do not respond to radiotherapy, and various methods of treatment have therefore been suggested.

Intracavity radiation use to be generated as a point source of radioactive material in the tip of a catheter surrounded by an equally distensible balloon, so that the bladder became a perfect sphere with this point source at the exact centre (*Fig.* 6). A second method was to distend the balloon with radioactive fluid (*Fig.* 7). This gave a more even distribution of radioactivity throughout the bladder wall, but both of these procedures suffered from the disadvantage that a balloon was essential, since the radioactive fluid must be recovered in toto. Otherwise it might have been preferable to instill the fluid free in the bladder to surround the tumours and intensify the radioactive dose at the pedicle of each tumour. The use of a bag, however, compresses each tumour against the bladder wall and thereby gives the same radioactive dose to the adjacent bladder as to the surface cells of the tumour. In fact, the adjacent bladder mucosa receives a considerably higher dose than the pedicle of a soft tumour compressed against the bladder wall. In Bristol, a series of cases were tried with a suspension of radioactive colloidal gold introduced into the bladder. A magnetic field was induced which could attract the gold to one particular part of the bladder wall carrying the tumour. Despite the ingenuity of this idea, the end results were disappointing.

The use of cytotoxic drugs within the bladder, first in the form of Podophyllum, then Thiotepa (Mitchell, 1971) was used, and, more recently,

Epodyl, in the treatment of low-grade multiple tumours (Riddle and Wallace, 1971). The dosage of Epodyl, however, is still empirical and the exact amount, and the frequency with which the treatment should be given, is still a matter of trial and error. Nevertheless, many dramatic improvements have been

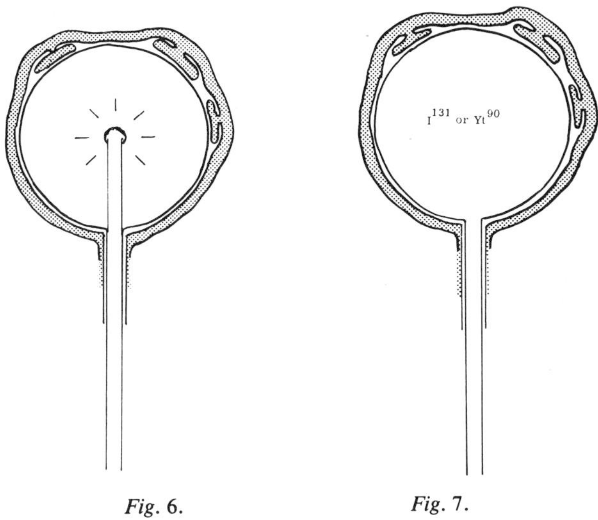

Fig. 6.   *Fig.* 7.

Fig. 6. Point source of radioactivity in the centre of a spherical balloon, to irradiate tumours of the bladder wall in multiple papillomatosis.

Fig. 7. Radioactive fluids in a distensible balloon, used in the treatment of multiple papillomatosis.

achieved with this form of therapy. It is essential that the entire bladder wall comes freely into contact with the cytotoxic drug, as it was found that the self-retaining balloon on the catheter used to introduce the Epodyl could, in fact, protect the bladder mucosa around the neck of the bladder from contact with the drug. The result of this was a persistence of tumour around the neck of the bladder and in the proximal urethra. The moral of this is presumably not to use a balloon catheter for intravesical cytotoxic therapy.

Helmstein's bladder distension has produced some remarkable improvements in neoplasm of the bladder (Helmstein, 1965). It has been used in the urinary tract for both the multiple papillomatosis as well as for the palliative treatment of the unpleasant T3, T4 tumours. The principle of this method of treatment is the insertion of a balloon into the bladder, which is distended to a pressure half-way between the patient's systolic and diastolic pressures. This is sustained under prolonged epidural anaesthesia for a period of 6 hours, producing ischaemia of the mucosa of the bladder wall and necrosis of more rapidly dividing cells, such as those of a neoplasm. In addition to this ischaemic effect, it is claimed hypothetically that a necrotic bladder tumour produces, in the host, an enhanced immune response against the original tumour. Many transient improvements have been claimed; but, as yet, there are no established cures, even in the case of multiple papillomatosis.

The third major problem in the management of neoplasm of the bladder is the care of the T3, T4 tumour which, if accurately staged from the clinical and endoscopic examination, would indicate a tumour beyond the reach of operative surgery. In Bristol, Symes (Consultant in Immunology) and Feneley (Urologist) have both been working on the effects of sensitized pig lymphocytes on these advanced tumours (*see* p. 325). Some of the results have been remarkable, and the most dramatic of all was a man whose tumour had fungated suprapubically into an extremely unpleasant discharging mass, occupying most of the bladder area of the suprapubic skin. Within 2 months of pig lymphocyte therapy, this man's proliferative tumour had vanished from the skin. On endoscopy of the bladder and on bimanual examination under anaesthetic, biopsies were taken from random areas and no tumour could be confirmed. This T4 tumour, as would be expected, eventually recurred 15 months after treatment, and was then rapidly progressive, the patient dying 4 months later, but at least he had been given 15 months of remarkably comfortable life.

Another method of treating bladder tumours of T3, T4 stage which received increasing interest about 2 years ago, was local hyperthermic perfusion of the bladder, a temperature being selected which will not damage normal healthy mucosa, but will necrose the more sensitive cells of a neoplasm (Hall et al., 1974). Unfortunately, at present this seems to be limited by the access of the heat to the tumour itself; as would be expected, reports seem to indicate that it is in fact only the surface of the tumours that shows the necrotic change.

In the management of T3, T4 tumours, the work of Shuttleworth and his colleagues at St Thomas's Hospital, using radiotherapy under hyperbaric oxygen, has given results statistically better than those of radical surgery, which, in these advanced cases, inevitably carries a high operative mortality (Shuttleworth, 1977).

Phototherapy, using a haematoporphyrin derivate and white light, is still very much in the experimental stage, but the first clinical trials have been carried out at St Mary's Hospital, Paddington.

Finally, the use of cytotoxic drugs is at present attracting increasing interest for the T3, T4 tumour. At Leeds, a cocktail of four cytotoxic drugs is being used in combination (Smith, 1977), while a further series recently reported from the Royal Marsden Hospital has concentrated on the use of Methotrexate alone, with some very encouraging results.

Progress in the last 10 years in the field of urothelial tumours has involved, primarily, a clearer understanding of the natural history of the disease, with convincing proof of the value of histological grading, which has now been shown to be consistent throughout all parts of the same bladder tumour. New carcinogens have been identified and other possible carcinogens are under suspicion. As regards therapy, there has been the development of the stimulating new concepts of immunotherapy, phototherapy, hyperthermia, and the use of cytotoxic drugs, so that even the problems of carcinoma in situ, the multiple papillomatosis, and the T3, T4 tumours have prospects of an improved prognosis.

REFERENCES

Cole P., Monsen R. R., Haning H. et al. (1971) Smoking and cancer of the lower urinary tract. *N. Engl. J. Med.* **284**, 129.

Hall R. R., Schade R. O. K. and Swinney J. (1974) Effects of hyperthermia on bladder cancer. *Br. Med. J.* **2**, 593.

Helmstein K. (1965) Hydrostatic pressure therapy—a new approach to the treatment of carcinoma of the bladder. *Opusc. Med. (Stockh.)* **11**, 328.

Johansson S., Angervall L., Bengtsson U. et al. (1974) Uroepithelial tumours of the renal pelvis associated with abuse of phenacetin-containing analgesics. *Cancer,* **33**, 743.

Miller A., Mitchell J. P. and Brown N. J. (1969) The Bristol Bladder Tumour Registry. *Br. J. Urol. suppl.* to No. 1, **41**, 1.

Mitchell R. J. (1971) Intravesical Thiotepa in the treatment of transitional cell bladder carcinoma. *Br. J. Urol.* **43**, 185.

Riddle P. R. and Wallace D. M. (1971) Intracavitary chemotherapy for multiple non-invasive bladder tumours. *Br. J. Urol.* **43**, 181.

Rose G. A. and Wallace D. M. (1973) Observations on urinary chemiluminescence of normal smokers and non-smokers and of patients with bladder cancer. *Br. J. Urol.* **45**, 520.

Shuttleworth K. E. D. (1975) Treatment of bladder tumour with radiotherapy and hyperbaric oxygen. Personal communication. In the press.

Smith P. H. (1977) Treatment of bladder tumours by cytotoxic therapy. Personal communication at informal meeting at The Institute of Urology, 7 October 1977.

Wallace D. M., Chisholm G. D. and Hendry W. F. (1975) T.N.M. classification of urological tumours (U.I.C.C.)—1974. *Br. J. Urol.* **47**, 1.

ADOPTIVE IMMUNOTHERAPY FOR URINARY BLADDER CANCER, USING TUMOUR-IMMUNE PIG LYMPH NODE CELLS

M. O. SYMES MD

Introduction

Adoptive immunity was a term coined by Medawar to denote the transfer of immunity by immunologically competent cells rather than serum.

The capacity for accelerated tumour rejection could be transferred from an animal which had rejected a particular tumour, to a second isogenic host, by parenteral injection of draining lymph node cells from the primary host (Mitchison, 1954). Such adoptive immunity was specific for the genotype of the tumour.

To apply this technique in man, cells would have to be transferred to the patient from an animal which had rejected the tumour to be treated. This poses a number of problems.

1. The choice of donor animal. The pig was selected, as it is readily available, free from infection, cheap and, most important, possesses a long chain of lymph nodes at the root of the mesentery. Thus it is possible to immunize these nodes by implantation of multiple tumour fragments between the leaves of the mesentery. The immune nodes are harvested 7 days later and a cell suspension prepared therefrom is injected into the arterial blood supply of the tumour to be treated.

2. The transferred pig cells will be rejected by the patient, thus terminating their anti-tumour action. The pig cells are immune to the tumour, whereas the patient is not sensitized to pig species antigen. So it may be expected that the anti-tumour action of the pig cells will be more rapid in onset than the rejection response of the patient. Therefore, significant tumour damage may result before the pig cells are rejected. Evidence of an anti-tumour effect will be presented later, but no evidence of immediate hypersensitivity to pig species

antigen has been noted in over 100 patients so far treated. As a precaution against this complication the pig cells are injected under general anaesthesia.

3. As the pig lymph node cells are immunized against human species antigens as well as any tumour-associated transplantation antigens that may be present on the tumour cells, there is a theoretical risk of inducing graft versus host disease in the patient. Graft versus host disease, characterized in man by a skin rash, lymphadenopathy, and fever following lymphocyte infusion, has *never* been observed in our patients. This is probably due to the rejection of the pig cells by the patient (*see above*); intra-arterial injection of the pig cells, which facilitates their contact with and reaction against the tumour; and the treatment of patients with large tumours. Only patients with clinical stage T3 or T4 histologically invasive lesions are considered suitable for this therapy. The ability of large tumours to 'absorb' the immunological attack of adoptively transfered cells and thus protect the host against the development of graft versus host disease has been demonstrated in mice by Symes (1967).

4. In theory it would be attractive to immunize the pig solely against tumour-associated transplantation antigens, thus rendering the pig cells specifically anti-tumour in their immunological action. This approach cannot be used, due to difficulty in isolating such antigens and the fact that they are not always present. A more important consideration is the 'weak' nature of tumour antigens, which elicit a poor immune response. By contrast, species antigens are strong and lead to a vigorous immune reaction. The latter is necessary if a useful anti-tumour effect is to be obtained, particularly when treating large neoplasms.

Studies in experimental animals

Woodruff and his colleagues (Woodruff, Symes and Stuart, 1963; Woodruff, Symes and Anderson, 1963) treated intraperitoneal transplants of the genetically non-specific Landschutz ascites tumour growing in F_1 Hybrid mice. The mice received tumour cells on day 0, sub-lethal whole body irradiation on day 4, and rat spleen cells or thoracic duct lymphocytes i.p. on day 5. Only tumour-immune rat cells delayed tumour growth, as measured by the time of appearance of the malignant ascites and the death of the animals.

Furthermore, thoracic duct lymphocytes were significantly more effective than spleen cells. In these experiments whole body irradiation was given as an immunosuppressant, designed to allow the rat cells longer to mediate their anti-tumour action. However, as explained above, this would also increase the liability of the tumour bearing host to develop graft versus host disease. Therefore, in subsequent experiments whole body irradiation was omitted. Alexander et al. (1966) also obtained growth inhibition of primary rat fibrosarcomata by adoptive transfer of lymphocytes from immunized sheep.

The necessity for immunized cells in order to produce an anti-tumour effect was further emphasized by the experiments of Prichard-Thomas and Symes (1978). They induced pulmonary metastases in A-strain mice by i.v. injections of A-strain mammary carcinoma cells. Three days later the mice received *local* thoracic irradiation and 7 days later pig cells i.v. The pig cells were either non-immune or tumour-immune, and only the latter reduced the number of metastases assessed on day 14. It was also shown that the pig cells had to be immunized against mouse tissue. Immunization against a human tumour was ineffective in inducing anti-tumour activity. The administration of pig cells without prior thoracic irradiation had no anti-tumour effect. Irradiation concentrated the injected pig cells in the lungs, as shown by experiments using ^{51}Cr labelled cells. The importance of localizing the transferred cells at the site of the tumour also influenced the design of the experiments by Woodruff and his colleagues wherein cells were given i.p. to treat ascites tumours.

Clinical studies

Two clinical studies have been carried out involving the treatment of transitional cell carcinoma of the urinary bladder by intra-arterial injection of tumour-immune pig lymph node cells.

In the first (Symes et l., 1978a), a series of 24 patients presented with recurrent invasive tumour following radical radiotherapy. Following pig lymph node cell therapy, as the only treatment, there was a remission of symptoms in 11 patients, and in 10 this was associated with a reduction in tumour size as assessed, radiologically, cystoscopically, and on pelvic examination under anaesthesia. At the same time, histological examination of pre- and post-treatment biopsies confirmed the presence of increased tumour necrosis following treatment. One of the patients is alive and well 4 years after treatment and 6 others lived for 1 year or more.

In the second study (Symes et al., 1978b), 23 patients were matched according to age, sex, T stage, and histological grade. The patients were divided into three groups which received tumour-immune pig lymph node cells followed 6 weeks later by 4000 rad, pig cells + 5500 rad, or 5500 rad alone. A further 14 matched patients received pig cells and/or 5500 rad.

There was no difference in the remission rates or survival times between the 16 patients receiving pig cells + 5500 rad and the 15 receiving 5500 rad alone.

However, a remission was observed in all 6 patients receiving pig cells + 4000 rad, compared with 6/9 remissions in the matched patients receiving pig cells + 5500 rad and 4/8 in those treated by 5500 rad alone. A remission was defined as relief of symptoms, a reduction in tumour size, and histological evidence of increased tumour necrosis. The median survival time, $21 \cdot 5$ months, in the patients receiving pig cells + 4000 rad was significantly greater than that in the other two groups of patients—$9 \cdot 0$ and $11 \cdot 0$ months respectively, ($P{<}0 \cdot 025$, $P{<}0 \cdot 05$).

REFERENCES

Alexander P., Delorme E. J. and Hall J. G. (1966) *Lancet* **1**, 1186.
Mitchison N. A. (1954) *Proc. R. Soc. Lond. (Biol.)* **142**, 72.
Pritchard-Thomas S. and Symes M. O. (1978) *Cancer Immunol. Immunother.* In the press.
Symes M. O. (1967) *Br. J. Cancer* **21**, 178.
Symes M. O., Eckert H., Feneley R. C. L. et al. (1978a) *Urology* In the press.
Symes M. O., Eckert H., Feneley R. C. L. et al. (1978b) *Br. J. Urol.* In the press.
Woodruff M. F. A., Symes M. O. and Anderson N. F. (1963) *Br. J. Cancer* **17**, 482.
Woodruff M. F. A., Symes M. O. and Stuart A. E. (1963) *Br. J. Cancer* **17**, 320.

VITAL AND MORBIDITY STATISTICS

M. CLARKE MB, DPH, MFCM

POPULATION

The size of the population has remained virtually static since mid-1973. Of the population estimated at mid-1976 to be 46·42 million, 10·52 million (23 per cent) were aged under 15 years, 10·17 million (22 per cent) were aged 15 – 29 years, 8·29 million (18 per cent) were aged 30 – 44 years and 9·42 million (20 per cent) were aged between 45 years and the normal age of entitlement to a retirement pension, i.e. 65 years for men and 60 years for women. Of the 8·03 million (17 per cent) above the respective retirement ages, 2·40 milion (5 per cent of the total population) were aged 75 years and over.

Males exceed females by 5 – 6 per cent at birth, a difference which starts to fall after the age of 20 and in the age group 50 – 54 years there were fewer men than women. The difference then increased to about 90 men for each 100 women in the age group 60 – 64 years, 70 – 100 in the age group 70 – 74 years and 42 – 100 in the age group 80 – 84 years. The much higher proportion of women in the older age groups reflects the higher mortality rates for men in middle age and later, and at ages over 80 the loss of males in the First World War.

The further decline in annual births, by 19 000 to 550 000 in 1976, and the rise in deaths, to 560 000, due mainly to an epidemic of influenza in the first quarter of the year, led to a small natural decrease in population, the first recorded occasion that deaths have exceeded births in a calendar year (D.H.S.S., 1977).

BIRTHS

In 1976 the crude birth rate for England and Wales fell to 11·9 live births per 1000 population of all ages: this is the lowest figure recorded and may be compared with 15·0 in 1955 and 14·4 in 1933. The post-war peak figure was 18·6 in 1964. The fertility rate (births per 1000 women aged 15 – 44) was 61, which is just in excess of the rate in 1933.

The marked decline in the proportion of married couples who have their first child within a few years of marriage has continued. This is due partly to a fall in pre-marital conception, but there is evidence to suggest that some of the delay may result from deliberate postponement of the starting of a family (D.H.S.S., 1977).

An analysis of a sample of the births that occurred in England and Wales during the period 1970 to 1975 showed that the annual decline of 25 per cent between 1970 and 1975 comprised little change in the numbers of legitimate births among women with husbands in Social Classes I and II (professional and intermediate occupations) but marked declines in the other Social Classes. Births fell by about one-quarter in Social Class IIIN (skilled non-manual occupations)· leading to a decline of about 10 per cent for the non-manual group as a whole. A drop of about one-quarter also occurred in Social Class IIIM (skilled manual occupations) and the largest fall—about one-third—occurred in Social Classes IV and V (partly skilled and unskilled manual occupations). Of the 549 000 legitimate births in 1975, 26 per cent were in Social Classes I and II, 10 per cent in Social Class IIIN, 39 per cent in Social Class IIIM and 20 per cent in Social Classes IV and V; the remaining 5 per cent were to women whose husbands were students or men of inadequately described occupation.

Results of the 1971 Census of Population showed that the smallest average family size for women who were nearing the end of their reproductive years was in Social Class IIIN, about 2·0 compared with the national average of about 2·3 for women married once only and married in the 1950s. The highest average family size, about 2·7, was in Social Class V. The remaining groups showed variations of a few per cent from the national average (Pearce and Britton, 1977).

Illegitimate births showed a further small decline in 1976 to 54 000, some 9 per cent of total live births. Over one-third of the illegitimate births occurred to girls aged under 20 years, and nearly one-third each to those aged respectively 20 – 24 years and over 25 years. Abortions outside marriage have been numerically greater than illegitimate births over the last four years and it is clear that abortions under the 1967 Abortion Act have played an important part in limiting fertility in this group. Abortion has been of little importance in limiting fertility in married women under 30, but it grows in importance at older ages and higher parities (Thompson, 1976).

The number of pre-marital conceptions, defined for statistical purposes as 'births occurring within 8 months of marriage', also showed a further decline in 1976 to 35 000 compared with 40 000 in 1975, 46 000 in 1974 and just over 70 000 in 1970. The number of such births has halved in 6 years. By contrast the 26 000 births to remarried women, 5 per cent of all births, were slightly higher than in the previous year, the continued increase in births to this group reflecting the greater numbers who divorce and remarry.

DEATHS

The 560 317 deaths in England in 1976 slightly exceeded the previous peak number of 555 889 in 1972. The crude mortality rate of 12·1 per thousand has been exceeded only once in the past 20 years, namely in 1963 when a moderate influenza epidemic was accompanied by severe cold in the first quarter of the year. These two factors, influenza and temperature, dominate annual variations in the national death rate. A third factor which has a more gradual effect is change in the age structure of the population. Allowance is made for this in the Standardized Mortality Ratio (SMR) which rose from 93 in 1975 to 95 in 1976 (1968 = 100). The explanation for the adverse mortality statistics of 1976 lies in the occurrence of a major influenza epidemic late in the first quarter of the year. The death rate in the first quarter was the highest for almost a decade and had not been exceeded since 1963.

One half of all deaths are ascribed to circulatory disorders of which the main components are ischaemic heart disease (26 per cent) and cerebro-vascular disease (13 per cent). One-fifth of all deaths are caused by some form of cancer, of which the commonest is cancer of the trachea, bronchus and lung (6 per cent). The third largest group of deaths are those attributed to respiratory disease, of which the various forms of pneumonia (9 per cent) and bronchitis, emphysema and asthma (4 per cent) are the main components. The contribution of each of these major groups of causes to total mortality has altered little over the past 20 years. However, the proportions assigned to malignant neoplasms rose from 18 per cent to 21 per cent and those for respiratory diseases rose from 12 per cent to 14 per cent, with a corresponding decline for all other diseases combined. Thus mortality is increasingly becoming concentrated in these three major groups.

Amongst males the death rate from lung cancer is now (1971 – 1975) falling in all age groups below 70 years. The greatest increase in death rates for men is found in the group aged 80 – 84, while the greatest improvement has occurred in the 35 – 44 years age group. Amongst women the death rate is rising in all age groups over 45, below this age some reductions in the rate are seen. Lung cancer accounts for 40 per cent of male deaths from cancer and 12 per cent of female cancer deaths. The second commonest site among male cancer deaths is the stomach (10 per cent), with the prostate (7 per cent) third. Among female deaths from cancer, the commonest site is the breast (20 per cent) followed by the lung and then the intestine (11 per cent).

Maternal mortality from child bearing increased from 62 deaths in 574 818 births in 1975 to 68 deaths in 555 722 births in 1976. The increase was not due to the major killers of some years ago—toxaemia, haemorrhage and abortion—as in total these accounted for 22 deaths in 1976 compared with 29 deaths in 1975. The increase appears to have occurred in other causes of mortality during the delivery and puerperium.

REFERENCES

Department of Health and Social Security (1977) *On the State of the Publich Health. Annual Report of the Chief Medical Officer of the Department of Health and Social Security for the Year 1976.* London, H.M.S.O.
Pearce D. and Britton M. (1977) The decline in births: some socioeconomic aspects. *Population Trends* 7. Office of Populations, Censuses and Surveys, London, H.M.S.O.
Thompson J. (1976) Fertility and abortion inside and outside marriage. *Population Trends* 5. Office of Populations, Censuses and Surveys, London, H.M.S.O.

STILLBIRTHS AND INFANT MORTALITY

This was a year of substantial reduction in infant and perinatal mortality. There were 550 383 live births and 5 399 stillbirths, giving a stillbirth rate of 9·6 per thousand total (live and still) births (*Table* 1). The reduction in the stillbirth rate since 1975, when it was 10·3, slightly exceeds the average annual improvement of the previous 5 years (0·5) and follows on a year when the rate was reduced by 0·8. Greater improvement occurred in infant mortality, with the number of deaths under one year falling from 8950 in 1975 to 7834 to give an infant mortality rate of 14·2 per thousand live births. The reduction of the rate from 15·7 in 1975 almost equals the combined improvement of the previous 3 years and is substantially greater than in any corresponding period for the previous 20 years. Deaths in the first week of life (4468) amounted to 57 per cent of all infant deaths, a proportion that has remained remarkably constant in recent years.

Table 1. LIVE BIRTH RATE, STILL BIRTH RATE, ILLEGITIMATE BIRTHS, MATERNAL MORTALITY RATE AND PERCENTAGE OF BIRTHS IN NHS HOSPITALS AND IN ALL INSTITUTIONS, ENGLAND, 1974 – 76

Year	Live birth rate per 1000 popu-lation	No. of live births	No. of still-births	Stillbirth rate per 1000 total births	Illegitimate births per 100 live births	Maternal mortality rate including abortions (all types) per 1000 total births	Percentage of births In all institu-tions	In NHS hospitals
1974	13·0	603 153	6741	11·1	8·8	0·12	95·6	93·9
1975	12·2	568 900	5918	10·3	9·1	0·12	96·6	95·0
1976	11·9	550 383	5399	9·6	9·2	0·13	97·4	95·9

(Source: D.H.S.S., 1977.)

The improvement in the perinatal mortality rate (stillbirths and first week deaths) from 19·3 to 17·6 per thousand total births is double the average annual improvement of the previous 5 years and is the greatest for almost 30 years.

International comparison of infant and perinatal mortality rates is bedevilled not only by differences in definition and registration practice, but also by the difficulty of obtaining up-to-date statistics. It is therefore not possible to assess the impact on our international position of the improvements made in 1976 in our infant and perinatal mortality rates as other countries may have made similar progress. At least 9 developed countries, however, had perinatal mortality rates lower than the 1976 England and Wales rate in 1973, while the Swedish rate was 13·2 in 1974 (D.H.S.S., 1977).

SICKNESS BENEFIT CLAIMS

Employed and self-employed persons who pay contributions under the Social Security Act can claim sickness benefit if they are incapacitated from working because of illness. After 6 months of entitlement, sickness benefit is replaced by invalidity benefit. This was introduced in September 1971 and is designed to be more suitable for prolonged incapacity. Invalidity benefit consists of invalidity pension, at the same rate as the standard retirement pension, and invalidity allowance. For the calendar year 1976, the number of new claims for sickness and invalidity benefits were about 10·7 million. This is a substantial rise on the figure of 9·6 million for the year 1975. Because of industrial action by staff employed by the Department, the figure of 10·7 million is partly based upon estimates but, allowing for the uncertainties in the estimates, a substantial rise in new claims did occur.

New claims for sickness and invalidity benefit in males expressed as rates per 1000 persons at risk during 1974/75 numbered 387 (standardized to the age distribution of the population at risk for 1962/63), a marked fall from the comparable rate of 421 in the previous year. The decline in the rate of new claims was present in all age groups. Days of benefit per person at risk similarly decreased from 16·6 in 1973 – 74 to 15·2 in 1974 – 75, the reduction in the main occurring in those over 40 years of age (D.H.S.S., 1977).

RESIDENTIAL FACILITIES FOR THE ELDERLY

By 1974 16·8 per cent of the population was over the normal retirement ages of 65 for men and 60 for women, compared with only 9·4 per cent in 1931. During the next 30 years we will see relatively little increase in the numbers of 65 – 74-year-olds in the population, but there will be a marked increase in the numbers aged 75 and over. This is in part explained by the large numbers of births in the period 1890 – 1914. Similarly following the large numbers of the very old in the 1990s, society will then experience a reduction in the numbers of the over 75-year-olds as the lower numbers of births from the 1930s move into old age (Davis, 1976). The consequences of the more immediate population changes are likely to be quite dramatic in terms of health and social services. While only 4 per cent of those over the age of 65 are in either hospital, social service or private and voluntary homes, the proportion increases from 2 per cent in those aged 65 – 74, to 6 per cent, and 19 per cent in the subsequent two decades, while in those aged 95 years and over 51 per cent are in institutional care. In terms of health and social services it is therefore of crucial importance what proportion of those aged 65 + are old or very old. It has been estimated that in Leicestershire, an area with 105 000 people ver the age of 65 in 1971, that the number of hospital and social service places for those over 65 will need to be increased from 4500 to 5500 if present services and admission policies are to be maintained (Clarke et al., 1977).

Less than 10 per cent of the elderly in care are in acute beds at any one time, while a further 30 per cent are in geriatric and psychiatric beds. The remaining 60 per cent are cared for in homes for the elderly. When the hospital service alone is considered (excluding psychiatric hospitals), 25 per cent of discharges of those over 65 years are from general medical beds, with general surgery dealing with 22 per cent and geriatrics with 18 per cent. Thirty-seven per cent of all discharges and deaths from general medical beds are of patients over 65 years, while the figures for general surgery and geriatrics are 24 and 96 per cent respectively. When the average number of beds used daily by patients aged over 65 are considered, 52 per cent are in geriatrics; 14 per cent general medicine; 10 per cent general surgery and the rest are in the remaining specialties (D.H.S.S., 1975). In order to deal with the predicted demand from, and on behalf of the very old, in the next few years a great deal of energy, resource and imagination in the organization of statutory and non-statutory services will be needed if a collapse of services is to be avoided.

REFERENCES

Clarke M., Hughes A. O., Palmer R. L. et al. (1977) Elderly in residential care: patterns of disability. In the press.
Davis N. (1977) Britain's Changing Age Structure 1931 – 2011. *Population Trends* 3. OPCS London, H.M.S.O.
Department of Health and Social Security (1975) *Hospital In-patient Enquiry, Preliminary Tables, 1973*. London, H.M.S.O.

APPENDICITIS

The death rate for appendicitis has declined from about 70 per million population in 1940 to around 7 per million in 1973. It appears that this reduction in the death rate reflects both improvements in treatment together with a reduction in incidence of acute appendicitis. In the first national study of morbidity undertaken in 1955/6 (G.R.O., 1962), about 40 people in every

10 000 consulted their G. P. in one year with a diagnosis for appendicitis. In the National Morbidity Study undertaken in 1970/1 (O.P.C.S., 1974) the number had declined to about 19 in every 10 000. Hospital discharge rates for patients with a main diagnosis of appendicitis have decreased in a similar manner from around 27 discharges for every 10 000 of the population in 1957 to about 18 in every 10 000 population in 1973 (Donnan and Lambert, 1976). Between 96 and 99 per cent of discharges with a principal diagnosis of appendicitis had operations during this time. Death rates from appendicitis are between 1 and 3 per milion until middle age, while after the age of 45 rates increase markedly until in both sexes over the age of 75 the rates are between 30 and 40 deaths per million each year. The Standardized Mortality ratio (SMR) for appendicitis in 1930/2 was 181 for Social Class I males and 76 for Social Class V males. By 1970/2 the situation had reversed with Social Class I males having an SMR of 60 and Social Class V males having an SMR of 117. Mortality rates do not vary consistently by region in England and Wales, but there are differences in the hospital discharge rates. The Manchester region and Wales have consistently higher, almost double, the discharge rates of the East Anglian and Sheffield regions (Donnan and Lambert, 1976). Fairbairn and Acheson (1969), in a study of the extent of organ removal in the Oxford area, reported that for men the appendicectomy was the second most common operation to have undergone by the age of 75, the first being tonsillectomy. For women, appendicectomy was the third most common, the first two being respectively tonsillectomy and hysterectomy. Approximately 12 per cent of both men and women would have had their appendix removed by the age of 75 in the Oxford Record Linkage area. When these authors reviewed appendicectomies by age, they showed that the picture was similar in both sexes, but the peak frequency of operation was reached rather earlier in men (10 – 14 years) than in women (15 – 19 years). Subsequently, the frequency of the operation declined until about the age of 35; from then on it remains at a steady state until 70.

Variations in the diagnosis and treatment of appendicitis may be involved in the apparent changes in incidence over time and between places. For example, when hospital discharge rates for appendicitis and an abdominal pain are combined, the total for each age group is very similar in 1957 and 1972 for both sexes, although the proportion contributed by abdominal pain is much greater in 1972 than in 1957. The change applies mainly to the age groups 5 – 14 and 15 – 44 years and is especially marked in females. Howie (1966) in a study of death from appendicitis and appendicectomy in Scotland, reported that in 45 per cent of cases that he reviewed the appendix was either normal or showed only changes of early mild appendicitis. A more recent study (Gilmore et al., 1975) of over 4000 appendicectomies in England reported that 22 per cent of specimens removed at operation were normal. Several series mentioned by Donnan and Lambert in Western countries give a similar figure of about 25 per cent of 'normal' appendices, although in a study by Lichtner and Pflanz (1971) of appendices removed at operation in Hanover, only one-quarter of the appendices removed showed any abnormality on examination by a pathologist. This high operation rate in Germany is almost certainly the cause of the high mortality rate in that country which occurs in patients over the age of 50. Howie in his study estimated that for the young adult patient the mortality of removing the normal appendix at 1 in 5000 seemed to be less than the mortality of failing to remove an abnormal appendix where the mortality was between 1 in 850 and 1 in 2300. The study by Howie failed to confirm the findings of Lee (1957), that the mortality rate from appendicitis was higher in non-teaching hospitals than in teaching hospitals. The finding by Lee and his colleagues may well have resulted from the varying case mix entering teaching and non-teaching hospitals.

REFERENCES

Donnan S. P. B. and Lambert P. M. (1976) Appendicitis: incidence and mortality. *Population Trends* 5. Office of Populations, Censuses and Surveys, London, H.M.S.O.

Fairbairn A. S. and Acheson E. D. (1969) The extent of organ removal in the Oxford area. *J. Chronic. Dis.* **22**, 111.

General Register Office (1962) *Morbidity Statistics from General Practice. Studies on Medical and Population Subjects,* No. 14. London, H.M.S.O.

Gilmore O. J. A., Browett J. P., Griffin P. H. et al. (1975). Appendicitis and mimicking conditions. *Lancet* **2**, 421.

Howie J. G. R. (1966) Death from appendicitis and appendicectomy. *Lancet* **2**, 1334.

Lee J. A. H., Morrison S. L. and Morris J. N. (1957) Fatality from 3 common surgical conditions in teaching and non-teaching hospitals. *Lancet* **2**, 785.

Lichtner S. and Pflanz M. (1971) Appendectomy in the Federal Republic of Germany: epidemiology and medical care patterns. *Med. Care* **9**, 311.

Office of Populations, Censuses and Surveys (1974) *Morbidity Statistics from General Practice, 2nd National Study 1970 – 71. Studies on Medical and Population Subjects, No. 26.* London, H.M.S.O.

Index